THE YEA
ANAESTHESIA AND

VOLUME

THE YEAR IN
ANAESTHESIA AND
CRITICAL CARE

VOLUME 2

EDITED BY

**JENNIFER HUNTER, TIM COOK,
HANS-JOACHIM PRIEBE, MICHEL STRUYS**

CLINICAL PUBLISHING

OXFORD

Clinical Publishing

an imprint of Atlas Medical Publishing Ltd

Oxford Centre for Innovation
Mill Street, Oxford OX2 0JX, UK

Tel: +44 1865 811116
Fax: +44 1865 251550
E mail: info@clinicalpublishing.co.uk
Web: www.clinicalpublishing.co.uk

Distributed in USA and Canada by:
Clinical Publishing
30 Amberwood Parkway
Ashland OH 44805 USA
tel: 800-247-6553 (toll free within US and Canada)
fax: 419-281-6883
email: order@bookmasters.com

Distributed in UK and Rest of World by:
Marston Book Services Ltd
PO Box 269
Abingdon
Oxon OX14 4YN UK
tel: +44 1235 465500
fax: +44 1235 465555
e mail: trade.orders@marston.co.uk

A catalogue record for this book is available from the British Library

ISBN-13 978 1 84692 051 6
ISBN-10 1 84692 051 5
Also available in hardback
ISBN-13 978 1 84692 003 5
ISSN 1745-9508

The publisher makes no representation, express or implied, that the dosages in this book are correct. Readers must therefore always check the product information and clinical procedures with the most up-to-date published product information and data sheets provided by the manufacturers and the most recent codes of conduct and safety regulations. The authors and the publisher do not accept any liability for any errors in the text or for the misuse or misapplication of material in this work

Project Manager: Prepress Projects Ltd, Perth, UK
Printed by T G Hostench SA, Barcelona, Spain

Contents

Editors

Tim M Cook, BA, MBBS, FRCA
Consultant in Anaesthesia and Intensive Care, Department of Anaesthesia, Royal United Hospital, Bath, UK

Jennifer M Hunter, MB, CHB, PHD, FRCA
Professor of Anaesthesia, University Department of Anaesthesia, Royal Liverpool University Hospital, Liverpool, UK

Hans-Joachim Priebe, MD, FRCA, FFARCSI
Professor of Anaesthesia, Department of Anaesthesia, University Hospital, Freiburg, Germany

Michel M R F Struys, MD, PHD
Professor in Anaesthesia and Research Coordinator, Department of Anaesthesia, Ghent University Hospital, Ghent, Belgium

Contributors

Joseph E Arrowsmith, MBBS, MD, FRCP, FRCA
Consultant in Cardiothoracic Anaesthesia, Papworth Hospital, Cambridge, UK

Rebecca Cusack, MRCP
Consultant Intensive Care Medicine, Southampton General Hospital, Southampton, UK

Amy M Fahrenkopf, MD, MPH
Instructor of Pediatrics, Harvard Medical School, Pediatric Hospitalist, Children's Hospital Boston, Boston, Massachusetts, USA

Ronnie Glavin, MPHIL, MB, CHB, FRCA, FRCP
Educational Contributor, Scottish Clinical Simulation Centre, Stirling Royal Infirmary, Stirling, UK

Peter A Goldstein, MD
Associate Professor, Department of Anesthesiology, Weill Medical College, Cornell University, New York, USA

Carin Hagberg, MD
Professor, Director of Neuroanaesthesia and Advanced Airway Management, Department of Anethesiology, University of Texas, Houston Medical School, Houston, Texas, USA

Paul Holder, BSc, MB, ChB, FRCA
Specialist Registrar, Department of Anaesthesia and Intensive Care, Aberdeen Royal Infirmary, Aberdeen, UK

Gabriella Iohom, FCARCSI, PhD
Consultant Anaesthetist and Lecturer in Anaesthesia and Intensive Care Medicine, Cork University Hospital, Cork, Ireland

Girish P Joshi, MBBS, MD, FFARCSI
Professor of Anesthesiology and Pain Management, Director of Perioperative Medicine and Ambulatory Anesthesia, University of Texas, Southwestern Medical Center, Dallas, Texas, USA

Nicholas C Lam, MD
Assistant Professor, Director of Regional Anesthesia, Department of Anesthesiology, University of Texas, Houston Medical School, Houston, Texas, USA

David G Lambert, PhD
Professor of Anaesthetic Pharmacology, Division of Anaesthesia, Critical Care and Pain Management, University of Leicester, Leicester Royal Infirmary, Leicester, UK

Christopher P Landrigan, MD, MPH
Assistant Professor of Pediatrics and Medicine, Harvard Medical School; Research Director, Children's Hospital Boston; Director, Sleep and Patient Safety Programme, Brigham and Women's Hospital, Boston, Massachusetts, USA

Sarah L M Mitchell, MB, ChB, FRCA
Consultant Anaesthetist, Royal Liverpool and Broadgreen University Hospital Trust, Liverpool, UK

Georg Mols, MD, DEAA
Professor of Anaesthesia, Department of Anaesthesia and Critical Care Medicine,
Freiburg, Germany

Jerry Nolan, FRCA, FCEM
Consultant in Anaesthesia and Critical Care Medicine, Royal United Hospital,
Bath, UK

Barbara Philips, MD, FRCA, DipICM
Senior Lecturer/Honorary Lecturer Intensive Care Medicine, St George's Hospital
Medical School, London, UK

Peter J Simpson, MD, FRCA
Consultant Anaesthetist, Frenchay Hospital, Bristol, UK

Robert J Sneyd
Associate Dean and Professor of Anaesthesia, Peninsula Medical School,
University of Plymouth, Plymouth, UK

Jasmeet Soar, MA, MB, BChir, FRCA
Consultant in Anaesthetics and Intensive Care Medicine, Southmead Hospital,
Bristol, UK

Ranjit Verma
Consultant Anaesthetist, Derby City General Hospital, Derby, UK

Tim Walsh, BSc(Hons), MBChB(Hons), FRCP, FRCA, Msc, MD
Consultant in Anaesthetics and Critical Care, Edinburgh Royal Infirmary,
Edinburgh, UK

Stephen T Webb, MB, BCh, BAO, FRCA
Specialist Registrar in Anaesthesia and Intensive Care Medicine, Royal Victoria
Hospital, Belfast, UK

Nigel R Webster, PhD, MB, ChB, FRCA, FRCP, FRCS
Professor, Academic Unit of Anaesthesia and Intensive Care, Institute of Medical
Sciences, Aberdeen, UK

Foreword

SIR PETER SIMPSON

Continuing Medical Education and Professional Development (CEPD) for practising clinicians is the cornerstone of our ability to provide high-quality, safe patient care and the major advances that continue to be made in anaesthesia and critical care must play a key part in this. Furthermore, formal performance assessment and revalidation, if not already in place, are just around the corner for all of us. Whatever the statutory requirements, we owe it to our patients and the quality and safety of the care we provide for them to ensure that we keep up to date in all areas of our practice, giving due consideration to new drugs and techniques that might improve patient outcomes still further. We may feel that with the ever-increasing workload and demands of complex patient care, we have no time to update our knowledge and skills, preferring to employ techniques with which we are familiar, supported by the sound clinical knowledge and judgement that we have acquired over many years. However, the development of anaesthetic techniques, equipment and pharmacology does not stand still and equally the sophistication of diagnostic tools for our patients means that we are able to obtain much better and more timely information than in the past. In some ways, the more we know, the more difficult it is to make a balanced judgement on the optimal care of a patient. Yet, how much more informative it is to know the actual jugular venous Po_2 or intracranial pressure than simply to make a judgement based on clinical interpretation?

The demands made of anaesthetists both in theatre, in pain management and in critical care mean that being able to find sufficient time to attend CEPD meetings, particularly outside one's own local environment, let alone overseas, is increasingly difficult. This means that for many of us there is limited opportunity to concentrate and learn in an undisturbed way and, importantly, to hear the views of experts in their chosen field. Inevitably, we rely to a great extent on information supplied in academic journals and textbooks together, increasingly, with the use of the Internet.

Without an enormous amount of time and a range of available journals, it is often difficult to obtain a balanced view about new areas of anaesthesia and critical care. What we really need is an expert to assess the current topic in question and to produce an objective commentary and judgement on the various papers that have been written during recent months. This is exactly the principle on which *The Year in Anaesthesia and Critical Care* is based. It provides an alternative concept of book-based CEPD, which concentrates on extracting information from a number of recent papers and assessing it in a meaningful and readable way. New books appear on a regular basis but most are either orientated towards examinations and assessment processes during training, or are specialist textbooks in a particular field of either anaesthesia, pain management or critical care. Few are aimed at CEPD for established career-grade clinical anaesthetists, but this, with its now established format and concept, is such a book.

No book of this kind should attempt to be comprehensive, and the editors have selected four key sections of recent development: perioperative care, clinical pharmacology, monitoring and equipment, and critical care. Each section begins with an excellent and objective editorial section, which includes an overview and summary of the subject area, individual comment and references. Key subjects within these four sections are then reviewed in more detail by experts in the field, who concentrate on a number of key publications that have occurred during the year, looking at the main findings and recommendations of each and then co-ordinating these to provide more detailed response and comment. The reader is thus able to have expert opinion and comment at two levels – both for the individual detailed subject area and more generally in the field, which is the subject of the particular section of the book. Laid out as it is, in sections and sub-sections, each with comprehensive headings, it is both easy to read and concentrate upon and importantly, one only needs to read a small section at a time to gain relevant information. Interruptions do not disturb one's flow of thought and learning unduly.

There is no doubt that the opportunity to concentrate on specific topic areas rather than the need to be comprehensive in terms of subject content makes for a much more readable and interesting book. Even at the level of studying for examinations, key comment and review by experts do much to help one's understanding of a subject and the research and scientific basis behind new developments and techniques. While this selective approach is exemplified in all parts of the book, the section on perioperative care serves to illustrate the theme and its value. The section concentrates on four very relevant, topical, but unconnected areas: perioperative blood component therapy and haemostasis, perioperative respiratory care, ambulatory anaesthesia and perioperative cardioprotection. For clinical anaesthetists wishing to read material to increase their knowledge, this combination has all the right ingredients. It develops themes about which they may already know a considerable amount but wish to be updated, leads them through new ideas and techniques and, finally, provides a detailed look at a more specialist area of work that would be of interest even if they were not acutely involved with it. It provides the opportunity to read about the advantages and disadvantages of new developments at length and to reason through recent research and publications that inform the choice of technique. Each author introduces new concepts that all clinicians should consider and allows us to obtain a balanced view, particularly in subject areas where our experience is limited and inevitably biased.

Although review articles are also an excellent way of keeping up to date and enhancing one's knowledge, inevitably they concentrate on specific topics and contain much of the authors' own opinions rather than looking at the variety of views from others and allowing the reader to exercise their own judgement. This book allows an objective discussion and comment to be made about all the articles written around a certain subject by others and then allows the reader to make a balanced judgement based upon the recommendations made. For continuous education to have an impact on one's opinion and clinical practice, one must be allowed to judge for oneself and not simply feel spoon-fed by others' opinions. The innovative format of this book and the ease with which one can read and concentrate on it makes it an ideal opportunity to enhance one's education in anaesthesia, critical care and pain management and the breadth of subjects covered will, I am sure, have widespread appeal.

Part I

Perioperative care

Unsettled issues in the field of perioperative care

HANS-JOACHIM PRIEBE

Introduction

Numerous advances have been made in the field of perioperative care during the past couple of years. Part I of this edition of the *Year in Anaesthesia and Critical Care* focuses on four areas of perioperative care: perioperative blood component therapy and haemostasis (Chapter 1), perioperative respiratory care (Chapter 2), perioperative cardioprotection (Chapter 3) and ambulatory and outpatient anaesthesia (Chapter 4). The following introduction to the section on perioperative care will concentrate on some aspects of perioperative cardioprotection and respiratory care that have recently received special attention – be it because they carry the potential for considerable impact on perioperative care or because the issues are far from being settled and provide ground for ongoing debate and controversy. Although this outline can only briefly address very few aspects of perioperative care, and, by necessity, will have to ignore the vast majority of topics relevant to perioperative care, it will reflect the broad scope of perioperative care.

Perioperative cardioprotection

In patients with coronary artery disease, the incidence of perioperative myocardial ischaemia and infarction remains high and is associated with adverse outcomes [1]. Consequently, the quest for cardioprotective strategies continues. Various approaches have been taken.

Myocardial conditioning

Rapid restoration of coronary blood flow following coronary artery occlusion is of the utmost importance in limiting myocardial injury. However, as reperfusion *per se* elicits myocardial injury, additional strategies are sought to attenuate reperfusion injury following myocardial ischaemia.

Ischaemic preconditioning

One such widely publicized strategy is ischaemic preconditioning, the phenomenon of cardioprotection by controlled brief periods of myocardial ischaemia prior to a subsequent prolonged period of myocardial ischaemia |2,3|. Although numerous experimental studies have demonstrated a cardioprotective effect of ischaemic preconditioning protocols, and despite evidence that human myocardium can be preconditioned |4–6|, the concept has not been adopted in routine clinical practice for various theoretical as well as practical limitations |7,8|.

Most studies were performed in animals with normal hearts and in patients with normal myocardial performance. Experimental and clinical evidence for a cardioprotective effect of ischaemic preconditioning in diseased hearts is limited. Intentionally eliciting ischaemia in an already damaged myocardium is valid reason for concern. Furthermore, except for cardiac surgery and coronary interventions, it is impossible to predict the beginning of a sustained period of myocardial ischaemia. This is a major limitation because the effectiveness of ischaemic preconditioning is crucially dependent on the exact timing of the brief episodes of myocardial ischaemia prior to the subsequent prolonged period of myocardial ischaemia. Even if applied in cardiac surgery, intermittent clamping and unclamping of either the aorta or coronary arteries may provoke distal embolization of atherosclerotic plaque material. Lacking these drawbacks, current cardioplegic techniques are likely to provide equivalent, if not superior, cardioprotection. The rather brief period (20–30 s) of severe myocardial ischaemia during coronary artery balloon angioplasty and stent placement and the use of distal perfusion catheters make ischaemic preconditioning during percutaneous coronary intervention unnecessary. Thus, the benefit of ischaemic preconditioning in diseased hearts in routine clinical practice remains to be determined.

Pharmacological preconditioning

Another strategy for cardioprotection is pharmacological preconditioning. A number of pharmacological substances are possible triggers or effectors of ischaemic preconditioning |7|. Amongst the substances that simulate ischaemic preconditioning without actually inducing myocardial ischaemia, and which have been investigated in humans, are adenosine, adenosine agonists, the K_{ATP} channel opener nicorandil, delta opioids and nitrates |7|. Under most experimental and certain clinical conditions |9,10|, the cardioprotective effect of pharmacological preconditioning (66–85% reduction in infarct size) is similar to that initially reported for ischaemic preconditioning (75% reduction in infarct size) |6|. However, not all clinical studies confirm effective cardioprotection by pharmacological preconditioning per se |7,8|.

Anaesthetic preconditioning

Anaesthetic-induced cardioprotection is a special form of pharmacological preconditioning |11–16|. It describes the phenomenon whereby exposure of the myocardium to an anaesthetic drug (in most cases to volatile anaesthetics) prior to the onset of myocardial ischaemia attenuates the extent of myocardial infarction, myocardial stunning and ventricular dysrhythmias following coronary reperfusion. Anaesthetic and ischaemic preconditioning are similarly effective in protecting the myocardium against prolonged ischaemia |11|.

Our understanding of the mechanisms involved in anaesthetic preconditioning is primarily based on experimental investigations. For anaesthetic preconditioning to be effective, the beginning of a sustained period of myocardial ischaemia must be predictable. Consequently, all clinical studies that have thus far documented a cardioprotective effect of anaesthetic preconditioning were performed in patients undergoing cardiac surgery |17–24|. The clinical relevance of anaesthetic preconditioning in non-cardiac surgery remains to be determined. Even in cardiac surgery, the benefit of anaesthetic preconditioning is not uniformly accepted |25|.

Remote preconditioning

Remote preconditioning is one of two novel cardioprotective strategies that have recently been described (the other being postconditioning; see below). It refers to the phenomenon of myocardial protection (or protection of any organ) derived from prior brief periods of ischaemia and reperfusion of non-cardiac organs |8,26|. Remote preconditioning can be elicited by intermittent brief periods of cross-clamping of various arteries (renal, mesenteric and iliac arteries; infrarenal aorta) |27,28| or upper limb ischaemia (by intermittent inflation of a blood pressure cuff or use of a tourniquet) |29|. It may be as cardioprotective as ischaemic preconditioning |28|.

Remote preconditioning by intermittent occlusion of intra-abdominal vessels has the obvious clinical drawback of requiring laparotomy and carrying the risk of organ damage in patients with pre-existing organ dysfunction and vascular disease. Large clinical studies are required to determine ultimate feasibility and clinical benefit of this strategy.

Postconditioning

The phenomenon of cardioprotection by postconditioning was first described in 2003 in an open chest canine model of coronary artery occlusion and reperfusion |30|. Rather than allowing uninterrupted coronary artery reperfusion following occlusion, reperfusion is interrupted by brief sequences of coronary occlusions and reperfusion |31|. The initial experimental studies showed that, following a 1-h coronary artery occlusion, an algorithm consisting of three sequences of 30-s reperfusion of coronary blood flow followed by 30 s of reocclusion of the coronary artery before subsequent uninterrupted reperfusion for 3 h reduced myocardial infarct size to a similar extent as observed during ischaemic preconditioning |31,32|.

Pre- and postconditioning share several of the ligand triggers and intracellular pathways |33|. What remains to be determined are the exact mechanisms by which postconditioning protects the heart and the relationship between, and the overlap of, mechanisms involved in pre- and postconditioning |34|. The phenomenon of postconditioning has been observed in dogs, rabbits, mice and rats |31|, and recently in pigs |35|. There is now preliminary evidence for a cardioprotective effect of postconditioning in humans as well |36–38|.

Anaesthetic postconditioning

In the case of anaesthetic postconditioning, the volatile anaesthetic is introduced immediately upon reperfusion. Its cardioprotective effect has been documented |19,39–41|. Anaesthetic postconditioning has considerable potential advantages in the clinical setting: it is practically feasible; it could be provided to patients arriving in the hospital, the operating room or the cardiac catheterization laboratory with ongoing myocardial ischaemia; and it could be provided during coronary reperfusion following percutaneous coronary interventions or coronary artery bypass graft surgery, or possibly even organ transplantation. It remains to be determined whether the cardioprotective effects of anaesthetic pre- and postconditioning are additive |42| or not |41|, and whether one form is superior to the other |43|. The ultimate myocardial protective strategy may be a combination of all, that is of pre-, post-, remote and pharmacological conditioning |8|.

Intensive medical therapy

More than 1 million coronary artery stents were inserted in the United States in 2004 |44|, and approximately 85% of stent placements are presently performed electively in patients with stable coronary artery disease |45|. Whereas percutaneous coronary intervention (PCI) reduces mortality and the incidence of myocardial infarction in patients with acute coronary syndromes |46|, this is not necessarily the case in patients with stable coronary artery disease |47,48|. Considering the increasing rate of coronary stent placements in patients with stable coronary artery disease, the increasing evidence for a highly beneficial effect of optimized medical therapy on outcome in patients with stable coronary artery disease, and considering the markedly elevated perioperative risks associated with surgery in patients with coronary stents |49,50|, a critical evaluation of the benefits of PCI in addition to optimal medical therapy was needed.

The Clinical Outcomes Utilization Revascularization and Aggressive Drug Evaluation (COURAGE) randomized trial compared the effect of combined PCI and optimal medical therapy with optimal medical therapy alone on the risk of death and non-fatal myocardial infarction |51|. Included were patients with stable coronary artery disease, those with an initial Canadian Cardiovascular Society (CCS) class IV angina who subsequently stabilized under medical therapy, and those with a coronary artery stenosis of at least 70% in at least one proximal epicardial artery and objective electrocardiographic evidence of myocardial ischaemia, or at least one coronary artery stenosis of at least 80% accompanied by classic angina. Excluded were patients with persistent CCS class IV angina, a highly positive stress test, refractory heart failure or cardiogenic shock, an ejection fraction of less than 30%, revascularization within the previous 6 months, and a coronary anatomy unsuitable for PCI.

All patients randomized to either group received daily anti-platelet therapy with aspirin and clopidogrel, anti-ischaemic therapy with long-acting metoprolol, amlodipine and isosorbide mononitrate alone or in combination, and secondary prevention with angiotensin-converting enzyme inhibitors. In addition, all patients were aggressively treated pharmacologically to reduce serum concentrations of low-density lipoprotein (LDL) cholesterol and to increase serum concentrations of high-density lipoprotein (HDL) cholesterol by modification of lifestyle and/or medication.

The main finding of this trial was the following: PCI in addition to intensive medical therapy did not reduce myocardial infarction and mortality during a follow-up period of 2.5–7.0 years. The 4.6-year cumulative rates of myocardial infarction and death were 19% in the combined PCI and medical therapy group and 18.5% in the medical therapy alone group, with a mortality rate of approximately 8% in both groups (no significant differences). At 5 years, 74% and 72% of patients in the combined PCI and medical therapy group and in the medical therapy alone group, respectively, were free of angina.

Several limitations of this study need to be considered before drawing final conclusions. Of the 35 539 patients who were initially screened, only 3071 (8.6%) met all inclusion criteria, and 2287 (6.4%) consented to participate in the study (combined PCI and medical therapy group: $n = 1149$; medical therapy alone group alone: $n = 1138$). The low number of patients enrolled in the study compared with that initially screened is of concern. Patients with severe ventricular dysfunction, a highly positive stress test or clinical instability were excluded.

Drug-eluting stents were used in only 31 (2.7%) of the 1149 patients in the PCI group, because they were not available until the late phase of patient recruitment. Although there are presently no good data to indicate that drug-eluting stents reduce the incidence of myocardial infarction and death in patients with stable coronary artery disease compared with bare metal stents |**52–58**|, on-label use of drug-eluting stents seems to reduce the rate of repeat revascularization |**55,57**|. It is thus conceivable that more frequent use of drug-eluting stents might have resulted in a lower rate of repeat revascularization and angina and, in turn, a better outcome in the combined PCI and medical therapy group.

In addition, approximately one-third of patients in the medical group required coronary revascularization for control of angina and acute coronary syndromes during the median follow-up of 4.6 years. With PCI being effective in ameliorating angina and in treating acute coronary syndromes, it cannot be entirely excluded that the relatively high crossover rate from the combined PCI and medical therapy group to the medical therapy alone group might have biased the results in favour of medical therapy alone, which might have contributed to the similar degree of symptom control and cardiovascular event rate at 5 years. However, during the same time period additional revascularization was also necessary in 21.1% of patients in the PCI group.

This is the first trial that routinely used stents in combination with what is presently considered optimal medical therapy. Despite the limitations, this study strongly suggests that even in the presence of objective evidence of baseline myocardial ischaemia and extensive coronary artery disease, PCI added to intensive medical therapy does not necessarily reduce the incidence of major cardiovascular events compared with intensive medical therapy alone during the several subsequent years. The findings may partly be explained by differences in atherosclerotic plaque morphology associated with stable coronary artery disease compared with acute coronary syndromes |1,59|. Myocardial ischaemia and anginal symptoms are usually associated with stable plaques. These plaques tend to have thick fibrous caps, small lipid cores and considerable amounts of smooth muscle cells and collagen, but few macrophages |60,61|. They ultimately undergo inward (constrictive) remodelling with narrowing of the coronary lumen that is readily detected by coronary angiography. As the potential for acute rupture is relatively low, stable plaques are less likely to cause acute coronary syndromes.

By contrast, vulnerable plaques tend to have thinner fibrous caps, larger lipid cores, fewer smooth muscle cells, more macrophages and less collagen. They undergo outward (expansive) remodelling with less narrowing of the coronary lumen. As a result, vulnerable plaques do not usually cause significant coronary stenosis and clinical symptoms before rupture and subsequent precipitation of an acute coronary syndrome. In other words, coronary lesions that cause acute coronary syndromes are not necessarily severely stenotic (and not necessarily readily detectable by coronary angiography), and severely stenotic lesions (readily detectable by coronary angiography) that cause anginal symptoms are not necessarily unstable. As stable plaques are less likely to trigger an acute coronary event, it should not come as a total surprise that focal management of even severe coronary artery stenoses by coronary artery revascularization (be it by PCI or surgically) does not reduce the incidence of major cardiovascular events. Following PCI, vulnerable plaques will continue to exist unchanged. Presumably by improving endothelial function and plaque stability, lipid-lowering therapy more successfully reduces the incidence of cardiac events than the severity of the stenosis |62|.

Consistent with the results of previous studies |63,64|, the observed clinical event rates associated with optimal medical therapy were lower than projected in the trial design |51|. This finding is in agreement with a meta-analysis showing that PCI is ineffective in reducing major cardiovascular events compared with medical management |65|. This may reflect reduced plaque vulnerability due to aggressive medication and intervention for cardiac risk factors. Existing clinical practice guidelines acknowledge the effectiveness of intensive medical therapy and, accordingly, state that even in patients with symptomatic, extensive, multivessel coronary artery disease, PCI can be safely deferred in patients with stable coronary artery disease, if optimal medical therapy is provided |66,67|. Short-term pretreatment with atorvastatin in patients with acute coronary syndromes undergoing early invasive strategy conferred an 88% risk reduction of 30-day major adverse cardiac events |68|. Preoperative use of lipid-lowering therapy in patients undergoing coronary artery bypass graft surgery was associated with improved survival to hospital discharge compared with patients not receiving lipid-lowering therapy |69|.

The Coronary Artery Revascularization Prophylaxis (CARP) trial failed to demonstrate a long-term benefit of prophylactic preoperative coronary revascularization (by PCI or coronary artery bypass graft surgery) |70|. Consistent with the results of the COURAGE trial |51|, lack of benefit by preoperative coronary revascularization may partly be explained by the long-term aggressive medical therapy in revascularized as well as non-revascularized patients. All of this adds further evidence for a benefit of aggressive perioperative medical therapy in patients with stable coronary artery disease, and for the lack of added benefit from preoperative coronary revascularization. Aggressive perioperative medical therapy may well be one of the most important, if not *the* most important, cardioprotective intervention.

Anti-platelet drug therapy

Dual anti-platelet therapy with aspirin and a thienopyridine reduces ischaemic cardiac events and deaths after coronary stenting and is, therefore, recommended in the European Society of Cardiology |71| and the American College of Cardiology/ American Heart Association practice guidelines for the treatment of patients undergoing percutaneous coronary intervention and for the medical treatment of patients with non-ST-segment-elevation acute coronary syndromes |72–74|. However, dual anti-platelet therapy is often prematurely discontinued by patients and healthcare providers, resulting in greatly increased risk of stent thrombosis, myocardial infarction and death |75,76|. Interruption of aspirin accounted for up to 15% of recurrent acute coronary syndromes in patients with established stable coronary artery disease |77|.

The recent science advisory from the American Heart Association, the American College of Cardiology, the Society for Cardiovascular Angiography and Interventions, the American College of Surgeons and the American Dental Association emphasizes the importance of 12 months of dual anti-platelet therapy after placement of a drug-eluting stent |78|. Amongst the various recommendations made by the science advisory, the following are the most relevant for the perioperative care of patients with coronary artery stents:

- Before implantation of a stent, the physician should discuss the need for dual antiplatelet therapy. In patients not expected to comply with 12 months of thienopyridine therapy, whether for economic or other reasons, strong consideration should be given to avoiding a DES [drug-eluting stent].

- In patients who are undergoing preparation for percutaneous coronary intervention and are likely to require invasive or surgical procedures within the next 12 months, consideration should be given to implantation of a bare-metal stent or performance of balloon angioplasty with provisional stent implantation instead of the routine use of a DES.

- Healthcare providers who perform invasive or surgical procedures and are concerned about periprocedural and postprocedural bleeding must be made aware of the potentially catastrophic risks of premature discontinuation of thienopyridine therapy. Such professionals who perform these procedures should contact the patient's cardiologist if issues regarding the patient's antiplatelet therapy are unclear, to discuss optimal patient management strategy.

- Elective procedures for which there is significant risk of perioperative or postoperative bleeding should be deferred until patients have completed an appropriate course of thienopyridine therapy (12 months after DES implantation if they are not at high risk of bleeding and a minimum of 1 month for bare-metal stent implantation).

- For patients treated with DES who are to undergo subsequent procedures that mandate discontinuation of thienopyridine therapy, aspirin should be continued if at all possible and the thienopyridine restarted as soon as possible after the procedure because of concerns about late-stent thrombosis.

The corresponding recommendations by the European Society of Cardiology are similar, but do not specifically address the management of anti-platelet medication in the perioperative period |71|:

- *following bare metal stent implantation in stable coronary artery disease*: administration of ticlopidine or clopidogrel in addition to aspirin for 3–4 weeks (I A);

- *following placement of drug-eluting stents*: clopidogrel administration for 6–12 months (I C);

- *following coronary brachytherapy*: clopidogrel administration for 12 months (I C);

- *following non-ST-segment-elevation acute coronary syndrome*: clopidogrel administration for 9–12 months (I B).

(*Recommendation class I* = evidence and/or general agreement that a given diagnostic procedure/treatment is beneficial, useful and effective. *Levels of evidence*: A, data derived from multiple randomized clinical trials or meta-analyses; B, data derived from a single randomized clinical trial or large non-randomized studies; C, data derived from retrospective studies or registries.)

As yet, there is no evidence for a benefit of 'bridging' stent patients with glycoprotein IIb/IIIa or anti-thrombin drugs. It remains to be seen whether poor responsiveness ('resistance') to aspirin |79| and clopidogrel |80| correlates with adverse clinical events.

Safe and effective perioperative management of dual anti-platelet therapy is an integral part of perioperative cardioprotection. The management will have to balance the risk of bleeding associated with continuation of anti-platelet therapy against the ischaemic risks associated with discontinuation of anti-platelet drugs |49,50,75,81,82|.

Perioperative respiratory care

Clinicians continue to struggle with several perioperative respiratory management issues, mostly because evidence-based data supporting one approach over the other are missing. Whenever 'hard' data are missing, clinical 'experience' tends to lead the way – with often unpredictable outcomes.

Prediction of postoperative complications

Postoperative pulmonary complications – the most important ones being atelectasis, pneumonia, respiratory insufficiency and exacerbation of pre-existing pulmonary disease – are as frequent and clinically relevant as postoperative cardiac complications |83|. However, the issue of perioperative pulmonary morbidity and mortality receives considerably less attention than its cardiac 'counterpart'.

The impact of clinical factors on postoperative pulmonary complications and the benefit of preoperative respiratory testing remain a matter of continued debate. Scientifically valid conclusions on the basis of existing data are limited by preponderance of observational rather than hypothesis-driven studies, inadequate sample sizes, non-uniform definitions and non-blinded assessment of postoperative pulmonary complications, and questionable statistical analyses.

The American College of Physicians recently addressed this issue and developed a guideline to 'guide clinicians on clinical and laboratory predictors of perioperative pulmonary risk before non-cardiothoracic surgery' and to 'evaluate the efficacy of strategies to reduce the risk for postoperative complications' |83|. The guideline specifically applies to adult patients undergoing non-cardiothoracic surgery. It is based on two systematic reviews of the literature |84,85|. Based on an extensive review of the literature, the American College of Physicians made six recommendations |83|:

1   'All patients undergoing non-cardiothoracic surgery should be evaluated for the presence of the following significant risk factors for postoperative pulmonary complications in order to receive pre- and postoperative interventions to reduce pulmonary risk: chronic obstructive pulmonary disease, age older than 60 years, American Society of Anesthesiologists (ASA) class of II or greater, functionally dependent and congestive heart failure.' Obesity and mild or moderate asthma were not identified as significant risk factors for postoperative pulmonary complications.

2   'Patients undergoing the following procedures are at higher risk for postoperative pulmonary complications and should be evaluated for other concomitant risk factors and receive pre- and postoperative interventions to reduce pulmonary complications: prolonged surgery (>3 hours), abdominal surgery, thoracic surgery, neurosurgery, head and neck surgery, vascular surgery, aortic aneurysm repair, emergency surgery, and general anesthesia.'

3   'A low serum albumin level (<35 g/L) is a powerful marker of increased risk for postoperative pulmonary complications and should be measured in all patients who are clinically suspected of having hypoalbuminaemia; measurement should be considered in patients with 1 or more risk factors for perioperative pulmonary complications.'

4   'All patients who after preoperative evaluation are found to be at higher risk for postoperative pulmonary complications should receive the following postoperative procedures in order to reduce postoperative pulmonary complications: (1) deep breathing exercises or incentive spirometry and (2) selective use of a nasogastric tube (as needed for postoperative nausea or vomiting, inability to tolerate oral intake, or symptomatic abdominal distension).'

5   'Preoperative spirometry and chest radiography should not be used routinely for predicting risk for postoperative pulmonary complications.'

6   'The following procedures should not be used solely for reducing postoperative pulmonary complication risk: (1) right-heart catheterization and (2) total parenteral nutrition or total enteral nutrition (for patients who are malnourished or have low serum albumin levels).'

The major *procedure*-related factors (surgical site, duration of surgery, anaesthetic technique and emergency surgery) were associated with higher likelihoods of postoperative complications than the major *patient*-related factors (advanced age, ASA physical class ≥2, functional dependence, chronic obstructive pulmonary disease and congestive heart failure).

The data regarding the value of *spirometry* in predicting increased risk for postoperative pulmonary complications in non-cardiothoracic surgeries were found to be inconsistent. While spirometry is frequently used to diagnose restrictive or obstructive pulmonary disease, such diagnoses do not seem to result in reliable individual preoperative risk stratification. In addition, there is no convincing evidence that information derived from spirometry is clinically more relevant than that derived from patient history and physical examination. Evidence did not support a benefit of preoperative spirometry in preoperative pulmonary risk stratification and, thus, does not support the routine preoperative use of spirometry even in the presence of major patient- or procedure-related risk factors.

Preoperative *chest radiography* in patients older than a particular age is frequently part of institutional practice guidelines. However, chest radiography rarely provides information not already expected from medical history and physical examination. Not surprisingly then, even pathologic preoperative chest radiographs rarely influenced perioperative management |86|. Only limited evidence supports the use of chest radiography in patients with cardiopulmonary disease, older than 50 years of age, scheduled for upper abdominal, thoracic or abdominal aortic aneurysm surgery. Based on the systematic reviews, the American College of Physicians concluded that 'preoperative pulmonary function testing or chest radiography may be appropriate in patients with a previous diagnosis of chronic obstructive pulmonary disease or asthma' |83|. Large randomized controlled studies will be necessary to evaluate the impact of these guidelines on outcome.

Prediction of difficult mask ventilation

Despite technical advances in airway equipment, airway problems remain a major concern |87|. Whereas a large body of literature addresses the prediction of difficult intubation |88|, only very few studies have looked at predictive factors of difficult mask ventilation |89,90|. This is the more surprising as successful mask ventilation may become a life-saving rescue intervention in cases of failed intubation. In turn, inability to mask ventilate carries the potential for considerable morbidity and mortality.

Of 22 660 prospectively studied attempts at mask ventilation in adults during a 24-month period at a university hospital, 37 (0.16%) were of grade 4 (impossible to ventilate) and 313 (1.4%) of grade 3 (difficult to ventilate) |91|. The combination of grade 3 or 4 mask ventilation and difficult intubation occurred in 84 (0.37%) attempts. Independent predictors of grade 3 mask ventilation (difficult to ventilate) were body mass index (BMI) of ≥ 30 kg/m^2, a beard, Mallampati classification III or IV, age ≥ 57 years, severely limited mandibular protrusion and a history of snoring. Independent predictors of grade 4 mask ventilation (impossible to ventilate) were a history of snoring and a thyromental distance of less than 6 cm. Independent predictors of the combination of grade 3 or 4 mask ventilation and difficult intubation were limited or severely limited mandibular protrusion, thick/obese neck anatomy, history of sleep apnoea, history of snoring and a BMI of ≥ 30 kg/m^2.

Of considerable clinical relevance is the answer to the question: what happened in those 37 patients in whom mask ventilation was impossible? Intubation was uncomplicated in 26 (70%) and difficult in 10 (27%) cases, and impossible (requiring emergent cricothyrotomy) in only one case (approximately 3%). It is comforting to know that, although impossible mask ventilation may be associated with difficult intubation, endotracheal intubation will still be possible in the vast majority of cases. However, the rather low incidence of complete inability to ventilate by mask (0.16%), and the finding that only one of 37 patients that could not be ventilated by mask required surgical airway access, may reflect an effective *a priori* decision for awake fibreoptic intubation in patients with anticipated difficult ventilation and intubation.

As difficult mask ventilation can occur as unexpectedly as difficult intubation, the (comforting) finding of ultimately successful intubation in almost all patients despite the inability to ventilate by mask, re-emphasizes the utmost importance of effective pre-oxygenation (reflected by an expired oxygen concentration of preferably ≥ 90% during a tight mask fit). Effective pre-oxygenation will 'bridge' the time between recognizing the inability to ventilate by mask and ultimately gaining access to the airway.

As a beard was found to be a risk factor for difficult mask ventilation, the authors feel obliged to inform their patients of this risk. Of the various risk factors for difficult mask ventilation identified, a beard was the only one that can be modified. This poses the question as to whether patients should be advised to preoperatively shave their beard.

The finding of limited or severely limited mandibular protrusion as being an independent predictor of difficult or impossible mask ventilation, re-emphasizes – in accordance with the American Society of Anesthesiologists Task Force on Management of the Difficult Airway |92| – the relevance of an evaluation of mandibular protrusion as part of a standard preoperative physical examination.

The investigation triggers a couple of general remarks on studies trying to identify predictors of adverse outcome. Undoubtedly, this study identified certain features that were *associated* with difficult airway management. For example, independent predictors of the combination of difficult or impossible mask ventilation and difficult intubation in 84 cases were limited mandibular protrusion, thick/obese neck anatomy, history of sleep apnoea, history of snoring and a BMI of ≥ 30 kg/m². However, these predictors were also present in 9.8% ($n = 1348$), 11% ($n = 1455$), 4.8% ($n = 682$), 27% ($n = 3560$) and 64% ($n = 9039$), respectively, of approximately 14 000 cases of unproblematic mask ventilation and intubation. Put differently, almost all patients who had predictors of difficult or impossible ventilation by mask and difficult intubation were, in fact, easy to manage.

This finding underlines an important principle: as long as the adverse outcome we are trying to predict is relatively rare (in this case, impaired mask ventilation and difficult intubation in just 84 (0.37%) of 22 660 attempts), then even in the presence of independent risk factors, outcome will not be adversely affected in almost all of these patients. Such very low positive predictive values will considerably limit the clinical usefulness of any predictor or predictive tests |93|.

The publication by Kheterpal *et al.* |91| raises an intriguing question regarding the timing of administration of the muscle relaxant in routine clinical practice. It is a commonly taught practice (often a dictum) to withhold muscle relaxants until effective mask ventilation has been established (with the curious exemption of rapid sequence induction). In the case of failed mask ventilation, the patient should be awoken (following a failed attempt at intubation or without such an attempt) and fibreoptic endotracheal intubation performed. The findings by Kheterpal *et al.* seem to contradict such conventional wisdom. First, a considerable number of patients are likely to have received muscle relaxants before effective mask ventilation had been established. This is suggested by 4775 (21.1%) cases of mask ventilation grade 2, defined as 'ventilated by mask with oral airway/adjuvant with or without muscle relaxant'. Second, of the 37 patients with impossible mask ventilation, only one patient had not received a muscle relaxant before the first attempt at intubation |94|. This patient was intubated without difficulty. Four patients had received a non-depolarizing muscle relaxant before failure of mask ventilation was observed. One of these required emergency cricothyrotomy. The remaining 32 patients received succinylcholine after inability to mask ventilation had been noted and before the first attempt at intubation.

One is tempted to interpret the findings as showing that the 97% intubation success rate following inability to ventilate by mask was due to the early administration of the muscle relaxant, either before or immediately after recognition of inability to ventilate by mask. It is highly questionable that endotracheal intubation could have been that successfully performed in the absence of muscle relaxation, or that these patients could have safely been awoken. These findings would support the view (including my own) that the earliest possible administration of the muscle relaxant may well be the most effective tactic |95,96|.

Ventilatory strategy

Controversy continues as to the optimal perioperative ventilatory strategies in patients with normal lungs |97,98| (see also Chapter 2). The main objective of an optimal ventilatory strategy is to keep the regional end-inspiratory stretch – an indicator of ventilatory stress – as low as possible, thereby reducing the potential for alveolar injury and inflammation |97,98|. Present guidelines strongly support the use of tidal volumes (V_T) of 6 ml/kg predicted body weight in patients with acute lung injury (ALI) and acute respiratory distress syndrome (ARDS) |99|.

Comparable guidelines for patients without acute lung injury (ALI) or ARDS are lacking. The results of smaller randomized controlled trials of perioperative ventilatory strategies during major surgery have been inconsistent |97|. There is, however, preliminary evidence for a lung-protective effect of a ventilation strategy with a V_T of less than 10 ml/kg predicted body weight and positive end-expiratory pressure (PEEP) compared with a more conventional strategy with a V_T higher than 10 ml/kg and no PEEP |97–104|. When trying to put these findings into proper clinical perspective, it is important to realize that existing evidence for a lung-protective effect of lower tidal volumes in patients with normal lungs is mostly based on retrospective studies, and on surrogate markers of outcome (such as inflammatory mediators), rather than on clinical outcome variables |97|.

When patients with predisposing factors for the development of acute or ventilator-induced lung injury (e.g. pulmonary oedema or inflammation, restrictive lung disease, lung resection or cancer surgery) subsequently receive 'hits' such as sepsis, aspiration or transfusion, they may develop the clinical picture of ALI/ARDS |97|. According to this multiple 'hit' theory, large tidal volumes may constitute the primary hit (thereby inducing or exacerbating pulmonary inflammation) or a subsequent hit. By this reasoning, all surgical patients are at risk of developing ventilation-induced lung injury and would thus 'deserve' lung-protective ventilation.

Taking the various factors into consideration, it appears sensible to recommend avoiding high tidal volumes (i.e. > 10 ml/kg predicted body weight) and plateau airway pressures (i.e. $> 15-20$ cmH$_2$O), even in surgical patients without any evidence of lung disease |97|. PEEP of at least 5 cmH$_2$O should be applied to avoid atelectasis and maintain oxygenation. There is, however, no sound scientific basis on which to base a recommendation for a reduction in tidal volumes to less than 10 ml/kg predicted body weight when plateau pressure is not higher than 16 cmH$_2$O |97| (see also Chapter 2). However, even in the absence of a high airway plateau pressure, cyclic recruitment and derecruitment of small airways or lung units may contribute to lung injury |105|.

By the same reasoning, in patients with increased risk for the development of acute or ventilator-induced lung injury (due to either underlying risk factors or exposition to subsequent 'hits'), it seems equally sensible to recommend a lower V_T of 6 ml/kg predicted body weight |101|. Higher PEEP may be required to counteract the adverse effect of lower tidal volumes and plateau pressures on the formation of atelectasis.

It is, of course, to be expected that at comparable tidal volumes, long-term mechanical ventilation with or without extrapulmonary 'hits' will be more injurious than short-term ventilation without such 'hits'. Rather than applying a fixed ventilatory strategy to all patients during anaesthesia, the strategy should take into account the underlying medical condition of the patient and the type of surgery, and be individualized accordingly |97,98| (see also Chapter 2).

Extubation strategy

Whereas detailed guidelines exist for the airway management during induction of anaesthesia |92|, no such guidelines exist for the period during and immediately following tracheal extubation. This is surprising because tracheal extubation is merely the logical consequence of tracheal intubation, and the need for continued control of the airway persists after extubation. Furthermore, the incidence of complications associated with extubation may be higher than the incidence during intubation |106|. Eighteen of the 156 perioperative claims for difficult airway management between 1985 and 1999 included in the ASA Closed Claims database were associated with extubation in the operating room |87|.

In most cases of problems occurring after extubation, supportive care will re-establish adequate oxygenation and ventilation, but sometimes reintubation becomes unavoidable. As reintubation will usually be more difficult than the initial intubation (due to the frequently emergent nature, the accompanying hypoxaemia and cardiovascular instability, the lack of patient cooperation, insufficient time for adequate preparation, and limited access to the airway), and as airway emergency and repeated intubation attempts have been associated with adverse outcome (including death and brain damage) |87,107|, an effective extubation strategy should have a low reintubation rate. In addition, it should allow oxygenation and ventilation and facilitate reintubation in case of failure to tolerate extubation.

The ASA Task Force on Difficult Airway Management recommends a preformulated strategy for extubation of the difficult airway |92|. The extubation strategy of the difficult airway should be adjusted to the type of surgery, the medical condition of the patient, and the experience and preference of the anaesthetist. It should include (a) consideration of the merits of extubation in the awake versus the unconscious state; (b) consideration of clinical factors that may impair respiration after extubation; (c) a preformulated airway management plan in case the patient is unable to tolerate extubation; and (d) consideration of the use of a device that can facilitate reintubation.

The airway exchange catheter (AEC) is such a device. It is introduced through the endotracheal tube before extubation and is left *in situ* after removal of the endotracheal tube until the need for reintubation is considered minimal. By maintaining access to the airway, it facilitates reintubation in case of failure to tolerate extubation. Endotracheal reintubation via an indwelling AEC was successful in 92–100% of cases |**108–110**|. Compared with patients without an indwelling AEC in place at the time of reintubation, the first-pass success rate for reintubation was significantly higher (87% vs. 17%), episodes of severe hypoxaemia (6% vs. 19%) and multiple intubation attempts were fewer (10% vs. 77%), oesophageal intubation was less frequent (0% vs. 18%), and there was less need for additional rescue airway devices and techniques and surgical airways (6% vs. 90%) |**110**|. Nevertheless, although complications during AEC-facilitated reintubation may be relatively infrequent, they do occur and may be severe. In addition, of a total of 329 patients with known or suspected difficult airway who had been extubated over an AEC during a 9-year period, 87 (26.4%) required reintubation |**110**|.

All in all, the concept of an AEC-facilitated 'staged' extubation strategy is an attractive one, on a theoretical basis as well as on the basis of demonstrated benefit in selected patients. In experienced hands, it has a satisfactory success rate without requiring overly sophisticated equipment and skills. Especially when using a paediatric-size AEC, patient tolerance seems to be excellent, vocalization is preserved, and the risks of airway trauma and pulmonary aspiration are small |108–110|. Since tolerance of extubation cannot reliably be predicted, it is reassuring to know that an AEC facilitates reintubation in the vast majority of patients with difficult airway. Even if the initial attempt at reintubation fails in the presence of severe respiratory insufficiency, a jet-stylet-type AEC allows capnography, oxygen insufflation and jet ventilation, thereby 'bridging' the time required to obtain additional airway equipment and qualified help. By maintaining access to the airway, an indwelling AEC may justify an earlier trial of extubation without taking unnecessary risk, thereby avoiding 'prophylactic' continuation of endotracheal intubation or tracheotomy. However, only well-designed, controlled prospective trials will be able to ultimately determine the most effective extubation strategy |111|.

Conclusion

It is hoped that improvement in perioperative cardioprotection by myocardial conditioning, intensive medical therapy, and safe and effective management of dual anti-platelet therapy; and improvement in perioperative respiratory care by reliable preoperative respiratory risk stratification, reliable prediction of difficult mask ventilation, and correct choices of ventilatory and extubation strategies will result in improved patient outcome. Although intuitively to be expected, a causal relationship between the discussed approaches and interventions and improved ultimate outcome remains to be established by large, well-designed clinical trials.

This introduction has touched on just a very few aspects of perioperative care. The following chapters of Part I of *The Year in Anaesthesia and Critical Care* reflect the multitude and diversity of factors that govern the large field of perioperative care, all of which are affecting patient outcome.

Addendum

After completion of this editorial, the American College of Cardiology (ACC)/ American Heart Association (AHA) published their revised guidelines on perioperative cardiac evaluation and care for non-cardiac surgery |112,113|. The guidelines were developed in collaboration with the Society of Cardiovascular Anesthesiologists, and the Writing Committee was chaired by Professor Lee A. Fleisher, a prominent anaesthetist. Amongst other topics, the revised guidelines contain fully updated, highly relevant evidence-based recommendations for preoperative clinical assessment and cardiac testing, preoperative coronary revascularization, perioperative cardiac medication, and for the management of patients presenting with coronary artery stents. All recommendations are classified, and the level of evidence on which the classifications are based is reported. These revised guidelines constitute a large source of detailed information regarding all aspects of perioperative cardiac care and a critical analysis of data available on this clinically important subject. Detailed knowledge of these guidelines can be expected to improve the overall quality of perioperative patient management.

References

1. Priebe H-J. Perioperative myocardial infarction – aetiology and prevention. *Br J Anaesth* 2005; **95**: 3–19.

2. Murry CE, Jennings RB, Reimer KA. Preconditioning with ischemia: a delay of lethal injury in ischemic myocardium. *Circulation* 1986; **74**: 1124–36.

3. Kloner RA, Przyklenk K, Shook T, Cannon CP. Protection conferred by preinfarction angina is manifest in the aged heart: evidence from the TIMI 4 Trial. *J Thromb Thrombolysis* 1998; **6**: 89–92.

4. Vaage J, Valen G. Preconditioning and cardiac surgery. *Ann Thorac Surg* 2003; **75**: S709–14.

5. Valen G, Vaage J. Pre- and postconditioning during cardiac surgery. *Basic Res Cardiol* 2005; **100**: 179–86.

6. Pasupathy S, Homer-Vanniasinkam S. Surgical implications of ischemic preconditioning. *Arch Surg* 2005; **140**: 405–9.

7. Kloner RA, Rezkalla SH. Preconditioning, postconditioning and their application to clinical cardiology. *Cardiovasc Res* 2006; **70**: 297–307.

8. Ramzy D, Rao V, Weisel RD. Clinical applicability of preconditioning and postconditioning: the cardiothoracic surgeon's view. *Cardiovasc Res* 2006; **70**: 174–80.

9. Teoh LK, Grant R, Hulf JA, Pugsley WB, Yellon DM. The effect of preconditioning [ischemic and pharmacological] on myocardial necrosis following coronary artery bypass graft surgery. *Cardiovasc Res* 2002; **53**: 175–80.

10. Teoh LK, Grant R, Hulf JA, Pugsley WB, Yellon DM. A comparison between ischemic preconditioning, intermittent cross-clamp fibrillation and cold crystalloid cardioplegia for myocardial protection during coronary artery bypass graft surgery. *Cardiovasc Surg* 2002; **10**: 251–5.

11. Zaugg M, Lucchinetti E, Uecker M, Pasch T, Schaub MC. Anaesthetics and cardiac preconditioning. Part I. Signalling and cytoprotective mechanisms. *Br J Anaesth* 2003; **91**: 551–65.

12. Zaugg M, Lucchinetti E, Garcia C, Pasch T, Spahn DR, Schaub MC. Anaesthetics and cardiac preconditioning. Part II. Clinical implications. *Br J Anaesth* 2003; **91**: 566–76.

13. Tanaka K, Ludwig LM, Kersten JR, Pagel PS, Warltier DC. Mechanisms of cardioprotection by volatile anesthetics. *Anesthesiology* 2004; **100**: 707–21.

14. De Hert SG. The concept of anaesthetic-induced cardioprotection: clinical relevance. *Best Pract Res Clin Anaesthesiol* 2005; **19**: 445–59.

15. Bienengraeber MW, Weihrauch D, Kersten JR, Pagel PS, Warltier DC. Cardioprotection by volatile anesthetics. *Vascul Pharmacol* 2005; **42**: 243–52.

16. Howell S, Kimpson P. Protecting the heart in non-cardiac surgery. In: Hunter J, Cook T, Priebe HJ, Struys M, eds. *The Year in Anaesthesia and Critical Care,* Vol. 1. Oxford: Clinical Publishing, 2005; pp. 103–8.

17. Conzen PF, Fischer S, Detter C, Peter K. Sevoflurane provides greater protection of the myocardium than propofol in patients undergoing off-pump coronary artery bypass surgery. *Anesthesiology* 2003; **99**: 826–33.

18. De Hert SG, Van der Linden PJ, Cromheecke S, Meeus R, ten Broecke PW, De Blier IG, Stockman BA, Rodrigus IE. Choice of primary anesthetic regimen can influence intensive care unit length of stay after coronary surgery with cardiopulmonary bypass. *Anesthesiology* 2004; **101**: 9–20.

19. De Hert SG, Van der Linden PJ, Cromheecke S, Meeus R, Nelis A, Van Reeth V, ten Broecke PW, De Blier IG, Stockman BA, Rodrigus I. Cardioprotective properties of sevoflurane in patients undergoing coronary surgery with cardiopulmonary bypass are related to the modalities of its administration. *Anesthesiology* 2004; **101**: 299–310.

20. Bein B, Renner J, Caliebe D, Scholz J, Paris A, Fraund S, Zaehle W, Tonner PH. Sevoflurane but not propofol preserves myocardial function during minimally invasive direct coronary artery bypass surgery. *Anesth Analg* 2005; **100**: 610–16.

21. Cromheecke S, Pepermans V, Hendrickx E, Lorsomradee S, ten Broecke PW, Stockman BA, Rodrigus IE, De Hert SG. Cardioprotective properties of sevoflurane in patients undergoing aortic valve replacement with cardiopulmonary bypass. *Anesth Analg* 2006; **103**: 289–96.

22. Lee MC, Chen CH, Kuo MC, Kang PL, Lo A, Liu K. Isoflurane preconditioning-induced cardio-protection in patients undergoing coronary artery bypass grafting. *Eur J Anaesthesiol* 2006; **23**: 841–7.

23. Law-Koune JD, Raynaud C, Liu N, Dubois C, Romano M, Fischler M. Sevoflurane-remifentanil versus propofol-remifentanil anesthesia at a similar bispectral level for off-pump coronary artery surgery: no evidence of reduced myocardial ischemia. *J Cardiothorac Vasc Anesth* 2006; **20**: 484–92.

24. Tritapepe L, Landoni G, Guarracino F, Pompei F, Crivellari M, Maselli D, De Luca M, Fochi O, D'Avolio S, Bignami E, Calabrò MG, Zangrillo A. Cardiac protection by volatile anaesthetics: a multicentre randomized controlled study in patients undergoing coronary artery bypass grafting with cardiopulmonary bypass. *Eur J Anaesthesiol* 2007; **24**: 323–31.

25. Symons JA, Myles PS. Myocardial protection with volatile anaesthetic agents during coronary artery bypass surgery: a meta-analysis. *Br J Anaesth* 2006; **97**: 127–36.

26. Heusch G, Schulz R. Remote preconditioning. *J Mol Cell Cardiol* 2002; **34**: 1279–81.

27. Wolfrum S, Schneider K, Heidbreder M, Nienstedt J, Dominiak P, Dendorfer A. Remote preconditioning protects the heart by activating myocardial PKCepsilon-isoform. *Cardiovasc Res* 2002; **55**: 583–9.

28. Weinbrenner C, Nelles M, Herzog N, Sarvay L, Strasser RH. Remote preconditioning by infrarenal occlusion of the aorta protects the heart from infarction: a newly identified non-neuronal but PKC-dependent pathway. *Cardiovasc Res* 2002; **55**: 590–610.

29. Gunaydin B, Cakici I, Soncul H, Kalaycioglu S, Cevik C, Sancak B, Kanzik I, Karadenizli Y. Does remote organ ischaemia trigger preconditioning during coronary artery surgery? *Pharmacol Res* 2000; **41**: 493–6.

30. Zhao ZQ, Corvera JS, Halkos ME, Kerendi F, Wang NP, Guyton RA, Vinten-Johansen J. Inhibition of myocardial injury by ischemic postconditioning during reperfusion: comparison with ischemic preconditioning. *Am J Physiol Circ Physiol* 2003; **285**: H579–88.

31. Vinten-Johansen J, Zhao ZQ, Zatta AJ, Kin H, Halkos ME, Kerendi F. Postconditioning. A new link in nature's armor against myocardial ischemia-reperfusion injury. *Basic Res Cardiol* 2005; **100**: 295–310.

32. Halkos ME, Kerendi F, Corvera JS, Wang NP, Kin H, Payne CS, Sun H-Y, Guyton RA, Vinten-Johansen J, Zhao Z-Q. Myocardial protection with postconditioning is not enhanced by ischemic preconditioning. *Ann Thorac Surg* 2004; **78**: 961–9.

33. Gross ER, Gross GJ. Ligand triggers of classical preconditioning and postconditioning. *Cardiovasc Res* 2006; **70**: 212–21.

34. Garcia-Dorado D, Vinten-Johansen J, Piper HM. Bringing preconditioning and postconditioning into focus. *Cardiovasc Res* 2006; **70**: 167–9.

35. Iliodromitis EK, Georgiadis M, Cohen MV, Downey JM, Bofilis E, Kremastinos DT. Protection from postconditioning depends on the number of short ischemic insults in anesthetized pigs. *Basic Res Cardiol* 2006; **101**: 502–7.

36. Laskey WK. Brief repetitive balloon occlusions enhance reperfusion during percutaneous coronary intervention for acute myocardial infarction: a pilot study. *Catheter Cardiovasc Interv* 2005; **65**: 361–7.

37. Staat P, Rioufol G, Piot C, Cottin Y, Cung TT, L'Huillier I, Aupetit JF, Bonnefoy E, Finet G, Andre-Fouet X, Ovize M. Postconditioning the human heart. *Circulation* 2005; **112**: 2143–8.

38. Darling CE, Solari PB, Smith CS, Furman MI, Przyklenk K. 'Postconditioning' the human heart: multiple balloon inflations during primary angioplasty may confer cardioprotection. *Basic Res Cardiol* 2007; **102**: 274–8.

39. Feng J, Lucchinetti E, Ahuja P, Pasch T, Perriard JC, Zaugg M. Isoflurane postconditioning prevents opening of the mitochondrial permeability transition pore through inhibition of glycogen synthase kinase 3ß. *Anesthesiology* 2005; **103**: 987–95.

40. Chiari PC, Bienengraeber MW, Pagel PS, Krolikowski JG, Kersten JR, Warltier DC. Isoflurane protects against myocardial infarction during early reperfusion by activation of phosphatidylinositol-3-kinase signal transduction: evidence for anesthetic-induced postconditioning in rabbits. *Anesthesiology* 2005; **102**: 102–9.

41. Deyhimy DI, Fleming NW, Brodkin IG, Liu H. Anesthetic preconditioning combined with postconditioning offers no additional benefit over preconditioning or postconditioning alone. *Anesth Analg* 2007; **105**: 316–24.

42. Obal D, Dettwiler S, Favoccia C, Scharbatke H, Preckel B, Schlack W. The influence of mitochondrial K(ATP)-channels in the cardioprotection of preconditioning and postconditioning by sevoflurane in the rat in vivo. *Anesth Analg* 2005; **101**: 1252–60.

43. Lucchinetti E, da Silva R, Pasch T, Schaub MC, Zaugg M. Anaesthetic preconditioning but not postconditioning prevents early activation of the deleterious cardiac remodeling

programme: evidence of opposing genomic responses in cardioprotection by pre- and postconditioning. *Br J Anaesth* 2005; **95**: 140–52.

44. Rosamond W, Flegal K, Friday G, Furie K, Go A, Greenlund K, Haase N, Ho M, Howard V, Kissela B, Kittner S, Lloyd-Jones D, McDermott M, Meigs J, Moy C, Nichol G, O'Donnell CJ, Roger V, Rumsfeld J, Sorlie P, Steinberger J, Thom T, Wasserthiel-Smoller S, Hong Y, for the American Heart Association Statistics Committee and Stroke Statistics Subcommittee Heart Disease and Stroke Statistics – 2007 Update: a report from the American Heart Association Statistics Committee and Stroke Statistics Subcommittee. *Circulation* 2007; **115**: e69–e171.

45. Feldman DN, Gade CL, Slotwiner AJ Parikh M, Bergman G, Wong SC, Minutello RM. Comparison of outcomes of percutaneous coronary interventions in patients of three age groups (< 60, 60 to 80, and > 80 years) (from the New York State Angioplasty Registry). *Am J Cardiol* 2006; **98**: 1334–9.

46. Mehta SR, Cannon CP, Fox KA, Wallentin L, Boden WE, Spacek R, Widimsky P, McCullough PA, Hunt D, Braunwald E, Yusuf S. Routine versus selective invasive strategies in patients with acute coronary syndromes: a collaborative meta-analysis of randomized trials. *JAMA* 2005; **293**: 2908–17.

47. Hueb W, Soares PR, Gersh BJ, César LAM, Luz PL, Puig LB, Martinez EM, Oliveira SA, Ramires JAF. The Medicine, Angioplasty, or Surgery Study (MASS-II): a randomized, controlled clinical trial of three therapeutic strategies for multivessel coronary artery disease: one-year results. *J Am Coll Cardiol* 2004; **43**: 1743–51.

48. Henderson RA, Pocock SJ, Clayton TC, Knight R, Fox KAA, Julian DG, Chamberlain DA. Seven-year outcome in the RITA-2 trial: coronary angioplasty versus medical therapy. *J Am Coll Cardiol* 2003; **42**: 1161–70.

49. Howard-Alpe GM, de Bono J, Hudsmith L, Orr WP, Foex P, Sear JW. Coronary artery stents and non-cardiac surgery. *Br J Anaesth* 2007; **98**: 560–74.

50. Dalal R, D'Souza S, Shulman MS. Brief review: Coronary drug-eluting stents and anesthesia: [Article de synthese court: Les tuteurs coronariens actifs et l'anesthesie]. *Can J Anesth* 2006; **53**: 1230–43.

51. Boden WE, O'Rourke RA, Teo KK, Hartigan PM, Maron DJ, Kostuk WJ, Knudtson M, Dada M, Casperson P, Harris CL, Chaitman BR, Shaw L, Gosselin G, Nawaz S, Title LM, Gau G, Blaustein AS, Booth DC, Bates ER, Spertus JA, Berman DS, Mancini GBJ, Weintraub WS, for the COURAGE Trial Research Group. Optimal medical therapy with or without PCI for stable coronary disease. *N Engl J Med* 2007; **356**: 1503–16.

52. Curfman GD, Morrissey S, Jarcho JA, Drazen JM. Drug-eluting coronary stents: promise and uncertainty. *N Engl J Med* 2007; **356**: 1059–60.

53. Spaulding C, Daemen J, Boersma E, Cutlip DE, Serruys PW. A pooled analysis of data comparing sirolimus-eluting stents with bare-metal stents. *N Engl J Med* 2007; **356**: 989–97.

54. Stone GW, Moses JW, Ellis SG, Schofer J, Dawkins KD, Morice M-C, Colombo A, Schampaert E, Grube E, Kirtane AJ, Cutlip DE, Fahy M, Pocock SJ, Mehran R, Leon MB. Safety and efficacy of sirolimus- and paclitaxel-eluting coronary stents. *N Engl J Med* 2007; **356**: 998–1008.

55. Kastrati A, Mehilli J, Pache J, Kaiser C, Valgimigli M, Kelbæk H, Menichelli M, Sabaté M, Suttorp MJ, Baumgart D, Seyfarth M, Pfisterer ME, Schömig A. Analysis of 14 trials comparing sirolimus-eluting stents with bare-metal stents. *N Engl J Med* 2007; **356**: 1030–9.

56. Lagerqvist B, James SK, Stenestrand U, Lindbäck J, Nilsson T, Wallentin L. Long-term outcomes with drug-eluting stents versus bare-metal stents in Sweden. *N Engl J Med* 2007; **356**: 1009–19.

57. Mauri L, Hsieh W, Massaro JM, Ho KKL, D'Agostino R, Cutlip DE. Stent thrombosis in randomized clinical trials of drug-eluting stents. *N Engl J Med* 2007; **356**: 1020–9.

58. Maisel WH. Unanswered questions – drug-eluting stents and the risk of late thrombosis. *N Engl J Med* 2007; **356**: 981–4.

59. Hochman JS, Steg PG. Does preventive PCI work? *N Engl J Med* 2007; **356**: 1572–4.

60. Naghavi M, Libby P, Falk E, Casscells SW, Litovsky S, Rumberger J, Badimon JJ, Stefanadis C, Moreno P, Pasterkamp G, Fayad Z, Stone PH, Waxman S, Raggi P, Madjid M, Zarrabi A, Burke A, Yuan C, Fitzgerald PJ, Siscovick DS, de Korte CL, Aikawa M, Airaksinen KEJ, Assmann G, Becker CR, Chesebro JH, Farb A, Galis ZS, Jackson C, Jang I-K, Koenig W, Lodder RA, March K, Demirovic J, Navab M, Priori SG, Rekhter MD, Bahr R, Grundy SM, Mehran R, Colombo A, Boerwinkle E, Ballantyne, Insull W Jr, Schwartz RS, Vogel R, Serruys PW, Hansson GK, Faxon DP, Kaul S, Drexler H, Greenland P, Muller JE, Virmani R, Ridker PM, Zipes DP, Shah PK, Willerson JT. From vulnerable plaque to vulnerable patient: a call for new definitions and risk assessment strategies. *Circulation* 2003; **108**: 1664–72.

61. Waxman S, Ishibashi F, Muller JE. Detection and treatment of vulnerable plaques and vulnerable patients: novel approaches to prevention of coronary events. *Circulation* 2006; **114**: 2390–411.

62. Sdringola S, Loghin C, Boccalandro F, Gould KL. Mechanisms of progression and regression of coronary artery disease by PET related to treatment intensity and clinical events at long-term follow-up. *J Nucl Med* 2006; **47**: 59–67.

63. Hochman JS, Lamas GA, Buller CE, Dzavik V, Reynolds HR, Abramsky SJ, Forman S, Ruzyllo W, Maggioni AP, White H, Sadowski Z, Carvalho AC, Rankin JM, Renkin JP, Steg G, Mascette AM, Sopko G, Pfisterer ME, Leor J, Fridrich V, Mark DB, Knatterud GL, for the Occluded Artery Trial Investigators. Coronary intervention for persistent occlusion after myocardial infarction. *N Engl J Med* 2006; **355**: 2395–407.

64. de Winter RJ, Windhausen F, Cornel JH, Dunselman PHJM, Janus CL, Bendermacher PEF, Michels HR, Sanders GT, Tijssen JPG, Verheugt FWA, for the Invasive versus Conservative Treatment in Unstable Coronary Syndromes (ICTUS) Investigators. Early invasive versus selectively invasive management for acute coronary syndromes. *N Engl J Med* 2005; **353**: 1095–104.

65. Katritsis DG, Ioannidis JP. Percutaneous coronary intervention versus conservative therapy in nonacute coronary artery disease: a meta-analysis. *Circulation* 2005; **111**: 2906–12.

66. Gibbons RJ, Abrams J, Chatterjee K, Daley J, Deedwania PC, Douglas JS, Ferguson TB Jr, Fihn SD, Fraker TD Jr, Gardin JM, O'Rourke RA, Pasternak RC, Williams SV, Gibbons RJ, Alpert JS, Antman EM, Hiratzka LF, Fuster V, Faxon DP, Gregoratos G, Jacobs AK, Smith SC Jr. ACC/AHA 2002 guideline update for the management of patients with chronic stable angina – summary article: a report of the American College of Cardiology/American Heart Association Task Force on practice guidelines

(Committee on the Management of Patients with Chronic Stable Angina). *J Am Coll Cardiol* 2003; **41**: 159–68.

67. Smith SC Jr, Feldman TE, Hirshfeld JW Jr, Jacobs AK, Kern MJ, King SB III, Morrison DA, O'Neill WW, Schaff HV, Whitlow PL, Williams DO, Antman EM, Smith SC Jr, Adams CD, Anderson JL, Faxon DP, Fuster V, Halperin JL, Hiratzka LF, Hunt SA, Jacobs AK, Nishimura R, Ornato JP, Page RL, Riegel B. ACC/AHA/SCAI 2005 guideline update for percutaneous coronary intervention – summary article: a report of the American College of Cardiology/American Heart Association Task Force on Practice Guidelines (ACC/AHA/SCAI Writing Committee to Update the 2001 Guidelines for Percutaneous Coronary Intervention). *Circulation* 2006; **113**: 156–75.

68. Patti G, Pasceri V, Colonna G, Miglionico M, Fischetti D, Sardella G, Montinaro A, Di Sciascio G. Atorvastatin pretreatment improves outcomes in patients with acute coronary syndromes undergoing early percutaneous coronary intervention. Results of the ARMYDA-ACS Randomized Trial. *J Am Coll Cardiol* 2007; **49**: 1272–8.

69. Powell BD, Bybee KA, Valeti U, Thomas RJ, Kopecky SL, Mullany CJ, Wright RS. Influence of preoperative lipid-lowering therapy on postoperative outcome in patients undergoing coronary artery bypass grafting. *Am J Cardiol* 2007; **99**: 785–9.

70. McFalls EO, Ward HB, Mortitz TE, Goldman S, Krupski WC, Littooy F, Pierpont G, Santilli S, Rapp J, Hattler B, Shunk K, Jaenicke C, Thottapurathu L, Ellis N, Reda DJ, Henderson WG. Coronary-artery revascularization before elective major vascular surgery. *N Engl J Med* 2004; **351**: 2795–804.

71. Silber S, Albertsson P, Avilés FF, Camici PG, Colombo A, Hamm C, Jørgensen E, Marco J, Nordrehaug J-E, Ruzyllo W, Urban P, Stone GW, Wijns W. Guidelines for percutaneous coronary interventions: The Task Force for Percutaneous Coronary Interventions of the European Society of Cardiology. *Eur Heart J* 2005; **26**: 804–47.

72. Braunwald E, Antman EM, Beasley JW, Califf RM, Cheitlin MD, Hochman JS, Jones RH, Kereiakes D, Kupersmith J, Levin TN, Pepine CJ, Schaeffer JW, Smith EE III, Steward DE, Theroux P, Gibbons RJ, Alpert JS, Faxon DP, Fuster V, Gregoratos G, Hiratzka LF, Jacobs AK, Smith SC Jr. ACC/AHA 2002 guideline update for the management of patients with unstable angina and non-ST-segment elevation myocardial infarction: summary article: a report of the American College of Cardiology/American Heart Association Task Force on Practice Guidelines (Committee on the Management of Patients With Unstable Angina). *J Am Coll Cardiol* 2002; **40**: 1366–74.

73. Smith SC Jr, Feldman TE, Hirshfeld JW Jr, Jacobs AK, Kern MJ, King SB III, Morrison DA, O'Neill WW, Schaff HV, Whitlow PL, Williams DO. ACC/AHA/SCAI 2005 guideline update for percutaneous coronary intervention: a report of the American College of Cardiology/American Heart Association Task Force of Practice Guidelines (ACC/AHA/SCAI Writing Committee to update the 2001 Guidelines for Percutaneous Coronary Intervention). 2005. Available at: http://www.americanheart.org. Accessed August 2007.

74. Smith SC Jr, Allen J, Blair SN, Bonow RO, Brass LM, Fonarow GC, Grundy SM, Hiratzka L, Jones D, Krumholz HM, Mosca L, Pasternak RC, Pearson T, Pfeffer MA, Taubert KA. AHA/ACC guidelines for secondary prevention for patients with coronary and other atherosclerotic vascular disease: 2006 update: endorsed by the National Heart, Lung, and Blood Institute [published correction appears in Circulation 2006; **113**: e847]. *Circulation* 2006; **113**: 2363–72.

75. Collet J-P, Montalescot G. Premature withdrawal and alternative therapies to dual oral antiplatelet therapy. *Eur Heart J* 2006; 8 (Suppl.): G46–52.

76. Biondi-Zoccai GGL, Lotrionte M, Agostoni P, Abbate A, Fusaro M, Burzotta F, Testa L, Sheiban I, Sangiorgi G. A systematic review and meta-analysis on the hazards of discontinuing or not adhering to aspirin among 50 279 patients at risk for coronary artery disease. *Eur Heart J* 2006; **27**: 2667–74.

77. Ferrari E, Benhamou M, Cerboni P, Baudouy M. Coronary syndromes following aspirin withdrawal: a special risk for late stent thrombosis. *J Am Coll Cardiol* 2005; **45**: 456–9.

78. Grines CL, Bonow RO, Casey DE, Gardner TJ, Lockhart PB, Moliterno DJ, O'Gara P, Whitlow P. Prevention of premature discontinuation of dual antiplatelet therapy in patients with coronary artery stents: a Science Advisory from the American Heart Association, American College of Cardiology, Society for Cardiovascular Angiography and Interventions, American College of Surgeons, and American Dental Association, with representation from the American College of Physicians. *Circulation* 2007; **115**: 813–18.

79. Hovens MMCM, Snoep JD, Eikenboom JCJ, van der Bom JG, Mertens BJA, Huisman MV. Prevalence of persistent platelet reactivity despite use of aspirin: A systematic review. *Am Heart J* 2007; **153**: 175–81.

80. Angiolillo DJ, Fernandez-Ortiz A, Bernardo E, Alfonso F, Macaya C, Bass TA, Costa MA. Variability in individual responsiveness to clopidogrel. Clinical implications, management, and future perspectives. *J Am Coll Cardiol* 2007; **49**: 1505–16.

81. Chassot P-G, Delabays A, Spahn DR. Perioperative antiplatelet therapy: the case for continuing therapy in patients at risk of myocardial infarction. *Br J Anaesth* 2007; **99**: 316–28.

82. Spahn DR, Howell SJ, Delabays A, Chassot P-G. Coronary stents and perioperative anti-platelet regimen: dilemma of bleeding and stent thrombosis. *Br J Anaesth* 2006; **96**: 675–7.

83. Qaseem A, Snow V, Fitterman N, Hornbake R, Lawrence VA, Smetana GW, Weiss K, Owens DK, for the Clinical Efficacy Assessment Subcommittee of the American College of Physicians. Risk assessment for and strategies to reduce perioperative pulmonary complications for patients undergoing noncardiothoracic surgery: a guideline from the American College of Physicians. *Ann Intern Med* 2006; **144**: 575–80.

84. Smetana GW Lawrence VA, Cornell JE. Preoperative pulmonary risk stratification for noncardiothoracic surgery: systematic review for the American College of Physicians. *Ann Intern Med* 2006; **144**: 581–95.

85. Lawrence VA, Cornell JE, Smetana GW. Strategies to reduce postoperative pulmonary complications after noncardiothoracic surgery: systematic review for the American College of Physicians. *Ann Intern Med* 2006; **144**: 596–608.

86. Smetana GW, Macpherson DS. The case against routine preoperative laboratory testing. *Med Clin N Am* 2003; **87**: 7–40.

87. Peterson GN, Domino KB, Caplan RA, Posner KL, Lee LA, Cheney FW. Management of the difficult airway: a closed claims analysis. *Anesthesiology* 2005; **103**: 33–9.

88. Shiga T, Wajima Z, Inoue T, Sakamoto A. Predicting difficult intubation in apparently normal patients. A meta-analysis of bedside screening test performance. *Anesthesiology* 2005; **103**: 429–37.

89. Langeron O, Masso E, Huraux C, Guggiari M, Bianchi A, Coriat P, Riou B. Prediction of difficult mask ventilation. *Anesthesiology* 2000; **92**: 1229–36.

90. Yildiz TS, Solak M, Toker K. The incidence and risk factors of difficult mask ventilation. *J Anesth* 2005; **19**: 7–11.

91. Kheterpal S, Han R, Tremper KK, Shanks A, Tait AR, O'Reilly M, Ludwig TA. Incidence and predictors of difficult and impossible mask ventilation. *Anesthesiology* 2006; **105**: 885–91.

92. Caplan RA, Benumof JL, Berry FA, Blitt CD, Bode RH, Cheney FW, Connis RT, Guidry OF, Nickinovich DG, Ovassapian A, for the American Society of Anesthesiologists Task Force on Difficult Airway Management. Practice Guidelines for Management of the Difficult Airway: An Updated Report by the American Society of Anesthesiologists Task Force on Management of the Difficult Airway. *Anesthesiology* 2003; **98**: 1269–77.

93. Yentis SM. Predicting trouble in airway management. *Anesthesiology* 2006; **105**: 871–2.

94. Kheterpal S, Tremper KK. Impossible mask ventilation (Correspondence). *Anesthesiology* 2007; **107**: 171–2.

95. Calder I. Impossible mask ventilation (Correspondence). *Anesthesiology* 2007; **107**: 171.

96. Yentis SM. Impossible mask ventilation (Correspondence). *Anesthesiology* 2007; **107**: 171.

97. Schultz MJ, Haitsma JJ, Slutsky AS, Gajic O. What tidal volumes should be used in patients without acute lung injury? *Anesthesiology* 2007; **106**: 1226–31.

98. Putensen C, Wrigge H. Tidal volumes in patients with normal lungs. One for all or the less, the better (Editorial)? *Anesthesiology* 2007; **106**: 1085–7.

99. Dellinger RP, Carlet JM, Masur H, Gerlach H, Calandra T, Cohen J, Gea-Banacloche J, Keh D, Marshall JC, Parker MM, Ramsay G, Zimmerman JL, Vincent JL, Levy MM. Surviving Sepsis Campaign guidelines for management of severe sepsis and septic shock. *Crit Care Med* 2004; **32**: 858–73.

100. Michelet P, D'Journo XB, Roch A, Doddoli C, Marin V, Papazian L, Decamps I, Bregeon F, Thomas P, Auffray JP. Protective ventilation influences systemic inflammation after esophagectomy: a randomized controlled study. *Anesthesiology* 2006; **105**: 911–19.

101. Wrigge H, Uhlig U, Baumgarten G, Menzenbach J, Zinserling J, Ernst M, Dromann D, Welz A, Uhlig S, Putensen C. Mechanical ventilation strategies and inflammatory responses to cardiac surgery: a prospective randomized clinical trial. *Intensive Care Med* 2005; **31**: 1379–87.

102. Zupancich E, Paparella D, Turani F, Munch C, Rossi A, Massaccesi S, Ranieri VM. Mechanical ventilation affects inflammatory mediators in patients undergoing cardiopulmonary bypass for cardiac surgery: a randomized clinical trial. *J Thorac Cardiovasc Surg* 2005; **130**: 378–83.

103. Reis Miranda D, Gommers D, Struijs A, Dekker R, Mekel J, Feelders R, Lachmann B, Bogers AJ. Ventilation according to the open lung concept attenuates pulmonary inflammatory response in cardiac surgery. *Eur J Cardiothorac Surg* 2005; **28**: 889–95.

104. Choi G, Wolthuis EK, Bresser P, Levi M, van der Poll T, Dzoljic M, Vroom B, Schultz MJ. Mechanical ventilation with lower tidal volumes and positive end-expiratory pressure prevents alveolar coagulation in patients without lung injury. *Anesthesiology* 2006; **105**: 689–95.

105. Mols G, Priebe H-J, Guttmann J. Alveolar recruitment in acute lung injury. *Br J Anaesth* 2006; **96**: 156–66.

106. Asai T, Koga K, Vaughan RS. Respiratory complications associated with tracheal intubation and extubation. *Br J Anaesth* 1998; **80**: 767–75.

107. Mort TC. Emergency tracheal intubation: Complications associated with repeated laryngoscopic attempts. *Anesth Analg* 2004; **99**: 607–13.

108. Dosemeci L, Yilmaz M, Yegin A, Cengiz M, Ramazanoglu A. The routine use of pediatric airway exchange catheter after extubation of adult patients who have undergone maxillofacial or major neck surgery: a clinical observational study. *Crit Care* 2004; **8**: R385–90.

109. Loudermilk EP, Hartmannsgruber M, Stoltzfus DP, Langevin PB. A prospective study of the safety of tracheal extubation using a pediatric airway exchange catheter for patients with a known difficult airway. *Chest* 1997; **111**: 1660–5.

110. Mort TC. Continuous airway access for the difficult extubation: the efficacy of the airway exchange catheter. *Anesth Analg* 2007; **105**: 1357–62.

111. Biro P, Priebe H-J. Staged extubation strategy: is use of an airway exchange catheter the answer? *Anesth Analg* 2007; **105**: 1182–5.

112. Fleisher LA, Beckman JA, Brown KA, Calkins H, Chaikof E, Fleischmann KE, Freeman WK, Froehlich JB, Kasper EK, Kersten JR, Riegel B, Robb JF. ACC/AHA 2007 guidelines on perioperative cardiovascular evaluation and care for noncardiac surgery: executive summary: a report of the American College of Cardiology/American Heart Association Task Force on Practice Guidelines (Writing Committee to Revise the 2002 Guidelines on Perioperative Cardiovascular Evaluation for Noncardiac Surgery). *Circulation* 2007; **116**: 1971–96.

113. Fleisher LA, Beckman JA, Brown KA, Calkins H, Chaikof E, Fleischmann KE, Freeman WK, Froehlich JB, Kasper EK, Kersten JR, Riegel B, Robb JF. ACC/AHA 2007 guidelines on perioperative cardiovascular evaluation and care for noncardiac surgery: a report of the American College of Cardiology/American Heart Association Task Force on Practice Guidelines (Writing Committee to Revise the 2002 Guidelines on Perioperative Cardiovascular Evaluation for Noncardiac Surgery). *Circulation* 2007; **116**: e418–99 (available at http://circ.ahajournals.org/cgi/content/full/116/17/e418).

1

Perioperative blood component therapy and haemostasis

TIM WALSH

Introduction

Blood transfusion requirements are increasingly used as a quality measure for many types of surgery. Greater patient awareness of the potential risks of transfusions, ranging from transfusion reactions to the transmission of variant Creutzfeldt–Jakob disease (CJD), has led to increased efforts to perform surgery without transfusion or decrease the number of blood donor exposures. These trends are also needed for logistic reasons. The number of blood donors is decreasing, partly as a result of legislation limiting eligibility such as previous recipients of allogeneic blood, and partly because of changing public priorities. The introduction of testing for variant CJD could cause a large decrease in donations, because of public fears concerning the consequences of testing (for example, on insurance policies). The number of patients undergoing procedures with a high risk of blood loss may increase as the population grows older. Many blood services are experiencing reduced blood stocks despite increasing efficiency by moving stocks more actively and using strategies such as electronic issue direct from the blood bank. These measures are decreasing blood wastage rates but could be insufficient to maintain the supply chain.

Many techniques are available to anaesthetists that may modify blood loss and transfusion requirements. There are now a large number of investigations in the literature showing those interventions that work well in different patient groups, but many questions still remain. Few studies have compared drugs with similar effects (for example, different anti-fibrinolytics) or evaluated interactions between different strategies (for example, perioperative cell salvage and anti-fibrinolytics). There have been few cost-effectiveness studies to help clinicians make a business case for the development of new services or funding of new drugs (for example, a cell salvage service or preoperative medication with erythropoietin). Finally, as these drugs become more widely used in trials, concerns regarding their overall safety profile are emerging. This chapter reviews recent publications covering each of these issues.

Perioperative anti-fibrinolytic treatment

Anti-fibrinolytics in cardiac surgery

Cardiac surgery is a major consumer of blood stocks; some estimates suggest that 20–30% of all blood is used in this setting. Greater blood use is associated with greater infection rates, longer hospital and intensive care stays, increased rates of re-exploration, and higher mortality |1|. Although many observational studies have examined this association, it is always difficult to determine whether blood transfusions cause these adverse effects or whether this is a form of confounding by indication. In other words, does blood cause the problem or is it simply associated with other, more important, causes of morbidity? Still, it is beneficial to both patients and blood stocks to utilize interventions that are effective in reducing blood transfusions in cardiac surgery. This specialty is particularly focused on exposure to blood, because many patients were previously infected with HIV and hepatitis C, and because transfusion rates are one of the outcomes scrutinized in the public domain.

Anti-fibrinolytic drugs decrease blood loss in cardiac surgery. This has been shown in multiple trials and confirmed in a Cochrane systematic review, last updated in 2003 |2|. Specifically, the review concluded that no further trials were needed for aprotinin, but that large trials were needed to evaluate cost-effectiveness and to compare effectiveness with other drugs, namely tranexamic acid and aminocaproic acid (both lysine analogues). Aprotinin is considerably more expensive than the other drugs. It may also have more diverse clinical effects than the lysine analogues as it is a serine protease enzyme inhibitor acting at potentially multiple sites.

The use of anti-fibrinolytic drugs for high-risk cases is recommended in most cardiac surgery clinical guidelines, including a recent comprehensive guideline published by the Society of Cardiovascular Anesthesiologists |3|. As a result, assessments of the effectiveness and safety of these drugs is problematic in 'real life'. There are, broadly speaking, two approaches: first, to use large observational cohorts to examine the association between the drugs and relevant clinical outcomes, using appropriate statistical methods to adjust for confounding factors; and, second, to perform meta-analyses of the available trial data to produce pooled estimates of the incidence of important clinical outcomes. Several high-profile studies have been published on this subject over the past 2 years. These are presented below, followed by a commentary.

The risk associated with aprotinin in cardiac surgery

Mangano DT, Tudor IC, Dietzel C. *N Engl J Med* 2006; **354**: 353–65

BACKGROUND. It is well established from randomized controlled trials (RCTs) that aprotinin limits blood loss in cardiac surgery with cardiopulmonary bypass. There is also RCT evidence that tranexamic acid and aminocaproic acid reduce blood loss. These therapies are recommended in clinical guidelines and embedded in routine practice worldwide. Relatively few data exist concerning the incidence of adverse effects with these drugs. In this prospective observational cohort study of 4374 patients undergoing coronary revascularization, the authors evaluated the relative safety of aprotinin (1295 patients), aminocaproic acid (883) and tranexamic acid (822) versus no drug (1374 patients). The authors hypothesized that the use of anti-fibrinolytic drugs was unsafe and increased renal, cardiovascular and neurological complications. Complex statistical methods were used to adjust for relevant covariates, including 97 potential risk factors.

INTERPRETATION. In propensity-adjusted, multivariable logistic regression, use of aprotinin was associated with doubling of risk for dialysis-dependent renal failure for patients undergoing complex surgery (odds ratio [OR] 2.59; 95% confidence interval [CI] 1.36–4.95] and primary surgery (OR 2.34; 95% CI 1.27–4.31). Aprotinin was associated with a 55% greater risk of myocardial infarction or heart failure and a 181% increased risk of stroke or encephalopathy. No increased risk was observed for tranexamic or aminocaproic acid. All three drugs decreased blood loss to a similar extent (mean reduction in blood loss ranging from 676 to 827 ml; $P<0.001$ for all three drugs). The authors concluded that in view of the association between aprotinin and serious organ damage, the continued use of aprotinin is not prudent, and that tranexamic and aminocaproic acid are equally efficacious but safer alternatives.

Mortality associated with aprotinin during 5 years following coronary artery bypass graft surgery

Mangano DT, Miao Y, Vuylsteke A, *et al*. *JAMA* 2007; **297**: 471–9

BACKGROUND. Concerns regarding the short-term adverse effects of aprotinin have been raised by cohort studies. However, there are no data concerning whether possible short-term risks are associated with increased longer term mortality. This study reported long-term mortality at 6 weeks, 6 months and annually for 5 years after coronary artery bypass graft (CABG) surgery among 3876 patients followed up in the previous cohort study discussed above (*N Engl J Med* 2006; 354: 353–65). Fewer patients were included because 7 of the 69 study centres did not undertake long-term follow-up. Deaths after 5 years were compared using various complex multivariable statistical methods that adjusted for possible confounders.

INTERPRETATION. Aprotinin treatment was associated with significantly higher 5-year mortality (20.8%) compared with control (12.7%), aminocaproic acid (15.8%) and tranexamic acid (14.7%). After statistical adjustment for the many potential confounders, the higher 5-year mortality remained for aprotinin compared with the control group, whichever statistical model was used (covariate adjusted hazard ratio for death 1.48, 95% CI 1.19–1.85; adjusted odds ratio for death with propensity adjustment 1.48, 95% CI 1.13–1.93; $P=0.005$). This effect was observed for the entire cohort and for the subgroup who survived their index hospital admission. Neither aminocaproic nor tranexamic acid was associated with increased mortality. The authors concluded that their earlier findings appear to translate into an excess mortality with aprotinin use (Fig. 1.1).

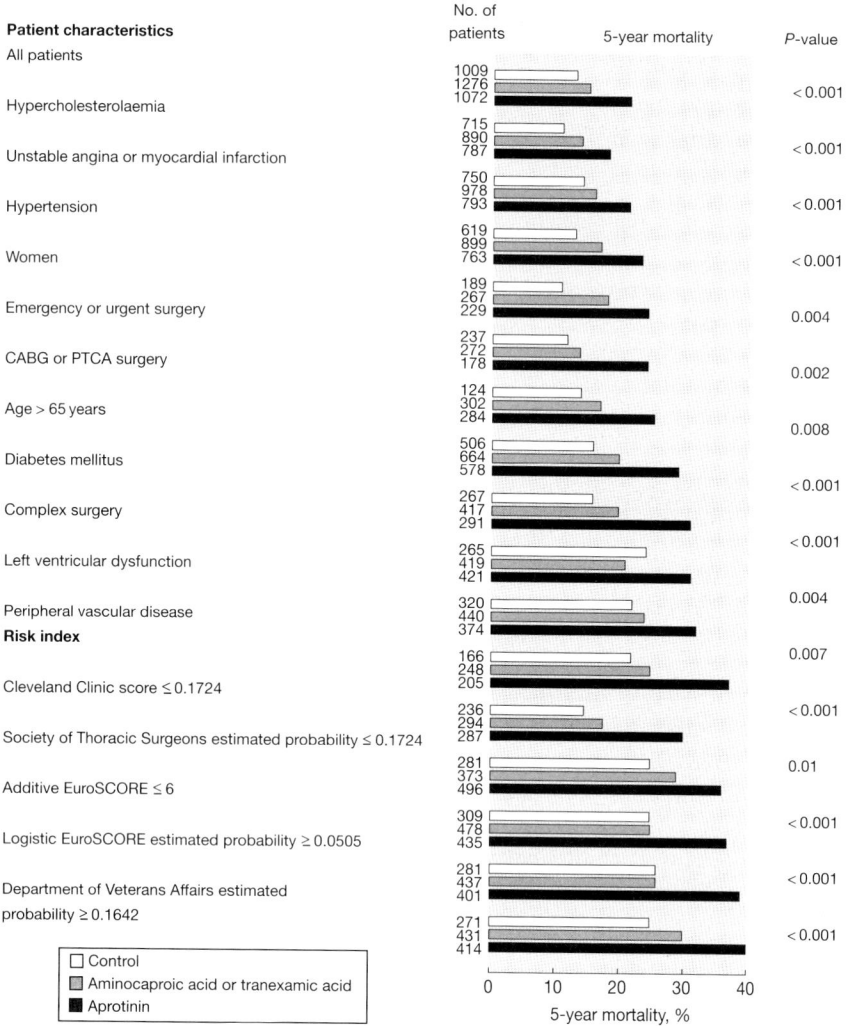

Patient characteristics	No. of patients	5-year mortality	*P*-value
All patients	1009 / 1276 / 1072		< 0.001
Hypercholesterolaemia	715 / 890 / 787		< 0.001
Unstable angina or myocardial infarction	750 / 978 / 793		< 0.001
Hypertension	619 / 899 / 763		< 0.001
Women	189 / 267 / 229		0.004
Emergency or urgent surgery	237 / 272 / 178		0.002
CABG or PTCA surgery	124 / 302 / 284		0.008
Age > 65 years	506 / 664 / 578		< 0.001
Diabetes mellitus	267 / 417 / 291		< 0.001
Complex surgery	265 / 419 / 421		0.004
Left ventricular dysfunction	320 / 440 / 374		0.007
Peripheral vascular disease	166 / 248 / 205		< 0.001
Risk index		
Cleveland Clinic score ≤ 0.1724	236 / 294 / 287		0.01
Society of Thoracic Surgeons estimated probability ≤ 0.1724	281 / 373 / 496		< 0.001
Additive EuroSCORE ≤ 6	309 / 478 / 435		< 0.001
Logistic EuroSCORE estimated probability ≥ 0.0505	281 / 437 / 401		< 0.001
Department of Veterans Affairs estimated probability ≥ 0.1642	271 / 431 / 414		< 0.001

Legend:
□ Control
▨ Aminocaproic acid or tranexamic acid
■ Aprotinin

5-year mortality, % (0 10 20 30 40)

Fig. 1.1 Long-term mortality by patient characteristics and risk indices. CABG, coronary artery bypass graft surgery; PCTA, percutaneous transluminal coronary angioplasty surgery. Complex surgery was defined as surgery under any of the following conditions: a history of coronary artery bypass grafting, valve surgery, non-coronary angioplasty or stenting, or other cardiac or vascular non-cardiac surgery, combined current heart surgery; or current surgery in emergency status or urgent status with evidence of congestive heart failure preoperatively. Adapted scores for risk indices are based on various in-hospital indices and scores (Cleveland Clinic score, Society of Thoracic Surgeons score, additive European system for cardiac operative risk evaluation (EuroSCORE), logistic EuroSCORE, and Department of Veterans Affairs score). *P* values were calculated using two-tailed χ^2 comparisons among the three groups. Source: Mangano *et al.* (2007).

A propensity score case–control comparison of aprotinin and tranexamic acid in high-transfusion-risk cardiac surgery

Karkouti K, Beattie WS, Dattilo KM, *et al. Transfusion* 2006; **46**: 327–38

BACKGROUND. There are relatively few data directly comparing aprotinin (widely considered the most effective blood-sparing drug in cardiac surgery) with tranexamic acid (a cheaper alternative). The authors hypothesized that aprotinin would be superior to tranexamic acid. They used prospectively collected data on 10870 patients undergoing cardiac surgery with cardiopulmonary bypass (CPB) in a single centre over 5 years. Of these, 586 patients received aprotinin and the remaining patients received tranexamic acid. The authors then used propensity scoring to try to match patients who received aprotinin with those who received tranexamic acid. They used 20 variables to try to match important differences between patients other than the anti-fibrinolytic drug received. The outcomes were stroke, acute renal failure requiring dialysis, acute deterioration in renal function, acute myocardial infarction, infection and in-hospital death.

INTERPRETATION. The propensity-matching model generated 449 aprotinin patients matched to 449 tranexamic acid patients. Seventy-five to eighty per cent of patients were transfused (with 30–35% of patients receiving ≥ 5 red cell units), confirming that a high-risk group for transfusion was studied. There were no statistically or clinically significant differences in the use of red blood cells, fresh-frozen plasma (FFP) or platelets between the propensity-matched groups, although differences trended towards higher platelet and FFP use with aprotinin. There was no difference in myocardial infarction, stroke, infection or in-hospital mortality. Aprotinin use was associated with higher risk of deterioration in renal function (24% vs. 17%; $P = 0.01$) and a trend to higher acute renal failure requiring dialysis (5.6% vs. 3.1%; $P = 0.08$). This association was strongest for patients with pre-existing renal dysfunction. The authors acknowledged the many potential limitations in the study design. They nevertheless concluded that their data raise concerns that aprotinin could adversely affect renal function, particularly in patients with pre-existing renal dysfunction.

Meta-analysis comparing the effectiveness and adverse outcomes of antifibrinolytic agents in cardiac surgery

Brown JR, Birkmeyer NJO, O'Connor GT. *Circulation* 2007; **115**: 2801–13

BACKGROUND. There are ongoing questions regarding the safety and effectiveness of anti-fibrinolytic drugs in cardiac surgery. This group performed a systematic review and meta-analysis of available data. They compared outcomes for each drug versus control, and where possible compared drugs with each other.

INTERPRETATION. Randomized controlled trial data from 138 trials were evaluated for outcomes including total blood loss, transfusion of red cells, re-exploration, mortality, stroke, myocardial infarction, dialysis-dependent renal failure and renal dysfunction (defined as 0.5 mg/dl increase in serum creatinine concentration from baseline). All drugs had similar effectiveness for decreasing blood loss (226 to 348 ml per case) and for decreasing the proportion of transfused patients. Only high-dose aprotinin reduced re-exploration rates (relative risk [RR] 0.49; 95% CI 0.33–0.73). There were no detected risks or benefits of any drug for mortality, stroke, myocardial infarction or dialysis-dependent renal failure (Fig. 1.2). However, high-dose aprotinin increased the risk of renal dysfunction (RR 1.47; 95% CI 1.12–1.94) (Fig. 1.3). In head-to-head comparison, aprotinin reduced blood loss more by an average of <300 ml per case, but there was no difference in the number of patients transfused. Other outcomes were similar between the drugs.

Comment

These studies confirm that all anti-fibrinolytic drugs are effective in decreasing blood loss in cardiac surgery. The question is which is most effective and, perhaps more importantly, do side-effects occur that outweigh this benefit? Ideally, the

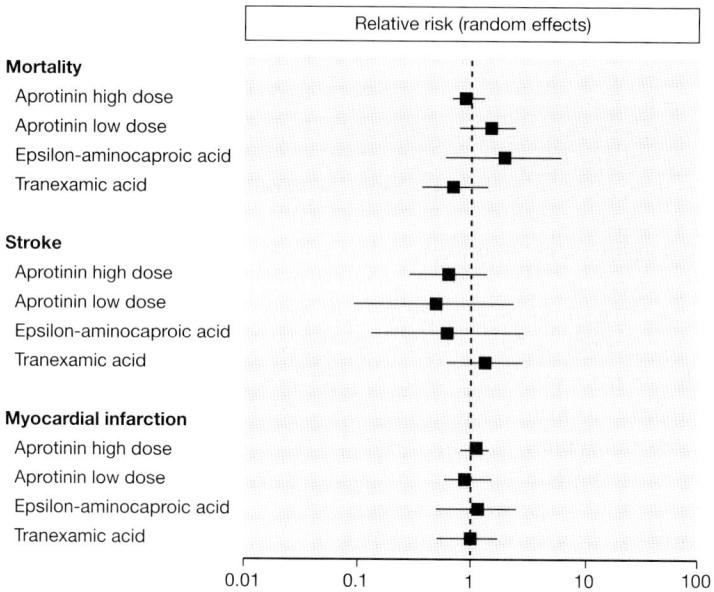

Fig. 1.2 Adverse outcomes by anti-fibrinolytic agent compared with placebo. The relative risks (RR) of adverse outcomes (mortality, stroke and myocardial infarction) by anti-fibrinolytic drug vs. placebo are plotted. The RR (square) and 95% CIs (horizontal bars) summarize the effect using a random-effects model. Effects left of 1.0 favour the anti-fibrinolytic drug over placebo; effects to the right favour placebo over anti-fibrinolytic drug. When the horizontal bars cross 1.0, the effect is not significantly different from the comparison group; this is the case for all agents and for all adverse events (mortality, stroke, myocardial infarction) plotted here. Source: Brown et al. (2007).

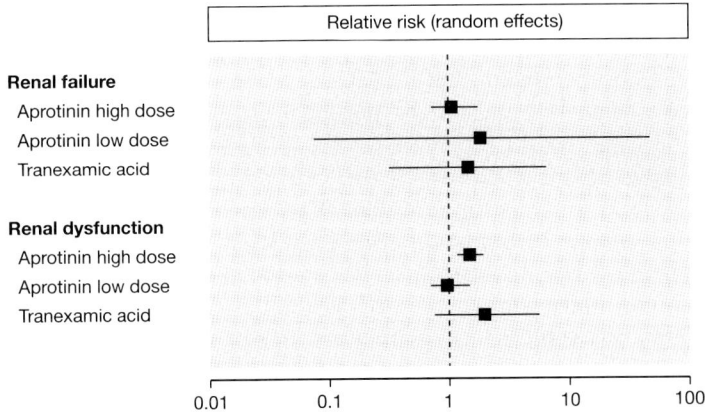

Fig. 1.3 Renal failure and dysfunction by anti-fibrinolytic drug compared with placebo. The relative risks (RR) of renal complications (dialysis-dependent renal failure and renal dysfunction defined as an increase in serum creatinine concentration of $\geq 0.5\,mg/dl$) by anti-fibrinolytic drug vs. placebo are plotted. The RR (square) and 95% CIs (horizontal bars) summarize the effect using a random effects model. The only statistically significant effect shown here is the increased risk of renal dysfunction with the use of high-dose aprotinin vs. placebo. Source: Brown *et al.* (2007).

safety profile would be determined in a large RCT powered to detect mortality, renal failure or the other outcomes described above. The problem is that these events are rare, so the trial would need to be very large and, therefore, unlikely to be funded or completed.

The two publications by Mangano and colleagues are striking and potentially worrying because, based on a very large number of patients, they appear to document a clear association between aprotinin use and harm, both when short- and long-term outcomes were evaluated. Although the study was not randomized, the data were collected prospectively, were apparently of high quality, and included many potentially important variables. There is some biological plausibility in the increased incidence of thrombotic complications, because aprotinin is an anti-fibrinolytic therapy given to a group of patients in whom the general therapeutic strategy is to use a variety of anti-coagulant and anti-platelet drugs to decrease coronary artery occlusion. In addition, aprotinin is known to have multiple incompletely understood biological actions and may be concentrated in renal tubules, which could explain the renal dysfunction.

The study by Karkouti and colleagues adds fuel to this fire by further suggesting a possible association with renal dysfunction, although the findings were less concerning for other outcomes. The key issue is whether the statistical handling of these observational data creates a fair comparison between the drug and the control groups. The methods used are well recognized, detailed and complex. Regression methods and the use of propensity matching essentially try to create a 'quasi-randomized' trial. The problem is that the groups can never be truly equal because clinicians chose to use a certain drug (or no drug) based on their experience and interpretation of available evidence. The comparisons could be considered unequivocal only if the included variables completely adjusted for clinician decisions, which can never be certain. Since surgeons and anaesthetists probably believed that blood sparing was most effective with aprotinin, they will probably have chosen it for the most difficult patients. This is bias by indication.

The meta-analysis by Brown uses data from RCTs, in which bias by indication was not present. These studies were mostly powered to detect decreased blood loss or transfusions, which is where the weakness of this approach to examine adverse effects arises. The completeness and consistency of reporting adverse outcomes vary, so it is difficult to be sure all were included. However, this potential reporting bias should have been distributed equally across different trial groups, so that, even if not all events were captured, this hopefully occurred equally. In addition, trials may not represent the 'real world' because patients excluded from protocols may be those more likely to suffer adverse effects in routine practice. The meta-analysis found no excess of thrombotic events or renal failure. Aprotinin in high dose seemed to decrease re-explorations but also increase renal dysfunction (but not renal failure).

What do these trials tell us about the use of anti-fibrinolytic drugs in CABG surgery? At present, we cannot be sure whether aprotinin has clinically important adverse effects compared with either placebo or the other drugs. A pragmatic view would be as follows. First, an anaesthetist/surgeon team should examine their own transfusion outcomes. For cases with low probability for transfusion (such as elective primary CABG), the safest practice is probably to avoid anti-fibrinolytics. Second, teams should identify and examine patients at high risk for transfusion and/or re-exploration (such as complex procedures or redo surgery). The use of anti-fibrinolytics should be evaluated in the context of the whole package of blood-sparing therapies. Specifically, cell salvage is of proven value in these cases, and the use of restrictive transfusion triggers postoperatively is safe. The choice between the three anti-fibrinolytic drugs is currently difficult, but a recent 'sting in the tail' following publication of these studies may make clinicians shy away from aprotinin until further data are available. A US Food and Drug Administration safety committee was reassured by safety data provided by Bayer (the manufacturer of Trasylol®) after publication of the above studies, but the company subsequently disclosed a large data set which may demonstrate 'increased risk for death, kidney failure, congestive heart failure and stroke'. |4|. At the time of writing, these data are still being analysed. A clearer answer is likely after analysis of these data and the completion and publication of the BART study, which will be the largest head-to-head comparison of all three drugs in preventing major bleeding complications in cardiac surgery |5|.

Note added in press. Bayer have withdrawn aprotinin following early stopping of the BART study by the data monitoring committee, because of higher mortality in the patients treated with aprotinin.

Anti-fibrinolytics in paediatrics

Tranexamic acid reduces intraoperative blood loss in paediatric patients undergoing scoliosis surgery

Sethna NF, Zurakowski D, Brustowicz, *et al. Anesthesiology* 2005; **102**: 727–32

BACKGROUND. Excessive bleeding often occurs during paediatric scoliosis surgery. The authors hypothesized that administration of tranexamic acid would reduce bleeding and transfusion requirements during scoliosis surgery. They randomly assigned patients to receive either 100 mg/kg of tranexamic acid before incision, followed by an infusion of 10 mg/kg/h during surgery, or a saline (placebo) control group. The primary outcome measures were blood loss and transfusion requirements.

INTERPRETATION. Forty-four patients were randomized. In the tranexamic acid group, blood loss was reduced by 41% compared with placebo (mean 1230 vs. 2085 ml; $P < 0.01$). The amount of blood transfused was less in the tranexamic acid group, but did not reach statistical significance (mean 615 ml vs. 940 ml; $P = 0.08$). The clinical effect was most marked in the patients with secondary scoliosis rather than idiopathic scoliosis. In a regression analysis, tranexamic acid was an independent predictor of blood loss, together with American Society of Anesthesiologists (ASA) physical class and preoperative platelet count. No adverse events were noted in any patient. The authors concluded that tranexamic acid is effective in reducing perioperative blood loss in paediatric scoliosis surgery.

Comment

Reducing or avoiding transfusions in children is highly desirable. Any long-term risks from transfusion (including variant CJD) have greater potential to affect those who will live for many years after exposure to blood. This was a well-performed single-centre study. The authors provide a power analysis based on their own data for blood loss during scoliosis surgery and studied the intended number of patients. They proved their hypothesis that bleeding would be reduced. The reduction in red cell transfusion volume was clinically but not statistically significant and could have been an effect of the small sample size. In addition, blood tends to be administered in fixed volumes and may behave less like a continuous variable, which could have contributed to the less impressive effects. It was interesting that the effect was greatest in the secondary scoliosis group, and the authors comment that this could be related to the high fibrinolytic activity described in Duchenne muscular dystrophy [6]. Although no adverse effects were described, this is not surprising in a small randomized trial. Clinicians using tranexamic acid in children should remain vigilant for complications, particularly thrombotic events. In addition, the interaction between tranexamic acid and other blood conservation strategies, particularly perioperative cell salvage, is not yet known.

Section summary

Anti-fibrinolytic drugs are effective in reducing blood loss in surgery. The papers reviewed show this for cardiac and paediatric scoliosis surgery. A recently published meta-analysis of 43 trials in orthopaedic surgical procedures also confirmed this effect |7|. In 23 trials, the odds ratios for allogeneic transfusion were 0.43 (95% CI 0.28–0.64) for aprotinin and 0.17 (95% CI 0.11–0.24%) for tranexamic acid. The recent publications concerning aprotinin show that we may not fully understand the clinical effects of these drugs. The meta-analysis in orthopaedic surgery was careful to point out that there were inadequate data concerning safety in this setting. These papers come at a time when allogeneic transfusions are safer than ever, but more expensive and in ever shorter supply. Few of these studies have evaluated the interaction of these drugs with other blood-sparing strategies, such as cell salvage. One recently published small RCT compared aprotinin, tranexamic acid and control in 180 patients undergoing first time CABG surgery, all of whom received cell salvage |8|. In this study, both drugs further decreased transfusion exposure compared with controls but aprotinin was superior to tranexamic acid.

Until more data are available, clinicians need to consider each patient individually, asking themselves questions such as: What is the risk of major bleeding in this case? How important is avoiding transfusion to this patient? Could I use other methods of blood conservation? Finally, is this patient at high risk of relevant complications such as renal failure or thrombosis?

Organizational changes to optimize blood use and reduce blood transfusions

There are many studies of individual strategies to reduce blood transfusions. However, few studies have evaluated the impact of organizational change. This section describes two recent publications, one in which several strategies were combined as a complex intervention; the other a simple evaluation of the potential effect of tailoring transfusions to individual patients.

A cluster randomized, controlled trial of a blood conservation algorithm in patients undergoing total hip arthoplasty

Wong CJ, Vandervoort MK, Vandervoort SL, *et al*. *Transfusion* 2007; **47**: 832–41

BACKGROUND. Many patients undergoing orthopaedic surgery require blood transfusion. Various individual strategies decrease transfusion requirements, including preoperative erythropoietin (EPO) therapy, preoperative donation and deposit of autologous blood, and restrictive transfusion triggers. Few studies have evaluated the impact of a combined strategy or protocol on transfusion requirements. In this study, a blood conservation algorithm (Fig. 1.4) was devised. It included oral iron and preoperative erythropoietin therapy for patients with a haemoglobin concentration (Hb)<130 g/l, preoperative autologous donation of 1–2 red cell units for patients with Hb > 130 g/l, and a restrictive transfusion trigger of 70 g/l postoperatively in asymptomatic patients. Using a cluster randomized design, the effectiveness of the algorithm was tested by comparing outcome in 14 hospitals with the algorithm and 15 hospitals without such algorithm. Data from 60 patients undergoing primary hip joint arthoplasty were included for each hospital.

INTERPRETATION. Before introduction of the algorithm (see Fig. 1.4), the mean allogeneic transfusion rate was 25.6% (range 14.9–47.4%) in the control and 25.2% (range 13.8–50.6%) in the intervention hospitals. After introduction of the algorithm, the allogeneic transfusion rates (mean 26.1% [range 3.3–43.3%] in the control vs. mean 16.5% [range 3.0–32.8%] in the intervention hospitals; $P = 0.02$) and the overall (allogeneic and autologous) transfusion rates (mean 39.7% in the control vs. mean 27.4% in the intervention hospitals; $P = 0.04$) were lower in the intervention hospitals. At the same time, the rate of autologous pre-donations (control hospitals 25.8% vs. intervention hospitals 27.1%) and the proportion of patients receiving autologous transfusions (control hospitals 15.9% [range 0–46.8%] vs. intervention hospitals 12.5%

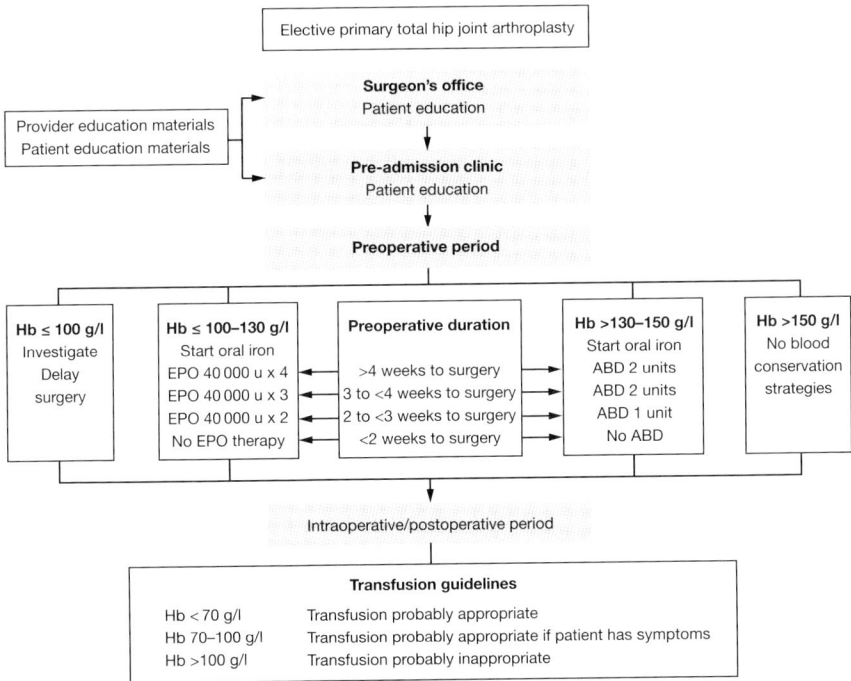

Fig. 1.4 Blood conservation algorithm for elective total hip joint arthroplasty. Source: Wong et al. (2007). ABD, autologous blood donation.

[range 3.3–29.1%]) were similar between hospitals. The major difference between the groups was the use of preoperative EPO (0.6% [range 0–5.1%] in control hospitals vs. 20.1% [range 3.7–36.7%] in intervention hospitals; $P<0.001$). Perioperative cell salvage was not part of the blood conservation strategy but was used more frequently in the control hospitals (19.6% vs. 1.3%). When allogeneic transfusions were used, the mean number of transfused units was similar in both groups (control group 2.1 per patient vs. intervention group 2.0 per patients). Hospital length of stay and incidence of major complications (highest incidence 3.3% in any centre) were similar. The authors concluded that a comprehensive approach to blood conservation can reduce allogeneic transfusion in patients undergoing primary hip joint arthoplasty.

Comment

This study is important because it evaluated the effect of an algorithm incorporating several individual components combined for a complex intervention (see Fig. 1.4). The cluster randomized design meant that the intervention was evaluated in the real world, and the authors comment that adherence to different components of the algorithm varied between centres in the intervention group, which is obvious from the data presented. Introduction of the algorithm clearly benefited patients: in the intervention hospitals: the absolute risk of allogeneic transfusion was 9.6% lower than in the control hospitals. This equates to avoiding blood transfusion in about 1 out of 10 patients. The authors comment that this rate could be even higher if clinicians followed it more universally. It is difficult to decide which part of the algorithm was most important, but the data suggest that it was the use of preoperative EPO in 20% of cases. The pattern of autologous predonation and transfusion was similar. The mean lowest postoperative Hb value was slightly higher in the algorithm group (94.1 g/l vs. 90.9 g/l; $P=0.04$), suggesting that postoperative anaemia was also less severe. Unfortunately, the authors did not include any data concerning the transfusion triggers actually used, so it is difficult to assess how closely this aspect of the algorithm was followed. Pre-transfusion Hb value was >100 g/l in 5.2% of transfusions in the intervention group and in 15.5% of transfusions in the control hospitals. This suggests significant non-compliance with restrictive transfusion triggers.

Surprisingly, there are no data on overall allogeneic blood use in the intervention and control hospitals. The authors state that: 'if allogeneic blood was given, the mean number of units was 2.1 in the *control* hospitals and 2.0 in the *intervention* hospitals.' Given that autologous use was similar, this does not suggest a major saving of allogeneic blood. From the data presented, I estimate that about 20 units of allogeneic units were saved per 100 cases managed with the algorithm. This, combined with greater transfusion avoidance, could be clinically important.

However, a key question is whether the strategy is cost-effective. Two of the key interventions were expensive: first, autologous donation, which was similar in intervention and control hospitals; second, preoperative EPO for anaemic patients, which was the major difference between groups (greater use in the intervention hospitals). Many centres have now abandoned autologous pre-donation because of high expense and evidence suggesting that it may increase overall exposure to blood transfusions. A Cochrane systematic review, updated in 2004, found that RCTs were of low quality and reported high overall transfusion rates |9|. Although the risk of allogeneic transfusion was decreased by 64% (RR 0.36; 95% CI 0.25–0.51), the risk of receiving any blood transfusion (allogeneic and/or autologous) was actually increased by preoperative autologous blood donation (ABD) (RR 1.33; 95% CI 1.10–1.61).

Preoperative EPO therapy is expensive, both in terms of drug costs and the need to deliver treatment to patients preoperatively. In this trial, EPO was provided free by manufacturers and a cost-effectiveness analysis was not included. Previous trials and systematic reviews have shown that EPO can decrease transfusion exposure and allogeneic blood use. However, it is unlikely to be cost-effective. Even as the costs of allogeneic blood increase, there will need to be a dramatic cost reduction in EPO before it is cost-effective when assessed against allogeneic blood savings. This is particularly true if baseline blood use is lowered with modern surgical and anaesthetic techniques, cell salvage for selected cases and more restrictive transfusion triggers. What is needed is more evidence for other benefits of EPO, such as improved recovery rates and quality of life; these are lacking in published studies. More work is also needed to examine which patients benefit most and what dosing schedule is most cost-effective. A recently published trial of patients presenting for orthopaedic surgery with a haematocrit of 30–39% found that two EPO doses were effective in achieving the preoperative target haematocrit of 40% in 63% of cases |10|. This is half of the widely recommended schedule of four doses of EPO.

Another unknown is the safety profile of perioperative EPO. As in the case of anti-fibrinolytics, rare adverse outcomes make this assessment difficult. In 2006, two large trials of long-term EPO therapy in patients with non-dialysis-dependent renal failure were published |11,12|. They failed to show any benefit but reported increased harm due to thrombotic events when anaemia was corrected to normal values. Given the current safety of allogeneic blood in terms of infections, it is difficult to be sure that EPO is safer than a blood transfusion.

A retrospective study evaluating single-unit red blood cell transfusions in reducing allogeneic blood exposure

Ma M, Echert K, Ralley F, et al. Transfusion Medicine 2005; **15**: 307–12

BACKGROUND. Most transfusion guidelines recommend single-unit transfusions followed by reassessment, but most clinicians still prescribe a minimum of two units of red cells when a transfusion decision is made. This single-centre study used retrospective analysis of adult patient data to assess the potential impact of single-unit transfusions. The authors used the observed change in haemoglobin (Hb) concentration per unit to assess likely savings if different transfusion triggers and targets (ranging from 7 to 9 g/dl) had actually been used.

INTERPRETATION. The authors evaluated 302 transfusion events; 78.5% were two-unit transfusions and the rest single-unit transfusions. Mean pre-transfusion Hb value was

7.74 g/dl. The authors estimated that, if the target Hb value was ≥9, ≥8, or ≥7 g/dl, a single-unit transfusion would have been sufficient in 42%, 80% and 98% of patients, respectively. They estimated that this could save 0.21, 0.57 or 0.82 red cell units per patient, respectively.

Comment

This was a simple study that made many assumptions based on purely retrospective data, but it gives a clear message. The traditional view that a single unit of red cells suggests no transfusion requirement and that two units is the minimum useful dose has no scientific basis. Recent studies indicating potential adverse effects from allogeneic blood exposure and equivalent outcomes when restrictive transfusion triggers are used suggest that the target Hb value for an individual patient should be documented and transfusions administered to achieve this target. Although many clinicians probably use a relatively low Hb value as transfusion trigger, they frequently still prescribe multiple red cell units. This may 'overshoot' the intended Hb value (if one was identified) and potentially increase the risk of complications, such as fluid overload. A cheap and simple change in practice of using single red cell units could have a significant impact on allogeneic blood use, reduce transfusion exposure and still maintain Hb concentration at the upper end of the 'safe' 7–10 g/dl range quoted in most guidelines.

Anaemia, transfusion triggers and outcomes

Preoperative hematocrit levels and postoperative outcomes in older patients undergoing non-cardiac surgery

Wu W-C, Schifftner TL, Henderson WG, et al. JAMA 2007; **297**: 2481–8

BACKGROUND. Anaemia is prevalent in elderly patients presenting for surgery. This group also has a high risk of cardiovascular complications, particularly after non-cardiac surgery. Although most elderly patients undergo preoperative Hb measurement, the influence of preoperative anaemia and polycythaemia on postoperative mortality and cardiovascular complications is poorly understood. This study investigated the association between preoperative haematocrit and outcome in patients aged > 65 years, using a large observational database (the Veterans Administration National Surgical Quality Improvement Program database).

INTERPRETATION. Data from 310 311 patients aged > 65 years who underwent non-cardiac surgery between 1997 and 2004 were included. The relation between preoperative haematocrit (measured within 3 months for 99%, and within 1 month for

79% of cases) and 30-day postoperative mortality was examined, adjusting for multiple patient- and surgery-related variables that also predicted mortality. Adjusted mortality increased by a mean of 1.6% (95% CI 1.1–2.2%) for every percentage point deviation from the normal haematocrit range of 39.0–53.9% (Table 1.1). A similar increased risk was observed for a composite outcome of 30-day mortality or cardiac event. In subgroup analysis, the association was limited to males and non-emergency surgery. Among surgical subspecialties, the mortality increase per percentage point deviation from the normal range was greatest for orthopaedic surgery (3.1% per 1% haematocrit deviation) (Table 1.2).

Comment

This study is subject to the limitations of any observational cohort study. There was a clear association for anaemia and polycythaemia with mortality and cardiovascular complications. However, it is not clear whether preoperative anaemia and polycythaemia cause harm, or if the association is explained by other confounding factors. Despite adjusting for 45 other wide-ranging independent associations (such as ASA physical class, complexity of procedure, type of surgery, various chronic disease states and a number of biochemical variables), it is impossible to know whether an abnormal haematocrit value *per se* causes adverse outcomes. This study did not include any data about perioperative transfusions or postoperative haematocrit values. It therefore does not tell us how to manage patients with anaemia or polycythaemia. At best, the study generates the hypothesis that preoperative anaemia is important, and emphasizes the need for more research. For non-cardiac surgery the prevalence of preoperative anaemia was 43%, so better evidence about perioperative anaemia management is relevant to many patients worldwide. The findings differ from a similar study in patients refusing blood transfusions, in which excess mortality was most prevalent in patients with cardiovascular disease [13]. As Wu and colleagues state, their data indicate the need for trials of different management strategies for patients with abnormal preoperative haematocrit values to determine whether modification of this risk factor alters outcomes.

Table 1.1 Thirty-day mortality risk per percentage point deviation from normal haematocrit range among different subgroups

Haematocrit (%)	No. of cases	Thirty-day crude mortality rates (%)	Thirty-day crude cardiac event rates (%)	Adjusted odds ratio for 30-day death (95% confidence interval)	Adjusted odds ratio for 30-day death or cardiac events (95% confidence interval)
<18.0	129	35.4	14.6	2.42 (1.55–3.79)	2.41 (1.55–3.73)
18.0–20.9	304	26.8	8.6	1.68 (1.22–2.30)	1.52 (1.12–2.07)
21.0–23.9	1292	16.6	4.9	1.09 (0.89–1.33)	1.11 (0.93–1.34)
24.0–26.9	5172	14.9	4.4	1.33 (1.16–1.52)	1.27 (1.13–1.44)
27.0–29.9	14339	11.2	3.7	1.25 (1.12–1.40)	1.25 (1.13–1.38)
30.0–32.9	24678	8.4	3.1	1.21 (1.08–1.35)	1.19 (1.08–1.31)
33.0–35.9	35742	5.8	2.5	1.22 (1.10–1.36)	1.20 (1.09–1.32)
36.0–38.9	51314	3.5	1.8	1.15 (1.04–1.28)	1.12 (1.03–1.23)
39.0–41.9	66487	2.2	1.3	1.04 (0.93–1.15)	1.10 (1.01–1.20)
42.0–44.9	61928	1.7	1.0	1.02 (0.91–1.13)	1.06 (0.97–1.17)
45.0–47.9	34354	1.5	0.9	1 [Reference]	1 [Reference]
48.0–50.9	11358	1.8	1.0	1.12 (0.94–1.32)	1.12 (0.97–1.30)
51.0–53.9	2577	3.1	1.4	1.48 (1.15–1.91)	1.42 (1.13–1.78)
≥54	637	5.6	2.9	1.56 (1.06–2.31)	1.55 (1.09–2.22)

The analysis was adjusted for American Society of Anesthesiologists class, serum albumin, emergency operation, disseminated cancer, functional status, work relative value unit, serum urea nitrogen, do-not-resuscitate order, surgical subspecialty, age, myocardial infarction in previous 6 months, white blood cell count, weight loss, ascites, dyspnoea, serum aspartate transaminase, impaired sensorium, platelet count, concurrent pneumonia, chronic obstructive pulmonary disease, congestive heart failure in previous 30 days, serum creatinine, serum sodium, serum bilirubin, dialysis, coma, steroid use, alkaline phosphatase, previous stroke with neurological deficit, bleeding disorder, surgical wound class, smoker, angina admission in prior 30 days, ventilator dependence, use of preoperative blood transfusion and acute renal failure. Source: Wu et al. (2007).

Table 1.2 Thirty-day mortality risk per percentage point deviation from normal haematocrit range among different subgroups

Patient subgroups	No. of cases	Death rate (%)	Adjusted odds ratio for 30-day death (95% confidence interval)
All cases	310311	3.9	1.02 (1.01–1.02)
Surgical subspecialties			
Orthopaedics	57636	3.5	1.03 (1.02–1.05)
Thoracic surgery	14051	7.3	1.01 (1.00–1.03)
General surgery	106340	5.0	1.01 (1.00–1.02)
Peripheral vascular surgery	47694	4.7	1.00 (0.99–1.02)
Clinical cohorts			
Age > 75 years	128269	5.2	1.02 (1.01–1.03)
Chronic obstructive pulmonary disease	60948	6.8	1.02 (1.01–1.03)
Any renal disease	57518	8.0	1.01 (1.00–1.02)
Any cardiac history	80459	6.1	1.00 (1.00–1.01)
Emergency cases	24773	16.1	1.00 (0.99–1.01)
Female	5605	3.4	0.99 (0.95–1.04)

The analyses were adjusted by the significant predictors of 30-day mortality listed in Table 1.1. For subgroup analyses, the corresponding variables defining distinct clinical cohorts were removed from the analyses of these cohorts. The normal haematocrit range was defined as haematocrit levels between 39% and 53.9% according to conventional definitions. Surgical subspecialty was determined by self-reported subspecialty of the attending surgeon who performed the surgery.

Source: Wu *et al.* (2007).

Silent myocardial ischaemia and haemoglobin concentration: a randomized, controlled trial of transfusion strategy in lower limb arthoplasty

Grover M, Talwalkar S, Casbard A, *et al. Vox Sanguinis* 2006; **90**: 105–12

BACKGROUND. Orthopaedic surgery patients frequently require blood transfusions. Although restrictive transfusion trigger values have become widely adopted, the optimum trigger value for patients with ischaemic heart disease is uncertain. This study used Holter monitoring to compare the effect of a restrictive and a liberal red cell transfusion strategy on the incidence of silent myocardial ischaemia (SMI) in patients without signs or symptoms of ischaemic heart disease (IHD) who underwent lower limb arthroplasty.

INTERPRETATION. In a multicentre controlled trial, 260 patients undergoing elective hip or knee replacement surgery were randomized to a restrictive (Hb value 8 g/dl) or liberal (Hb value 10 g/dl) transfusion trigger. Patients were monitored for SMI from 12 h preoperatively to 72 h postoperatively. The primary outcome was the ischaemic load, namely the mean time of SMI per hour over the monitored period. In the restrictive vs. liberal group, mean postoperative Hb value was 9.9 g/dl vs. 11.1 g/dl, transfusion rate 34% vs. 43%, and the incidence of SMI 19% vs. 24% (*P* = 0.41). There was no overall difference in the ischaemic load between the restrictive (median 0 min/h; range 0 to

4.2 min/h) and liberal group (median 0 min/h; range 0–19.5 min/h). Among patients who experienced SMI, the mean ischaemic load was smaller in the restrictive group than in the liberal group (0.5 min/h vs. 1.5 min/h; ratio 0.32; $P = 0.011$).

Comment

There is uncertainty regarding how to manage anaemic patients with IHD in the perioperative period. There are no adequately powered RCTs to guide decisions. Expert opinion, supported by the physiological rationale that reduced oxygen content is potentially harmful in the high oxygen extraction coronary circulation, is that higher transfusion triggers should be used for patients with coronary disease. Most guidelines suggest a Hb trigger of 8–9 g/dl, aiming for a concentration of 9–10 g/dl |14|. This advice is supported by cohort studies that found associations between Hb concentrations <9–10 g/dl and adverse outcomes in the critical care and perioperative settings |13,15|. In the Transfusion Requirements in Critical Care (TRICC) trial subgroup analysis, the survival curves of patients with IHD were superior in the liberal group (transfusion trigger <10 g/dl) than in the restrictive group (transfusion trigger <7 g/dl), although the difference was not statistically significant and the study was not powered for this analysis |16|. Grover and colleagues therefore set out to answer an important question in a group of patients who frequently suffer perioperative anaemia and have high transfusion rates. Unfortunately, this study does not provide definitive answers for several reasons: first, the study was powered for a higher mean rate of SMI (30%) than was observed; second, their intention was to recruit 660 patients to achieve adequate power, but recruitment was slower than anticipated and funding ran out before completion; third, the transfusion protocols did not achieve a clinically important separation of the groups, and the restrictive group had a relatively high mean Hb concentration. Therefore, although the study was designed to show equivalence between transfusion triggers for Hb values of 8 g/dl and 10 g/dl and the incidence of perioperative SMI, it does not prove this relationship. The authors also excluded patients with signs of more severe or unstable IHD, which is the group of greatest interest. However, the study does show that about 20% of patients undergoing major orthopaedic surgery experience SMI, and it probably excludes a large adverse effect from a moderately restrictive transfusion practice.

Section summary

The increasing trend to early postoperative discharge and limited follow-up after major surgery raises concerns that cardiovascular morbidity or other important consequences of anaemia may be missed. A recently published study showed that a cohort of orthopaedic patients took 1–2 months to recover from a mean Hb concentration of 10.4 g/dl at postoperative day 1 |17|. If surgeons and anaesthetists become more restrictive with transfusions (based on present recommendations), patients will be exposed to a significant period of postoperative anaemia. Similar observations have been made in critically ill patients managed with restrictive transfusion triggers in the intensive care unit (ICU). In a multicentre cohort study, 25% of intensive care survivors managed with a mean transfusion trigger of 7.8 g/dl had a Hb concentration <9 g/dl at ICU discharge |18|. Of these, 25% had documented IHD with a similar prevalence of anaemia. A third of the patients still had a Hb concentration <10 g/dl when discharged home |19|. Considering the previously reported association between postoperative anaemia and adverse outcomes (Wu *et al.* 2007), the findings of Grover and colleagues and those of the TRICC trial (the only large RCT comparing two transfusion triggers) should be interpreted with caution. More studies are needed to determine whether restrictive transfusion triggers are safe for all patients, or whether increased morbidity occurs as a consequence of postoperative anaemia. The FOCUS trial is an ongoing trial that may answer some of these questions. It will recruit 2600 patients undergoing hip fracture surgery, comparing a liberal with a symptomatic transfusion trigger. The outcomes are based on function and cardiovascular status. The trial protocol was recently published, and the results are eagerly awaited |20|.

Paediatrics

Transfusion strategies for patients in paediatric intensive care units

Lacroix J, Hebert P, Hutchison JS, *et al. N Engl J Med* 2007; **356**: 1609–19

BACKGROUND. The optimal haemoglobin (Hb) threshold for red cell transfusions in critically ill children is unknown. The authors hypothesized that a restrictive transfusion strategy using leuco-depleted red cells would be as safe as a liberal transfusion strategy. The authors randomized 637 stable critically ill children aged between 3 days and 14 years who had Hb concentrations <9.5 g/dl within 7 days of intensive care admission. A total of 320 patients were randomized to a Hb transfusion threshold of 7 g/dl and 317 to a threshold of 9.5 g/dl. The primary outcome was the proportion of patients who died during the 28 days after randomization, had concurrent dysfunction of two or more organ systems (termed MODS) or progression of MODS, as evidenced by worsening of one or more organ dysfunctions.

INTERPRETATION. Mean Hb values in the restrictive and liberal groups were 8.7 g/dl and 10.8 g/dl, respectively (mean difference 2.1 g/dl; $P<0.001$). In the restrictive group, 54% of patients did not receive transfusions compared with 2% in the liberal group ($P<0.001$). Patients in the restrictive group received 44% fewer transfusions, and the mean blood use was 0.9 vs. 1.7 transfusions per patient ($P<0.001$). New or progressive MODS developed in 38 patients in the restrictive group, compared with 39 in the liberal group (absolute risk reduction with the restrictive strategy 0.4%; 95% CI −4.6% to 5.4%). There were 14 deaths in each group and no difference in the measured adverse events, which included organ dysfunction, nosocomial infections, days of mechanical ventilation and ICU stay (Table 1.3). The authors concluded that in stable critically ill children a Hb transfusion trigger of 7 g/dl decreases transfusions without increasing adverse outcomes.

Table 1.3 Effects of restrictive and liberal transfusion strategies on outcomes in paediatric intensive care unit patients*

Variable	Restrictive strategy group	Liberal strategy group	Absolute risk reduction, odds ratio or difference in means (95% CI)	P-value
Primary outcome				
New or progressive MODS – no./total no. (%)†	38/320 (12)	39/317 (12)	0.4 (−4.6 to 5.5)	NI‡
Age (days)				
≤28	1/11 (9)	0	−9.1 (−26.1 to 7.9)	1.00
29–364	14/143 (10)	20/142 (14)	4.3 (−3.2 to 11.8)	0.28
>364	23/166 (14)	19/167 (11)	−2.5 (−9.6 to 4.7)	0.51
Country§				
Belgium	3/66 (5)	4/66 (6)	0.74 (0.16–3.43)	0.70
Canada	32/205 (16)	28/203 (14)	1.16 (0.67–2.00)	0.60
United Kingdom	2/26 (8)	5/23 (22)	0.30 (0.05–1.73)	0.17
United States	1/23 (4)	2/25 (8)	0.52 (0.04–6.18)	0.61
Severity of illness (PRISM score)†¶				
0 (lowest quartile)	3/64 (5)	4/64 (6)	1.5 (−6.3 to 9.4)	1.00
1–4 (second quartile)	13/128 (10)	11/111 (10)	−0.3 (−7.9 to 7.4)	0.94
5–7 (third quartile)	6/54 (11)	6/67 (9)	−2.2 (−13.0 to 8.7)	0.69
≥8 (highest quartile)	16/74 (22)	18/75 (24)	2.4 (−11.1 to 15.9)	0.73
Suspended protocol – no./total no. (%)	18/39 (46)	13/20 (65)	18.9 (−7.3 to 45.0)	0.17
Secondary outcomes				
Measures of severity of organ dysfunction ‖				
No. of dysfunctional organs	1.6 ± 1.4	1.5 ± 1.2	−0.1 (−0.26 to 0.13)	0.87
PELOD score**				
After randomization	9.8 ± 11.9	8.4 ± 10.9	−1.4 (−3.1 to 0.4)	0.16
On day 1	6.3 ± 6.8	5.2 ± 6.2	−1.1 (−2.1 to − 0.1)	0.09
Highest daily score after day 1	10.2 ± 13.3	8.9 ± 11.9	−1.2 (−3.2 to 0.8)	0.34

Variable	Restrictive strategy	Liberal strategy	Difference (CI)	P value
Change in score	3.8 ± 10.9	3.8 ± 9.9	−0.1 (−1.7–1.5)	0.97
Average daily score	5.0 ± 6.1	4.2 ± 5.1	−0.8 (−1.7−0.1)	0.13
Variable				
Clinical outcomes – no./total no. (%)†				
Death				
In ICU	11/320 (3)	8/317 (3)	−0.9 (−3.6 to 1.7)	
From any cause during 28-day study	14/320 (4)	14/317 (4)	0 (−3.2 to 3.2)	
Nosocomial infections	65/320 (20)	79/317 (25)	4.6 (−1.9 to 11.1)	
At least one adverse event	97/320 (30)	90/317 (28)	−1.92 (−9.0 to 5.2)	
Reactions to red cell transfusion	3/320 (1)	6/317 (2)	1.0 (−0.9 to 2.8)	
Duration of care (days)||				
Mechanical ventilation	6.2 ± 5.9	6.0 ± 5.4	−0.14 (−1.1 to 0.8)	0.76
ICU stay after randomization	9.5 ± 7.9	9.9 ± 7.4	0.46 (−0.7 to 1.7)	0.39

*Plus–minus values are means ± SD.

†The comparison between the restrictive-strategy group and the liberal-strategy group is given as an absolute reduction in risk.

‡Non-inferiority (NI) was checked only for the primary outcome (the number of patients who had new or progressive multiple organ dysfunction syndrome [MODS], including death, after randomization). The absolute risk reduction for new or progressive MODS in the restrictive strategy group compared with the liberal strategy group was 0.4% (two-sided 95% CI −4.6 to 5.5) by intention-to-treat analysis; we also calculated a two-sided 97.5% CI of −5.4 to 6.2. Some experts also consider that a per-protocol analysis should be done in a non-inferiority trial. In the per-protocol analysis, we excluded 11 patients who did not meet the 80% adherence criterion; the number of patients with the primary outcome was 37 of 319 (11.6%) in the restrictive strategy group and 38 of 307 (12.4%) in the liberal strategy group (absolute risk reduction 0.8%; two-sided 95% CI −4.3 to 5.9). In all analyses, the upper limit of the confidence interval was lower than the safety margin of error of 10% approved by consensus before the study was undertaken, which means that noninferiority was statistically significant.

§The comparison between the restrictive strategy group and the liberal strategy group is given as an odds ratio.

¶Scores on the Paediatric Risk of Mortality (PRISM) range from 0 to 76, with higher scores indicating a higher risk of death.

||The comparison between the restrictive strategy group and the liberal strategy group is given as a difference between the means.

**Scores on the Paediatric Logistic Organ Dysfunction (PELOD) assessment range from 0 to 71, with higher scores indicating more severe organ dysfunction. The PELOD score can be estimated over the entire stay in the ICU or over 1 day (daily PELOD). The change in the PELOD score is the difference between the daily PELOD score at study entry and the worst daily PELOD score thereafter. Patients whose PELOD score did not change or decreased after randomization were considered to have a change of 0.

Source: Lacroix *et al.* (2007).

Comment

This is a landmark study. The authors used a restrictive strategy similar to the TRICC study in critically ill adults, namely a transfusion trigger of 7 g/dl aiming to maintain a Hb concentration of 8–9.5 g/dl. They showed this was as safe as more liberal blood use. The main benefit was a dramatic reduction in blood exposure and blood use in critically ill children. The number needed to treat to avoid transfusions with the restrictive practice compared with liberal blood use was only two, which is a huge clinical effect. The authors had to choose a composite endpoint because mortality is low in paediatric ICUs, so a sufficiently powered trial for this endpoint was not feasible. The study was designed to show equivalence, and the authors predefined this as the upper limit of the 95% confidence interval for the primary outcome being < 10% higher in the restrictive groups compared with the liberal group. This value in the trial was +4.6% so the data suggested that, at worst, about 1 in 20 children might suffer worsening organ failures with the restrictive practice, but most likely this outcome was similar for the groups. The possibility remains that a restrictive transfusion strategy has adverse effects that were not detected in the study, but there is little to suggest this, especially as ICU length of stays were similar. As was the case after publication of the TRICC trial in adults, the next challenge will be to translate the findings of this study into clinical practice. Doing so will avoid unnecessary transfusions for many thousands of sick children.

Conclusion

There are proven interventions that clearly avoid transfusions in the perioperative period. Perhaps the most effective and cheapest of these remains a clear documentation of a transfusion trigger and a target haemoglobin range, achieved using tailored (single unit) transfusions whenever possible. We still lack a clear understanding of the risks of anaemia in older patients and those with cardiovascular disease. Until further trials are published, clinicians need to use their experience and physiological monitoring to judge what haemoglobin value is safe in the perioperative period. As the risk–benefit profile of anti-fibrinolytics is, if anything, less certain now than previously, it is best to use an individualized approach. Local audit of practice will identify those surgeries, surgeons or anaesthetists for whom blood losses and transfusion requirements are greater than departmental or national averages. In some cases, particularly high-risk surgeries such as complex or revision cardiac surgery and revision hip arthroplasty, the risk–benefit will probably favour the use of an anti-fibrinolytic and/or perioperative cell salvage whenever possible. This approach is also appropriate for patients who decline or wish to avoid blood transfusions. For more expensive therapies, such as preoperative EPO and/or autologous donation, cost-effectiveness is likely to become increasingly important given the financial constraints in many healthcare systems. At present, the safety and continued availability of allogeneic blood probably make these therapies unjustified in most health services. However, in the likely case that allogeneic blood becomes scarcer and more expensive, and/or the cost of EPOs decreases, the balance could shift. In anticipation of this situation we need to further improve our understanding of the safety of the various blood-sparing drugs and strategies. Several ongoing trials and studies will hopefully provide some clarification of these issues in the near future.

References

1. Speiss BD. Transfusion and outcome in heart surgery. *Ann Thorac Surg* 2002; **74**: 986–7.

2. Henry DA, Moxey AJ, Carless PA, O'Connell D, McClelland B, Henderson KM, Sly K, Laupacis A, Fergusson D. Anti-fibrinolytic use for minimising perioperative allogeneic blood transfusion. Cochrane Database of Systematic Reviews. 2007, Issue 4. Art. no. CD001886.DOI:10.1002/14651858.CD001886.pub2

3. Ferraris VA, Ferraris SP, Saha SP, Hessel EA, Haan CK, Royston BD, Bridges CR, Higgins RS, Despotis G, Brown JR, for the Society of Cardiovascular Anesthesiologists Special Task Force on Blood Transfusion. Perioperative blood transfusion and blood conservation in cardiac surgery: the Society of Thoracic Surgeons and The Society of Cardiovascular Anesthesiologists clinical practice guideline. *Ann Thorac Surg* 2007; **83** (5 Suppl.): S27–86.

4. Hiatt WR. Observational studies of drug safety – aprotinin and the absence of transparency. *N Engl J Med* 2006; **355**: 2172–3.

5. http://controlled-trials.com/isrctn/trial/APROTININ/0/15166455.html

6. Kannan S, Meert KL, Mooney JF, Hilman-Wiseman MS. Bleeding and coagulopathy changes during spinal fusion surgery: a comparison of neuromuscular and idiopathic scoliosis patients. *Pediatric Crit Care* 2002; **3**: 364–9.

7. Zufferey P, Merquiol F, Laporte S, Decousus H, Mismetti P, Auboyer C, Samama CM, Molliex S. Do antifibrinolytics reduce allogeneic blood transfusion in orthopedic surgery? *Anesthesiology* 2006; **105**: 1034–46.

8. Diprose P, Herbertson MJ, O'Shaughnessy D, Deakin CD, Gill RS. Reducing allogeneic transfusion in cardiac surgery: a randomized double-blind placebo-controlled trial of antifibrinolytic therapies used in addition to intra-operative cell salvage. *Br J Anaesth* 2005; **94**: 271–8.

9. Henry DA, Carless PA, Moxey AJ, O'Connell D, Forgie MA, Wells PS, Fergusson D. Preoperative autologous donation for minimising perioperative allogeneic blood transfusion. Cochrane Database of Systematic Reviews. 2001, Issue 4. Art. no. CD003602.DOI:10.1002/14651858.CD003602.

10. Rosencher N, Poisson D, Albi A, Aperce M, Barre A, Samama CM. Two injections of erythropoietin correct moderate anemia in most patients awaiting orthopedic surgery. *Can J Anesth* 2005; **52**: 160–5.

11. Drueke TB, Locatelli F, Clyne N, Eckardt KU, Macdougall IC, Tsakiris D, Burger HU, Scherhag A. Normalization of hemoglobin level in patients with chronic kidney disease and anemia. *N Engl J Med* 2006; **355**: 2071–84.

12. Singh AK, Szczech L, Tang KL, Barnhart H, Sapp S, Wolfson M, Reddan D. Correction of anemia with epoetin alfa in chronic kidney disease. *N Engl J Med* 2006; **355**: 2085–98.

13. Carson JL, Duff A, Poses RM, Berlin JA, Spence RK, Trout R, Noveck H, Strom BL. Effect of anaemia and cardiovascular disease on surgical mortality and morbidity. *Lancet* 1996; **348**: 1055–60.

14. Hebert PC, Fergusson DA. Do transfusions get to the heart of the matter? *JAMA* 2004; **292**: 1610–12.

15. Hebert PC, Wells G, Tweeddale M, Martin C, Marshall J, Pham B, Blajchman M, Schweitzer I, Pagliarello G. Does transfusion practice affect mortality in critically ill patients? Transfusion Requirements in Critical Care (TRICC) Investigators and the Canadian Critical Care Trials Group. *Am J Respir Crit Care Med* 1997; **155**: 1618–23.

16. Hebert PC, Yetisir E, Martin C, Blajchman MA, Wells G, Marshall J, Tweeddale M, Pagliarello G, Schweitzer I. Is a low transfusion threshold safe in critically ill patients with cardiovascular diseases? *Crit Care Med* 2001; **29**: 227–34.

17. Wallis JP, Wells AW, Whitehead S, Brewster N. Recovery from post-operative anaemia. *Transfusion Med 2005;* **15**: 413–18.

18. Walsh TS, Saleh E, Lee R, McClelland DB. Anaemia at hospital discharge among survivors of critical illness. *Intensive Care Med* 2006; **32**: 1206–13.

19. Walsh TS, Lee RJ, Maciver CR, Garrioch M, MacKirdy F, Binning AR, McClelland DB, for the Audit of Transfusion in Intensive Care in Scotland (ATICS) study group. Prevalence of anaemia at discharge from the intensive care unit: the impact of evidence-based transfusion practice. *Intensive Care Med* 2006; **32**: 100–9.

20. Carson JL, Terrin ML, Magaziner J, Chaitman BR, Apple FS, Heck DA, Sanders D, for the FOCUS Investigators. Transfusion trigger trial for functional outcomes in cardiovascular patients undergoing surgical hip fracture repair (FOCUS). *Transfusion* 2006; **46**: 2192–206.

2

Perioperative respiratory care

GEORG MOLS

Perioperative protective ventilation

Lung-protective ventilation is the mainstay of supportive therapy in acute lung injury (ALI) of critically ill patients. The injured lung can be further damaged by at least two mechanisms: first, by an atelectrauma through repeated collapse and reopening of alveoli due to ventilation at low end-expiratory airway pressures [1,2]; and, second, by alveolar overdistension through high end-inspiratory airway pressures and volumes. Lung-protective ventilation aims at avoiding both injurious stimuli by using high levels of positive end-expiratory pressure (PEEP) and low tidal volumes and plateau pressures. This concept is based on a large body of experimental and clinical data [1], and partly (as for the use of low tidal volumes) on clinical outcome data [3]. The reduction in tidal volume in ALI is also based on the 'baby lung' concept derived from systematic computerized tomography scans [4].

The concept of lung-protective ventilation is pathophysiologically sound in ALI. One may argue that what is beneficial for the injured lung should also be beneficial for the non-injured lung in the perioperative setting. For that reason, 'protective' ventilation has become increasingly popular in the operating theatre. However, the uncritical transfer of a therapeutic concept from one setting to a completely different one may be problematic. Lung-protective ventilation with small tidal volumes may be the most physiological and least injurious ventilatory strategy for the injured 'baby lung', to which large tidal volumes are very harmful. However, in the healthy lung the disadvantages of this strategy (e.g. formation of atelectasis, impaired oxygenation) may well outweigh any advantages. Thus, ventilation with small tidal volumes in various perioperative settings is a matter of debate.

Protective ventilation influences systemic inflammation after esophagectomy

Michelet P, D'Journo X-B, Roch A, et al. Anesthesiology 2006; **105**: 911–19

BACKGROUND. Lung-protective ventilation, including reduction of tidal volume and the use of PEEP, may reduce inflammation associated with one-lung ventilation, thoracotomy and oesophagectomy. The authors conducted a single-centre randomized study involving 52 patients. Protective ventilation included the use of PEEP 5 cmH₂O, except during the immediate postoperative period, and the reduction of tidal volume from 9 ml/kg predicted body weight towards 5 ml/kg during one-lung ventilation. During conventional ventilation, no PEEP was used and tidal volume was kept at 9 ml/kg. In both groups, no PEEP was used during postoperative controlled mechanical ventilation but during pressure support ventilation prior to extubation.

INTERPRETATION. The authors observed lower blood concentrations of several cytokines (IL-1β, IL-6, IL-8) in the group whose lungs were ventilated protectively compared with those ventilated conventionally. TNF-α, however, was below the threshold of detection throughout. Differences between strategies began to develop prior to one-lung ventilation, but reached statistical significance only during and after this time. Clinical variables such as Pao_2/Fio_2 and extravascular lung water index showed similar results. Extubation was achieved earlier with protective than with conventional ventilation.

Comment

Oesophagectomy is a high-risk surgical procedure that is associated with frequent respiratory complications. The reasons for these complications are manifold. First, complete change of upper gastrointestinal anatomy and lack of natural barriers against aspiration may cause small ongoing aspiration of gastric content in the postoperative period. Second, intraoperative trauma to the lungs may cause lung injury. To improve surgical access to the oesophagus, frequently a right-sided thoracotomy with (one-lung) ventilation of the left lung is performed. Intraoperatively, the right lung can be injured by surgical manipulation and the left lung by unphysiological ventilation. Third, prolonged collapse of the right lung may cause atelectasis. Finally, surgery itself causes inflammation. As a result, ALI occurs in about 24% of patients undergoing oesophagectomy |5|. Reduction of ventilator-associated injury may be one approach of reducing overall respiratory risk after oesophagectomy.

The study demonstrates the benefits of lung protective ventilation during oesophagectomy with regard to systemic inflammation and certain clinical endpoints. The study was underpowered to detect a difference in survival. However, even if protective ventilation were beneficial in terms of survival, such benefit may be overshadowed by negative factors like surgery itself. However, this is more of a methodological concern that should not distract from the demonstration of a beneficial effect of protective ventilation.

Contrary to usual quality assessment, the small size of the study can be considered a strength. As outcome after oesophagectomy is heavily dependent on surgical experience and skill, the effect of ventilatory strategy *per se* on outcome may be difficult to extract when patients are operated on by different surgeons. In this study, all patients were operated on by the same surgical team.

The results of the study are consistent with observations during protective ventilation in ALI. Although one-lung ventilation with underlying healthy lungs and the 'baby lung' in ALI represent different pathophysiological entities, the amount of ventilated lung tissue is reduced in both instances. Reduction of the tidal volume is, thus, a plausible strategy to reduce side-effects of mechanical ventilation.

In this study, the protective ventilatory strategy included the use of PEEP. Thus, it cannot be determined with certainty whether the beneficial effects were primarily due to the reduction in tidal volume or the use of PEEP. In addition, as most would consider the use of PEEP standard during ventilation, one could argue that the group whose lungs were ventilated without PEEP throughout received substandard care. Nevertheless, despite its limitations, the study makes a plausible case for the use of protective ventilation in oesophagectomy.

Intraoperative tidal volume as a risk factor for respiratory failure after pneumonectomy

Fernandez-Perez E, Keegan M, Brown D, et al. Anesthesiology 2006; **105**: 14–18

BACKGROUND. The authors retrospectively analysed perioperative data from 170 pneumonectomy patients. They performed multivariate logistic regression in an attempt to identify risk factors for the development of respiratory failure, defined as need for prolonged mechanical ventilation for more than 48 h after surgery.

INTERPRETATION. Thirty per cent of 170 patients developed respiratory failure, of whom 50% (15% of all patients) fulfilled the criteria of acute lung injury (ALI). Multivariate logistic regression revealed larger tidal volumes as the only independent risk factor for postoperative respiratory failure. Interestingly, and in contrast with previous reports |6|, administration of large amounts of fluids alone was not found to be a significant risk factor. However, large tidal volumes, in combination with excessive fluid administration, were identified as a second risk factor in multivariate logistic regression.

Comment

Pneumonectomy is associated with a very high incidence of perioperative respiratory failure. ALI/acute respiratory distress syndrome (ARDS) develops with an incidence of 6–7% |6,7|. Milder forms of respiratory failure are observed considerably more frequently |8|. Respiratory failure after pneumonectomy is a main predictor of adverse outcome, including mortality. As with oesophagectomy, multiple factors contribute to adverse outcome: thoracotomy itself, type and technique of surgery, fluid management, and possibly ventilatory strategy, especially during one-lung ventilation. Again, administering low tidal volumes, and in this way avoiding the injurious effect of high tidal volumes, may reduce perioperative risk. This approach is supported by experimental data showing reduced lung trauma associated with protective (one-lung) ventilation compared with conventional ventilation |9|.

Very similar to the situation during oesophagectomy (see above) and ALI |3|, this study provides evidence that large tidal volumes are harmful when only parts of the lung are ventilated. A large tidal volume was identified as the only single risk factor for the development of postoperative respiratory failure. The findings of this study are supported by a prospective study in patients undergoing thoracic surgery |10|. Patients were randomized to either conventional (10 ml/kg) or low (5 ml/kg) tidal volumes. Low tidal volumes were associated with less inflammation than higher ones. The study was underpowered for analysis of clinical endpoints. Increased inflammation as a consequence of large tidal volumes may partly explain the aetiology of postoperative respiratory failure associated with high tidal volumes, as observed in the study discussed here.

The main limitation of this study is the lack of detailed knowledge on exactly how the patients' lungs were ventilated during one-lung ventilation and thereafter. Study results and conclusion were based on the single largest recorded tidal volume during the perioperative period. However, tidal volumes during one-lung ventilation could not be reliably derived from the patients' records. In addition, the level of PEEP was not documented throughout the procedure. As PEEP is lung protective, this may have confounded the results. Although these limitations considerably reduce the impact of the findings, they should, nevertheless, not distract from the sound advice to use lower tidal volumes whenever not all alveoli are available for ventilation, for whatever reason.

Mechanical ventilation with lower tidal volumes and positive end-expiratory pressure prevents alveolar coagulation in patients without lung injury

Choi G, Wolthuis EK, Bresser P, et al. Anesthesiology 2006; **105**: 689–95

BACKGROUND. Forty patients scheduled for long duration surgery (> 5 h) were randomized to either ventilation with high tidal volume (12 ml/kg) and no PEEP or to ventilation with low tidal volume (6 ml/kg) and a PEEP of 10 cmH$_2$O. Bronchoalveolar lavage was performed after induction of anaesthesia and 5 h thereafter. The authors determined bronchoalveolar coagulation as a marker of inflammation.

INTERPRETATION. The authors observed a procoagulant shift in bronchoalveolar fluids of patients whose lungs had been ventilated with large tidal volume and no PEEP. This procoagulant shift was not observed in patients whose lungs were ventilated 'protectively'. Clinical variables did not differ between groups. The authors interpret their findings as indication for high tidal volumes being a 'primary hit' of multiple hits leading to ALI.

Comment

This study shows that the ventilatory strategy may have an impact on intra-alveolar coagulation. It provides further evidence for a beneficial effect of low tidal volumes in situations of reduced alveolar surface. This might beg the question: why not routinely reduce tidal volume? Two hours of mechanical ventilation with a conventional tidal volume of 10 ml/kg can induce considerable changes in the immune status of children without prior pulmonary pathology undergoing cardiac catheterization |11|. A proinflammatory reaction within the lungs was accompanied by a decrease in the activity of natural killer cells in peripheral blood. However, these findings were not associated with clinical signs of lung injury. In addition, the simultaneous administration of volatile anaesthetics or the catheterization may have contributed to the findings. Nevertheless, they question the commonly held belief that short-term intraoperative mechanical ventilation is generally harmless to healthy lungs.

It is important to be aware that in the study discussed here (Choi *et al.*), coagulation instead of inflammation was studied. The two are closely linked, but not the same. Thus, one has to question somewhat the authors' suggestion that the procoagulant shift may represent the first 'hit' in the initiation of inflammation. By contrast, no |12| or only minor inflammation |13| had previously been reported under similar clinical conditions. The procoagulatory shift may simply be an 'adaptive mechanism with host protective functions', as the authors rightly point out.

Overall, the study by Choi *et al.* importantly contributes to the understanding of the effects of mechanical ventilation, and it may trigger further research in this area. However, although it suggests that it might not be bad advice to routinely use lower tidal volumes and higher levels of PEEP in an effort to reduce the adverse effects of mechanical ventilation, it does not provide sufficient justification for routinely applying a ventilatory strategy intraoperatively that is considered the gold standard in severe lung injury. At the current state of knowledge, one is inclined to consider the findings as interesting with regard to pathophysiology, but less relevant for clinical practice.

Obesity

Obesity is an increasing problem in industrialized countries (especially the USA |14|) and developing countries |15|. Although morbid obesity (body mass index [BMI] > 40 kg/m^2) was not considered a major problem in Europe until recently, this is no longer the case |16|. Worldwide, anaesthetists are increasingly confronted with obesity in their daily clinical practice. Obesity is associated with increased respiratory and surgical complications. Respiratory complications include aspiration of gastric content, difficulties in ventilation and airway management, hypoxaemia, atelectasis and postoperative pneumonia |17,18|. The two publications discussed below address the issues of titration of PEEP and choice of anaesthetic technique in obese patients.

Positive end-expiratory pressure optimization using electric impedance tomography in morbidly obese patients during laparoscopic bypass surgery

Erlandsson K, Odenstedt H, Lundin S, et al. Acta Anaesthesiol Scand 2006; 50: 833–9

BACKGROUND. The authors used electric impedance tomography (EIT) in 15 morbidly obese patients (BMI $49 \pm 8 kg/m^2$) for the titration of PEEP during gastric bypass surgery. It is noteworthy that a continuous positive airway pressure (CPAP) of 10 cmH$_2$0 was used during preoxygenation, prior to induction of anaesthesia and muscle relaxation. Subsequently, the authors varied PEEP and tidal volume while recording EIT. PEEP was considered optimal when no impedance change (ΔZ) was observed during the recording. In addition to EIT, functional residual capacity (FRC) and other variables were measured before and after surgery.

INTERPRETATION. The impedance (ΔZ) of EIT during ventilation with different PEEP levels was the basis for adjusting PEEP (Fig. 2.1). A horizontal line was used as a surrogate for optimal PEEP, whereas an increasing or decreasing slope was interpreted as recruitment or derecruitment. By such definition, optimal PEEP was determined to be $15 \pm 1 cmH_2O$. At this PEEP level, FRC was 1706 ± 447 ml before and 2210 ± 540 ml after surgery. Surprisingly, Pao_2/Fio_2 ratio and shunt fraction remained unchanged. The authors drew three main conclusions: (1) EIT can be used to titrate PEEP in obese patients; (2) the chosen level of PEEP (15 cmH$_2$O) is higher than previously considered adequate in morbidly obese patients; and (3) CPAP prior to induction of anaesthesia may be helpful in maintaining a normal lung volume.

Comment

This publication by Erlandsson *et al.* reflects the increasing attention anaesthetists have paid to intraoperative respiratory management of patients at risk for respiratory

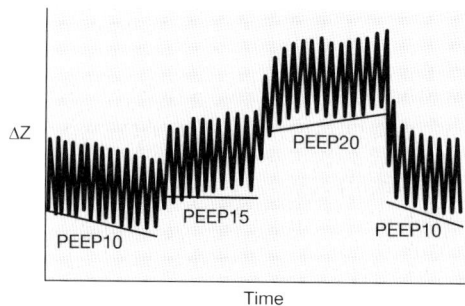

Fig. 2.1 Electric impedance tomography (EIT) tracing during different PEEP levels. A decreasing slope indicates derecruitment, an increasing slope recruitment. A horizontal line reflects constant FRC, interpreted as the point of optimal PEEP. Source: Erlandsson *et al.* (2006).

complications. EIT is an interesting method for clinical use for two reasons: it is (almost) non-invasive and it 'shows' the impact of ventilation on the distribution of intrapulmonary volume in real time. However, interpretation requires some experience |19,20|. Especially in obese patients, EIT is difficult to use, as admitted by the authors themselves.

Interpretation of the presented data deserves some comment. During ventilation with PEEP 15 cmH$_2$O (see Fig. 2.1), impedance was considered to be constant. However, close examination of the figure shows that impedance was not truly constant at any PEEP level. This may be the case only during longer periods of ventilation at one particular PEEP level (e.g. 15 cmH$_2$O). One might support the view that recruitment *per se* is beneficial. In such a case, constant impedance (reflecting constant lung volume) would not necessarily be beneficial and not necessarily reflect optimal PEEP. Most practitioners would support the view that a constant lung volume following full recruitment is the least traumatic for lung tissue |2|. However, experimental data suggest that an injured lung could not and should not be fully recruited when attempting lung protection |21|. The different views reflect the uncertainty with regard to the optimal ventilatory strategy.

The findings by Erlandsson *et al.* imply that we should be paying increased attention to alveolar recruitment in obese patients by using relatively high PEEP levels throughout the perioperative period, and by possibly using CPAP before induction of anaesthesia in an attempt to reduce the formation of atelectasis. Ultimately, direct correlation of functional data (such as those obtained by EIT) with morphological data on lung tissue will be required to determine the optimal ventilatory strategy. This remains a long way to go. Nevertheless, the publication by Erlandsson *et al.* shows that new methods of guiding ventilatory strategy are in the 'pipeline'.

Impact of spinal anaesthesia on perioperative lung volumes in obese and morbidly obese female patients

Regli A, von Ungern-Sternberg BS, Reber A, et al. Anaesthesia 2006; **61**: 215–21

BACKGROUND. Spirometric measures (vital capacity, VC; forced vital capacity, FVC; forced expiratory volume in 1s, FEV$_1$; peak expiratory flow rate, PEFR; mid-expiratory flow rate, MEF$_{25-75}$) were studied in 28 obese (BMI 30–40 kg/m^2) and 13 morbidly obese (BMI > 40 kg/m^2) patients scheduled for vaginal surgery before and after application of spinal anaesthesia with 10 mg of 0.5% hyperbaric bupivacaine, and postoperatively. All patients were premedicated with 7.5 mg midazolam orally. Spirometry was performed with the patient in the 30° head-up position during the preoperative visit, 10 min after application of spinal anaesthesia (60 min after premedication), and at 1, 2 and 3 h after surgery, by which time patients had been mobilized.

INTERPRETATION. Compared with preoperative values, all spirometric measures decreased by approximately 20–50% following initiation of spinal anaesthesia. They remained unchanged until 2 h after surgery and had improved only slightly by the time of mobilization at 3 h postoperatively. PEFR and MEF$_{25-75}$ decreased the most. Decreases in spirometric variables were significantly more pronounced in morbidly obese than in obese patients. There was no correlation between spirometric variables and motor blockade.

Comment

Obesity poses an increasing challenge to anaesthetists. Obese and, even more so, morbidly obese patients develop extensive atelectasis during general anaesthesia which persists for at least 24 h after removal of the endotracheal tube |22|. Spinal and epidural anaesthesia are often used in obese patients, with the assumption that the impairment of respiratory function would be less severe |23|. This study by Regli *et al.* clearly demonstrates that this assumption does not necessarily hold true (at least with regard to spirometric measures of respiratory function). However, it does not provide an explanation for the impairment in respiratory function. Principally, two mechanisms are to be considered: first, atelectasis by increased weight of adipose tissue; and, second, impaired expiratory effort as a result of the inevitable depressant effect of spinal and epidural anaesthesia on abdominal and thoracic muscle strength. Both mechanisms are likely to have been involved. An additional adverse effect of the premedication with midazolam cannot be ruled out.

The publication does not address the impact of lung volume reduction on pulmonary gas exchange. However, the 20–35% reductions in vital capacity alone make an adverse effect on gas exchange very likely. Overall, the data clearly indicate that spinal anaesthesia is not necessarily innocent in obese patients. They strongly suggest close postoperative observation of obese patients after spinal anaesthesia in the postanaesthesia care unit for several hours, ideally until the time of mobilization. The more obese the patient, the more important close postoperative observation becomes.

Miscellaneous

Pressure-controlled versus volume-controlled ventilation during one-lung ventilation for thoracic surgery

Unzueta MC, Casas JI, Moral MV. *Anesth Analg* 2007; **104**: 1029–33

BACKGROUND. Fifty-eight patients scheduled for thoracic surgery with one-lung ventilation were randomly allocated to initial volume-controlled or pressure-controlled ventilation. After 30 min of one-lung ventilation in the selected

ventilatory mode, the mode was changed. Pulmonary gas exchange and airway pressures were recorded during initial two-lung ventilation, during one-lung ventilation, after crossover and following reinstitution of two-lung ventilation.

INTERPRETATION. During one-lung ventilation at similar tidal volumes, oxygenation did not differ between ventilatory modes, and peak airway pressures were lower during pressure-controlled than during volume-controlled ventilation. The statistically significant differences in plateau pressures were clinically irrelevant.

Comment

In Europe, pressure-controlled ventilation with a decelerating inspiratory flow pattern is very popular for the treatment of patients suffering from ALI. Compared with volume-controlled ventilation, pressure-controlled ventilation is thought to have the following advantages: superior gas exchange and distribution, lower peak airway pressures and reduced incidence of ventilator-associated lung injury. However, such advantages have not uniformly been confirmed |24,25|. As *lack of proof of benefit* is not identical with *proof of lack of benefit,* pressure-controlled ventilation remains popular in European intensive care settings.

The crossover design used by Unzueta *et al.* did not allow assessment of any potential protective effect of pressure-controlled ventilation. Lack of superior oxygenation during pressure-controlled ventilation in this patient population resembles that observed in patients with ALI. However, an entirely different pathophysiology of impaired gas exchange underlies both conditions. During one-lung ventilation, ventilation–perfusion mismatch is iatrogenic, due to interrupting ventilation of one lung. By contrast, ventilation–perfusion mismatch during ALI results from morphological lung tissue changes at the lobular and alveolar level. As a consequence, higher airway pressures and higher PEEP may improve gas exchange in ALI, but not during one-lung ventilation.

Different peak airway pressures but comparable plateau pressures during both ventilatory modes require explanation. At first sight, lower peak airway pressures during pressure-controlled ventilation may be interpreted as reflecting a lesser mechanical stress on the respiratory system. However, whereas peak airway pressure is determined by both elastance and resistance, plateau pressure is exclusively determined by elastance (as long as inspiratory time is sufficient). Stated otherwise, the difference between peak and plateau airway pressure results predominantly from the resistive pressure drop across artificial and natural airways |26,27|. Consequently, peak airway pressure provides little information on the true respiratory stress or 'invasiveness' of a given ventilatory mode. Plateau pressure is better suited for this purpose. As plateau pressures were similar during pressure- and volume-controlled ventilation, the invasiveness of the two ventilatory modes seems to have been similar during one-lung ventilation. In conclusion, the findings by Unzueta *et al.* suggest that pressure-controlled ventilation offers no benefit compared with volume-controlled ventilation during one-lung ventilation.

The effect of bi level positive airway pressure mechanical ventilation on gas exchange during general anaesthesia

Yu G, Yang K, Baker AB, et al. Br J Anaesth 2006; **96**: 522–32

BACKGROUND. The lungs of 20 patients with normal body weight scheduled for coronary artery bypass grafting were ventilated with either biphasic positive airway pressure (BIPAP, a form of pressure-controlled ventilation) or intermittent positive pressure (IPPV, volume-controlled ventilation) with or without PEEP of $4\,cmH_2O$. Both ventilatory modes were applied in random order for 60 min each. Intrapulmonary shunt, dead space, and the distributions of ventilation (logSDV) and perfusion (logSDQ) were studied by the multiple inert gas elimination technique (MIGET) during each mode of ventilation and during spontaneous breathing before induction of anaesthesia. Anaesthesia was provided by target-controlled infusions of propofol and remifentanil and muscle relaxation by rocuronium.

INTERPRETATION. No significant differences in shunt, dead space or the distribution of ventilation (logSDV) were observed between ventilatory modes. Only logSDQ was slightly larger during IPPV (especially in the absence of PEEP) reflecting a similarly wider distribution of perfusion values. Notably, shunt did not differ between pre-induction and mechanical ventilation.

Comment

The findings of this study suggest that in the perioperative setting, the mode of ventilation is of minor importance. The distributions of ventilation and perfusion were studied by MIGET, a method providing much more insight into the lungs' functional status than the analysis of pulmonary gas exchange. Surprisingly, even with this sophisticated technique, except for logSDQ, no significant differences between ventilatory modes were observed. LogSDQ reflects the wideness of the distribution of perfusion. An ideal distribution would be narrow. However, as all other variables were similar between ventilatory modes, the overall impact of the ventilatory mode on the investigated variables was in fact minimal and most likely incidental.

This lack of differences between ventilatory modes deserves two comments: first, as even shunt did not differ between pre-induction and intraoperative periods, one might argue that the patient population was simply 'too' healthy to benefit from any particular form of ventilatory strategy. This possibility is supported by the fact that BMI was in the normal range in all patients. Routine clinical practice shows that patients with normal body weight and without pulmonary pathology can be ventilated with pretty much any kind of ventilatory mode without major adverse consequences. This is certainly not the case for obese patients and for those with pulmonary pathology.

Second, a valid comparison between different ventilatory modes is possible only at comparable airway pressures. Although peak, plateau and mean airway pressures can never be identical during IPPV and BIPAP ventilation, similarity in at least one of the airway pressures should be aimed for. Unfortunately, the authors provided few data on airway pressures. This prevents an ultimate assessment of the clinical relevance of the findings.

With these limitations in mind, and in agreement with the findings during pressure-controlled ventilation in one-lung ventilation discussed above (Unzueta *et al.*) and during ALI |24|, this study would support the view that the mode of ventilation is of minor importance.

Effects of propofol vs. sevoflurane on arterial oxygenation during one-lung ventilation

Pruszkowski O, Dalibon N, Moutafis M, *et al*. *Br J Anaesth* 2007; **98**: 539–44

BACKGROUND. Sixty-five patients undergoing lung lobectomy were anaesthetized with either propofol or sevoflurane. In addition, they received peridural analgesia with ropivacaine and sufentanil and muscle relaxation with atracurium. Depth of general anaesthesia was adjusted to a bispectral index (BIS) value of between 40 and 60.

INTERPRETATION. Oxygenation during one-lung ventilation did not differ between groups. BIS was 51 ± 4 in the sevoflurane and 46 ± 8 in the propofol group (no significant difference). Mean end-tidal sevoflurane concentration was $1.3\%\pm0.3\%$ and calculated propofol plasma concentration was $2.6\pm0.9\mu g/ml$.

Comment

Oxygenation during one-lung ventilation is often critical due to iatrogenic shunting of blood through the non-ventilated lung. Volatile anaesthetic drugs may further worsen oxygenation by interfering with hypoxic pulmonary vasoconstriction (HPV) |28,29|. As propofol does not inhibit HPV |28|, total intravenous anaesthesia with propofol may be advantageous. Published data regarding the clinical relevance of volatile anaesthetic-induced inhibition of HPV are contradictory. This may in part be due to the use of different concentrations of volatile anaesthetics. Ideally, the effects of volatile and intravenous anaesthetics on oxygenation during one-lung ventilation should be compared at equipotent anaesthetic concentrations.

In this study, sevoflurane does not seem to have affected HPV. This may be explained by a relatively low end-tidal concentration, made possible by the simultaneous provision of peridural analgesia. Use of BIS monitoring contributed to the 'safe' use of such low sevoflurane concentrations. Thus, this study does not suggest that impairment of HPV by volatile anaesthetics is generally of no clinical relevance. Rather, it indicates that with current practice of thoracic anaesthesia –

which includes the use of peridural analgesia to provide baseline analgesia, and the possible use of BIS monitoring to reduce the likelihood of intraoperative awareness in the presence of low end-tidal concentrations of volatile anaesthetics – volatile anaesthetic-induced inhibition of HPV is of no major clinical concern. Nevertheless, the question of why use volatile rather than intravenous anaesthetics at all during lung surgery may well be a legitimate one.

Impact of depth of propofol anaesthesia on functional residual capacity and ventilation distribution in healthy preschool children

von Ungern-Sternberg BS, Frei FJ, Hammer J, et al. Br J Anaesth 2007; **98**: 503–8

BACKGROUND. The pulmonary effects of two depths of sedation with propofol were studied in increasing order in 20 preschool children (mean age approximately 50 ± 13 months; mean weight 17.5 ± 3.9 kg). Patients were breathing spontaneously via a tight-fitting face mask. Chin lift was used to prevent upper airway collapse. Functional residual capacity (FRC), lung clearance index (LCI) and mean dilution number (MDN) as indicators of ventilation distribution and airway collapse were determined at the two depths of sedation.

INTERPRETATION. At the lesser and the greater depth of sedation, plasma propofol concentrations were $1.4 \pm 0.4\,\mu g/ml$ (mean $\pm$ SD) and $3.2 \pm 0.9\,\mu g/ml$, and BIS values 58 ± 7 and 36 ± 6, respectively. With increasing depth of sedation, absolute FRC and FRC per kilogram body weight decreased substantially from 364 ± 108 ml (20.7 ± 3.3 ml/ kg) to 310 ± 100 ml (17.7 ± 3.9 ml/kg), and tidal volume decreased from 128 ± 22 ml to 104 ± 26 ml, while the ratio of tidal volume to FRC remained constant. LCI and MDN increased simultaneously.

Comment

This elegant and straightforward study demonstrates that an increasing depth of sedation with propofol may have substantial pulmonary side-effects in children and may increase the risk of hypoxia. Compared with adults, children are *per se* at greater risk for hypoxia during sedation and anaesthesia due to their lower FRC and higher oxygen demand. Any additional reduction in FRC must be expected to become critical in children. The study by von Ungern-Sternberg *et al.* shows that this is exactly what may happen during increasing depth of propofol sedation. It additionally shows that propofol sedation may impair effectiveness of ventilation as reflected by altered distribution of ventilation.

The paper has several limitations. First, although carefully attended to, upper airway occlusion could not be entirely excluded as an explanation for the change in respiratory variables. Second, the two stages of sedation were studied in increasing but not random order. Presumably, this was done because of the difficulty in standardizing the depths of sedation. Owing to interindividual variability in pharmacokinetics, similar propofol plasma concentrations at a given depth of sedation would have been difficult to achieve if the deeper sedation been studied first. Nevertheless, this is an important limitation because the influence of time on the results cannot be ruled out with certainty |23|. FRC and other variables could have changed with the duration rather than the depth of sedation. Third, the methods applied do not allow an explanation of the mechanism(s) responsible for the observed respiratory changes.

However, despite the methodological concerns and the lack of explanation for the mechanisms involved, the findings show that increasing depth of sedation with propofol decreases FRC in preschool children and puts them at increased risk of hypoxia. This supports the common wisdom that no technique – in this case deep sedation without a safe airway – should be pushed beyond its limits.

Haemodynamic effects of sustained pulmonary hyperinflation in patients after cardiac surgery: open vs. closed chest

Nielsen J, Nygard E, Kjaergaard J, et al. *Acta Anaesthesiol Scand* 2007; **51**: 74–81

BACKGROUND. The effects of a manually applied, sustained inflation manoeuvre (peak airway pressure 40 cmH$_2$O for 15 s) were studied before and after chest closure in 10 patients undergoing conventional coronary artery bypass graft surgery via median sternotomy. Between both inflation manoeuvres, the lungs were ventilated without PEEP. Haemodynamics were measured with the PiCCO system and a pulmonary artery catheter before, at the end and after each manoeuvre. Similar filling of the heart was confirmed by echocardiography.

INTERPRETATION. During the inflation manoeuvre, cardiac output decreased from approximately 5.5 l/min to 3 l/min. One minute later, cardiac output had returned close to baseline value. Changes in mean arterial pressure were in the same directions, those in mean pulmonary artery and central venous pressure in the opposite directions. Most important, the haemodynamic responses to inflation were similar during open and closed chest.

Comment

During cardiopulmonary bypass, either no or only low airway pressure is applied to the lungs in order to avoid alveolar alkalosis in the basically not perfused lungs and to improve surgical access to the heart. Together with direct surgical manipulation, this results in atelectasis of large parts of the lungs. After having come off cardiopulmonary bypass and before transfer to the intensive care unit, the lungs are usually recruited by sustained inflation manoeuvre to improve pulmonary gas exchange and to avoid other sequelae of atelectasis. The sustained inflation manoeuvre is regularly accompanied by cardiovascular depression of usually brief duration; however, even brief cardiovascular depression immediately following cardiac surgery and cardiopulmonary bypass is of concern.

One would expect that pulmonary recruitment before chest closure to be haemodynamically better tolerated than after chest closure because (i) chest closure itself may induce haemodynamic impairment and (ii) the increase in pleural pressure and its transmission to the great vessels are blunted during an open chest. Contrary to this expectation, cardiovascular depression was found to be similar during open-and closed-chest surgery. The authors propose two opposing mechanisms during open- and closed-chest surgery that might have contributed to the comparable cardiovascular response to lung inflation: transmission of increased intrathoracic pressure to the great vessels during closed chest vs. increased stretching of alveolar capillaries (resulting in increased pulmonary vascular resistance) during open chest. The study design and available data do not allow verification of these proposed mechanisms. Nevertheless, the clinical implication of the findings is rather straightforward: recruit the lungs when you feel that it is indicated. You do not need to wait for chest closure. But be prepared for cardiovascular depression under both conditions.

Conclusion

What are the main 'take-home messages' of the various publications discussed? Recent findings |**34,35;** Choi *et al.*|, current understanding of the pathophysiology of ALI, and the concept of the 'baby lung' strongly support a ventilatory strategy of reducing the tidal volume in situations of reduced lung volume (e.g. during certain surgical procedures, one-lung ventilation or lung disease). This makes intuitive sense, because otherwise the reduction in the accessible lung volume will result in large alveolar tidal volumes, which, in turn, carry the potential for alveolar overdistension and subsequent lung injury.

The situation is less clear for intraoperative ventilation of lungs with normal volume (Choi *et al.*). The authors of a recent review article argued that, despite lack of scientific evidence, tidal volume should be lower than 10 ml/kg, even in the absence of lung injury |**30**|. An accompanying editorial recommended a ventilatory strategy adjusted to the patients' pathology and the surgical procedure |**31**|. These authors argued that very large tidal volumes (above 10 ml/kg) are obsolete nowadays and unsuited to recruit the lungs. In the face of very limited 'hard' data, it seems reasonable to recommend the use of low tidal volumes whenever lung volume is considerably reduced for whatever reason. Under all other circumstances, there is presently no conclusive evidence to support the recommendation of routinely reducing the tidal volume to well below 10 ml/kg.

In obese patients, alveolar recruitment and the need for possibly higher than usually applied PEEP levels are important (Erlandsson *et al.*). We must not underestimate the respiratory risk to obese and, particularly, of morbidly obese patients associated with spinal anaesthesia (Regli *et al.*). It may, thus, be advisable to monitor them in the postoperative care unit for several hours.

We have learned that pressure-controlled ventilation is not necessarily superior to volume-controlled ventilation during one-lung ventilation and general anaesthesia (Unzueta *et al.*, Yu *et al.*). This is similar to conditions during ALI. With current anaesthetic techniques for thoracic surgery, it is unlikely that volatile anaesthetics impair hypoxic pulmonary vasoconstriction to a degree that adversely affects oxygenation during one-lung ventilation (Pruszkowski *et al.*).

We have learned that deep sedation may critically impair respiration in children by reducing FRC (von Ungern-Sternberg *et al.*). Finally, we have learned that the adverse cardiovascular effects of sustained lung inflation following cardiac surgery and cardiopulmonary bypass are similar when performed during open- or closed-chest surgery (Nielsen *et al.*). All of the publications discussed here considerably contribute to a safer perioperative respiratory care.

References

1. Dreyfuss D, Saumon G. Ventilator-induced lung injury: lessons from experimental studies. *Am J Respir Crit Care Med* 1998; **157**: 294–323.

2. Mols G, Priebe H-J, Guttmann J. Alveolar recruitment in acute lung injury. *Br J Anaesth* 2006; **96**: 156–66.

3. The Acute Respiratory Distress Syndrome Network. Ventilation with lower tidal volumes as compared with traditional tidal volumes for acute lung injury and the acute respiratory distress syndrome. *N Engl J Med* 2000; **342**: 1301–8.

4. Gattinoni L, Mascheroni D, Torresin A, Marcolin R, Fumagalli R, Vesconi S, Rossi GP, Rossi F, Baglioni S, Bassi F, Nastri G, Pesenti A. Morphological response to positive end expiratory pressure in acute respiratory failure. Computerized tomography study. *Intensive Care Med* 1986; **12**: 137–42.

5. Tandon S, Batchelor A, Bullock R, Gascoigne A, Griffin M, Hayes N, Hing J, Shaw I, Warnell I, Baudouin SV. Peri-operative risk factors for acute lung injury after elective oesophagectomy. *Br J Anaesth* 2001; **86**: 633–8.

6. Licker M, de Perrot M, Spiliopoulos A, Robert J, Diaper J, Chevalley C, Tschopp J-M. Risk factors for acute lung injury after thoracic surgery for lung cancer. *Anesth Analg* 2003; **97**: 1558–65.

7. Kutlu CA, Williams EA, Evans TW, Pastorino U, Goldstraw P. Acute lung injury and acute respiratory distress syndrome after pulmonary resection. *Ann Thorac Surg* 2000; **69**: 376–80.

8. Miller DL, Deschamps C, Jenkins GD, A B, Allen MS, Pairolero PC. Completion pneumonectomy: factors affecting operative mortality and cardiopulmonary morbidity. *Ann Thorac Surg* 2002; **74**: 876–84.

9. Gama de Abreu M, Heintz M, Heller A, Szechenyi R, Albrecht DM, Koch T. One-lung ventilation with high tidal volumes and zero positive end-expiratory pressure is injurious in the isolated rabbit lung model. *Anesth Analg* 2003; **96**: 220–8.

10. Schilling T, Kozian A, Huth C, Buhling F, Kretzschmar M, Welte T, Hachenberg T. The pulmonary immune effects of mechanical ventilation in patients undergoing thoracic surgery. *Anesth Analg* 2005; **101**: 957–65.

11. Plötz FB, Vreugdenhil HAE, Slutsky AS, Zijlstra J, Heijnen CJ, van Vught H. Mechanical ventilation alters the immune response in children without lung pathology. *Intensive Care Med* 2002; **28**: 486–92.

12. Wrigge H, Uhlig U, Zinserling J, Behrends-Callsen E, Ottersbach G, Fischer M, Uhlig S, Putensen C. The effects of different ventilatory settings on pulmonary and systemic inflammatory responses during major surgery. *Anesth Analg* 2004; **98**: 775–81.

13. Wrigge H, Uhlig U, Baumgarten G, Menzenbach J, Zinserling J, Ernst M, Drömann D, Welz A, Uhlig S, Putensen C. Mechanical ventilation strategies and inflammatory responses to cardiac surgery: a prospective randomized clinical trial. *Intensive Care Med* 2005; **31**: 1379–87.

14. Ogden CL, Carroll MD, Curtin LR, McDowell MA, Tabak CJ, Flegal KM. Prevalence of overweight and obesity in the United States, 1999–2004. *JAMA* 2006; **295**: 1549–55.

15. Kellshadi R. Childhood overweight, obesity, and the metabolic syndrome in developing countries. *Epidemiological Reviews* 2007; **29**: 62–76.

16. Wiegand S, Maikowski U, Blankenstein O, Biebermann H, Tarnow P, Gruters A. Type 2 diabetes and impaired glucose tolerance in European children and adolescents with obesity – a problem that is no longer restricted to minority groups. *Eur J Endocrinol* 2004; **151**: 199–206.

17. Reber A. Atemwege und respiratorische Funktion bei Adipositas: Anästhesiologische und intensivmedizinische Aspekte und Empfehlungen. *Anaesthesist* 2005; **54**: 715–27.

18. Flier S, Knape JTA. How to inform a morbidly obese patient on the specific risk to develop postoperative pulmonary complications using evidence-based methodology. *Eur J Anaesthesiol* 2006; **23**: 154–9.

19. Victorino JA, Borges JB, Okamoto VN, Matos GFJ, Tucci MR, Caramez MPR, Tanaka H, Sipmann FS, Santos DCB, Barbas CSV, Carvalho CRR, Amato MBP. Imbalances in regional lung ventilation: a validation study on electrical impedance tomography. *Am J Respir Crit Care Med* 2004; **169**: 791–800.

20. Frerichs I, Hinz J, Herrmann P, Weisser G, Hahn G, Dudykevych T, Quintel M. Detection of local lung air content by electrical impedance tomography compared with electron beam CT. *J Appl Physiol* 2002; **93**: 660–6.

21. Chu EK, Whitehead T, Slutsky AS. Effects of cyclic opening and closing at low- and high-volume ventilation on bronchoalveolar cytokines. *Crit Care Med* 2004; **32**: 168–74.

22. Eichenberger A-S, Proietti S, Wicky S, Frascarolo P, Suter P, Spahn DR, Magnusson L. Morbid obesity and postoperative pulmonary atelectasis: an underestimated problem. *Anesth Analg* 2002; **95**: 1788–92.

23. Duggan M, Kavanagh BP. Pulmonary atelectasis: a pathogenetic perioperative entity. *Anesthesiology* 2005; **102**: 838–54.

24. Prella M, Feihl F, Domenighetti G. Effects of short-term pressure-controlled ventilation on gas exchange, airway pressures, and gas distribution in patients with acute lung injury/ARDS: comparison with volume-controlled ventilation. *Chest* 2002; **122**: 1382–8.

25. Rappaport SH, Shpiner R, Yoshihara G, Wright J, Chang P, Abraham E. Randomized, prospective trial of pressure-limited vs. volume-controlled ventilation in severe respiratory failure. *Crit Care Med* 1994; **22**: 22–32.

26. Guttmann J, Eberhard L, Fabry B, Bertschmann W, Wolff G. Continuous calculation of intratracheal pressure in tracheally intubated patients. *Anesthesiology* 1993; **79**: 503–13.

27. Guttmann J, Kessler V, Mols G, Hentschel R, Haberthür C, Geiger K. Continuous calculation of intratracheal pressure in the presence of pediatric endotracheal tubes. *Crit Care Med* 2000; **28**: 1018–26.

28. Schwarzkopf K, Schreiber T, Preussler N-P, Gaser E, Hüter L, Bauer R, Schubert H, Karzai W. Lung perfusion, shunt fraction, and oxygenation during one-lung ventilation in pigs: the effects of desflurane, isoflurane, and propofol. *J Cardiothorac Vasc Anesth* 2003; **17**: 73–5.

29. Loer S, Scheeren T, Tarnow J. Desflurane inhibits hypoxic pulmonary vasoconstriction in isolated rabbit lungs. *Anesthesiology* 1995; **83**: 552–6.

30. Schultz MJ, Haitsma JJ, Slutsky AS, Gajic O. What tidal volumes should be used in patients without acute lung injury? *Anesthesiology* 2007; **106**: 1226–31.

31. Putensen C, Wrigge H. Tidal volumes in patients with normal lungs: one for all or the less, the better? *Anesthesiology* 2007; **106**: 1085–7.

3

Perioperative cardioprotection

STEPHEN WEBB, JOSEPH ARROWSMITH

Cardiovascular complications are a significant cause of morbidity and mortality after both cardiac and non-cardiac surgery. It is increasingly accepted that the 'window' of cardiac risk persists long into the postoperative period and that non-fatal perioperative cardiac events are predictive of long-term (>18 months) morbidity and mortality [1]. The human and financial implications are enormous; as many as 10% of all patients undergoing non-cardiac surgery have, or are at risk of having, cardiovascular disease (CVD); a third of patients over 65 years of age have CVD and two-thirds of patients undergoing vascular surgery have clinically relevant CVD. Despite significant advances in risk assessment, diagnostic techniques and therapeutic interventions, myocardial ischaemia remains the most important potentially reversible risk factor for morbidity after non-cardiac surgery. An accumulating body of evidence suggests that perioperative cardioprotection may have significant short- and long-term benefits.

Preoperative cardiac risk assessment

The aims of preoperative cardiac risk assessment are straightforward – evaluation of the patient with known CVD, identification of patients with symptoms or signs of CVD and identification of patients who, by virtue of the type of surgery planned, are at high risk of perioperative cardiac complications. Guidelines produced jointly by the American College of Cardiology (ACC) and the American Heart Association (AHA) have sought to address the issue of perioperative cardiovascular evaluation and risk assessment [2,3]. Despite the fact that many of the ACC/AHA guideline recommendations are based on level B (i.e. single randomized trials or non-randomized trials) or level C (i.e. expert opinion or case studies) evidence, they have been widely accepted into clinical practice. Prospective application of existing guidelines in the setting of randomized trials will undoubtedly be reflected in future versions of the guidelines [4].

Consideration of the patient's functional status, the presence of cardiac risk factors (Table 3.1) and the type of surgery planned allows risk stratification, in terms of identification of low-risk patients who need no further investigation and high-risk patients who may benefit from further investigation (e.g. stress echocardiography or myocardial scintigraphy, coronary angiography) or risk modification (e.g. preoperative coronary revascularization, valve surgery). The management of

Table 3.1 The revised cardiac risk index (RCRI). Low risk, 0–1 points; intermediate risk, 2–3 points; high risk, > 3 points

Factor	Score
High-risk surgery	1
Coronary artery disease	1
Congestive heart failure	1
Cerebrovascular disease	1
Insulin-dependent diabetes mellitus	1
Serum creatinine > 2 mg/dl (160 μmol/l)	1

Source: Lee *et al.* |**5**|.

intermediate-risk patients, however, presents the clinician with a dilemma. The 2002 ACC/AHA updated guidelines recommend that *all* intermediate-risk patients undergoing major vascular surgery should undergo preoperative non-invasive cardiac testing. This recommendation is based on the assumption that non-invasive testing has high positive *and* negative predictive values – an assumption that may not hold true in certain groups |6|. Unfortunately, for the majority of patients in this group, this approach merely delays surgery without conferring any outcome benefit. Recent evidence suggests that (i) non-invasive testing should be reserved only for high-risk patients; (ii) preoperative myocardial revascularization does not reduce perioperative mortality in patients with significant but symptomatically stable coronary artery disease; and (iii) intermediate and high-risk patients should receive perioperative beta-blocker therapy |7|.

Should major vascular surgery be delayed because of preoperative cardiac testing in intermediate-risk patients receiving beta-blocker therapy with tight heart rate control?

Poldermans D, Bax JJ, Schouten O, *et al. J Am Coll Cardiol* 2006; **48**: 964–9

BACKGROUND. In their second multicentre investigation, the Dutch Echocardiographic Cardiac Risk Evaluation Applying Stress Echo (DECREASE-II) group assessed the value of preoperative non-invasive cardiac stress testing in intermediate-risk (one or two risk factors) patients receiving heart rate-targeted beta-blocker therapy prior to major vascular surgery. A total of 1476 patients scheduled for elective abdominal aortic or infra-inguinal arterial surgery at five centres were screened for the presence of cardiac risk factors – age > 70 years, angina pectoris, prior myocardial infarction (MI) on the basis of history or pathological Q-waves on electrocardiography, congestive heart failure or a history of decompensated congestive heart failure, drug treatment for diabetes mellitus, renal dysfunction (serum creatinine concentration > 160 μmol/l), prior stroke or transient ischaemic attack. A total of 770 (52%)

patients were randomized to either undergo ($n = 386$) or not undergo ($n = 384$) dobutamine stress echocardiography or dobutamine/dipyridamole stress perfusion scintigraphy. Stress testing stratified patients into one of three groups: those with no ischaemia, those with limited inducible ischaemia (1–4 ischaemic segments on echocardiography or 1–2 ischaemic walls on perfusion scintigraphy in a six-wall model) and those with extensive inducible ischaemia (> 4 ischaemic segments on echocardiography or > 2 ischaemic walls on perfusion scintigraphy). Patients in the latter group proceeded to coronary angiography and myocardial revascularization at the discretion of the attending physician. Beta-blocker therapy (oral bisoprolol or parenteral metoprolol) was commenced in all intermediate-risk patients at the time of screening and continued perioperatively, aiming for a heart rate of 60–65 beats/min. The primary endpoint was the combined incidence of cardiac death and non-fatal MI (increased serum concentration of cardiac troponin-T and new Q-waves) within 30 days after surgery. All patients were screened on an outpatient basis at 3-monthly intervals for cardiac events.

INTERPRETATION. The prevalence of angina pectoris or prior MI was similar in the groups undergoing and not undergoing testing. In the group undergoing testing, 287 (74%) demonstrated no ischaemia, 65 (17%) limited ischaemia, and 34 (8.8%) extensive ischaemia. In the last group, 12 (35%) proceeded to preoperative myocardial revascularization. There was no difference in the heart rates of patients allocated to testing or no testing throughout the perioperative period. There was no difference in the primary endpoint between the groups undergoing and not undergoing preoperative testing (9/386 [2.3%] vs. 7/384 [1.8%]; odds ratio [OR] 0.78, 95% confidence interval [CI] 0.28–2.1). Preoperative testing appeared to have no significant impact on 2-year outcome (4.3% vs. 3.1%; $P = 0.30$) (Fig. 3.1). Regardless of testing status, patients with a preoperative heart rate <65 beats/min had a significantly lower incidence of the primary endpoint than patients with a heart rate > 65 beats/min (1.3% vs. 5.2%; OR 0.24, 95% CI 0.09–0.66; $P = 0.003$) (see Fig. 3.1). The median [range] interval between screening and surgery was significantly greater in the testing group compared with the no testing group (53 [13–121] days vs. 34 [7–88] days; $P<0.001$).

Comment

The results of this study challenge existing guidelines by suggesting that non-invasive preoperative cardiac stress testing is of no benefit in intermediate-risk vascular surgical patients receiving beta-blocker therapy with optimal heart rate control. In discussing the results of two previous studies |8,9|, the authors speculate that the failure to demonstrate a favourable effect of metoprolol on cardiac morbidity following non-cardiac surgery may, at least in part, be attributable to inadequate heart rate control. The inference is that aggressive 'goal-directed' beta-blocker therapy is superior to non-invasive testing in this group of patients. Unfortunately, it is not possible to assess the impact of preoperative revascularization in intermediate-risk patients because of the small number of patients found to have extensive stress-induced ischaemia.

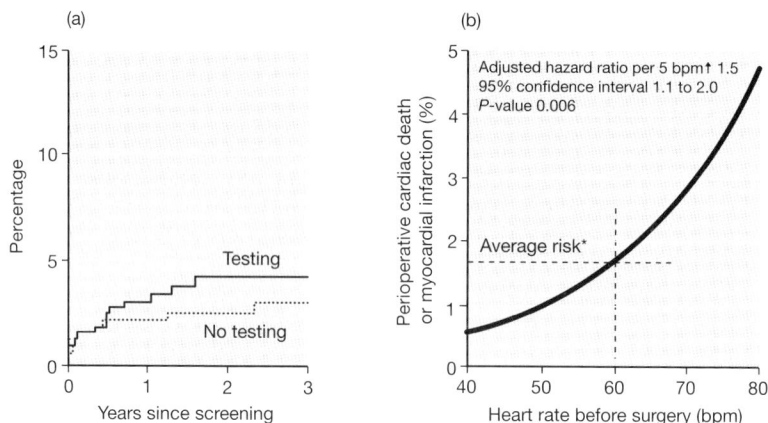

Fig. 3.1 Left: Incidence of cardiac death or myocardial infarction (MI) during 3-year follow-up, according to allocated strategy in patients with one or two cardiac risk factors. The incidence of cardiac death or MI was associated with the number of cardiac risk factors at screening (log-rank $P<0.001$). There was no significant difference in the long-term incidence of cardiac events between patients allocated to cardiac testing or no testing (log-rank $P = 0.30$). Right: The relation between heart rate and perioperative cardiovascular events in patients with one to two risk factors. The hazard ratio was adjusted for clinical risk factors. bpm, beats/min. Source: Poldermans et al. (2006).

N-Terminal pro-brain natriuretic peptide identifies patients at high risk for adverse cardiac outcome after vascular surgery

Mahla E, Baumann A, Rehak P, et al. Anesthesiology 2007; **106**: 1088–95

BACKGROUND. Brain natriuretic peptide (BNP) is released from cardiomyocytes in response to stretch and ischaemia. Plasma concentrations of BNP and its metabolite N-terminal pro-BNP (NT-proBNP) correlate well with the extent of stress-inducible myocardial ischaemia and are predictive of outcome in both stable and unstable coronary syndromes. While *preoperative* concentrations of BNP and NT-proBNP have been shown to be predictive of early and long-term outcome after non-cardiac surgery, they do not reflect the impact of anaesthesia, and the neurohumoral and circulatory changes that occur *during* and immediately *after* surgery. The purpose of this prospective study was to evaluate the prognostic value of preoperative vs. postoperative concentrations of NT -proBNP in predicting major adverse cardiac events (MACEs) in patients undergoing major elective vascular surgery. Patients with acute coronary syndrome, congestive heart failure, left ventricular ejection fraction <40%, aortic stenosis, atrial fibrillation or impaired renal function were excluded from the study. NT-proBNP was chosen in preference to BNP because of its longer half life (6–120 min vs. 20 min).

INTERPRETATION. Of the 287 patients screened during the 9-month study, 218 (76%) were studied. Perioperative management (i.e. continuation of cardiac medication, discontinuation of anti-platelet drugs, intraoperative anti-coagulation, blood transfusion, postoperative analgesia) was standardized according to the type of surgical procedure undertaken. Serum concentrations of NT-proBNP, cardiac troponin-T (cTnT) and high-sensitivity C-reactive protein (hs-CRP) were analysed in venous blood samples drawn before surgery and on the third, fourth or fifth postoperative day. The primary outcome variable was the combined endpoint of non-fatal MI, the requirement for emergency coronary revascularization or cardiac death. Forty-four patients (20%) experienced a total of 51 cardiac events during the follow-up period. Of the 30 patients (14%) who died, half were determined to have had a lethal cardiac event. Nineteen patients (9%) sustained an in-hospital MI. Median preoperative NT-proBNP concentrations were higher in patients who experienced postoperative major adverse cardiac events (551 pg/ml vs. 179 pg/ml; $P<0.001$) (Fig. 3.2), as was the median perioperative rise in NT-proBNP concentration (609 vs. 183 pg/ml; $P<0.001$). The area under the receiver operator characteristic (ROC) curve for postoperative NT-proBNP and cardiac events was 0.80 (95% CI, 0.72–0.87) with an optimum discriminate threshold of 860 pg/ml. The area under the corresponding ROC curve for preoperative NT-proBNP and cardiac events was 0.74 (95% CI, 0.64–0.82). Multivariate analysis revealed three independent predictors of MACE: postoperative NT-proBNP concentration $\geq$860 pg/ml (OR 19.8; $P<0.001$), surgical complications (OR 7.5; $P=0.010$) and preoperative creatinine concentration >1.2 mg/dl or 106 μmol/l (OR 3.4; $P=0.042$).

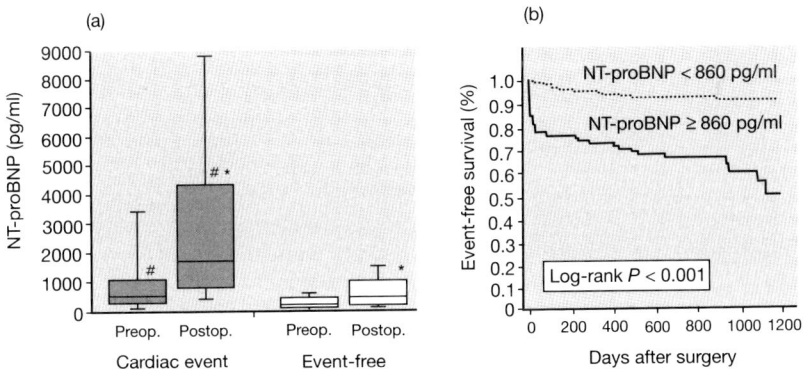

Fig. 3.2 (a) Box-and-whisker plots of preoperative (preop.) and postoperative (postop.) N-terminal pro-brain natriuretic peptide (NT-proBNP) levels in the 44 patients with cardiac events after index surgery (grey bars) compared with the 174 event-free patients (open bars). *$P<0.001$ vs. preoperative. #$P<0.001$ vs. event-free patients. (b) Overall event-free survival divided by postoperative N-terminal pro-brain natriuretic peptide (NT-proBNP) levels during the 24–30 months of postoperative follow-up among the 218 patients. Source: Mahla et al. (2007).

Comment

The ability of preoperative serum concentration of NT-proBNP to predict major adverse cardiac events (MACEs) following non-cardiac surgery is well established |10,11|. This is the first investigation to demonstrate that postoperative NT-proBNP concentration has, at least, the same prognostic value, and it is one of the few studies to look at *postoperative* risk stratification. Ninety per cent of patients with NT-proBNP <860 pg/ml remained free of major adverse cardiac events, whereas 50% patients with NT-proBNP ≥860 pg/ml sustained such an event. The obvious question is can the finding of elevated NT-proBNP before or after surgery be used to guide investigations and therapeutic interventions that might actually *alter* the likelihood of a subsequent major adverse cardiac event |12|? Further work is required, (i) to confirm these findings in patients with existing cardiac or renal dysfunction (specifically excluded from this study) and (ii) to assess the impact of anaesthetic management and targeted pharmacotherapy.

Preoperative myocardial revascularization

Preoperative myocardial revascularization has long been proposed as a strategy to protect against perioperative major adverse cardiac events in patients undergoing non-cardiac surgery |13|. Initial enthusiasm for this approach |14–19| was tempered by the finding that as many as one in five patients undergoing surgery after percutaneous coronary intervention (PCI) died |20|. The multicentre Coronary Artery Revascularization Prophylaxis (CARP) trial suggested that myocardial revascularization prior to elective vascular surgery does not reduce short- or long-term mortality in symptomatically stable patients with anatomically severe coronary artery disease |21|. Similarly, a subgroup analysis demonstrated that patients with critical limb ischaemia or intermittent claudication were not improved by coronary revascularization |22|. The 'completeness' of preoperative coronary revascularization may be an important factor. A multicentre Veterans Affairs Cooperative trial demonstrated that, in comparison with PCI, preoperative coronary artery bypass grafting (CABG) surgery was associated with a lower rate of perioperative myocardial infarction during subsequent vascular surgery (6.6% vs. 16.8%; $P = 0.024$) |23|. Existing guidelines suggest that 'prophylactic' preoperative myocardial revascularization should be reserved for patients in whom the intervention is indicated on symptomatic or prognostic grounds, irrespective of the need for non-cardiac surgery |24|.

Current recommendations call for dual anti-platelet therapy following coronary stenting – aspirin for life and clopidogrel for 3–12 months – according to the type of stent used |25|. As a consequence, an increasing number of patients presenting for surgery are taking anti-platelet therapy. While retrospective studies indicate that patients undergoing non-cardiac surgery after recent stent insertion are at high risk of perioperative major adverse cardiac events |20,26|, the minimum safe interval between PCI and elective surgery remains unknown. Equally uncertain is the best way to manage anti-coagulation in the perioperative period – balancing the risks of acute stent thrombosis and haemorrhagic complications |27|.

Coronary artery stenting and non-cardiac surgery – a prospective outcome study

Vicenzi MN, Meislitzer T, Heitzinger B, *et al. Br J Anaesth* 2006; **96**: 686–93

BACKGROUND. Conducted at three centres (two Austrian, one US), this prospective, observational study was designed to assess outcome in patients undergoing non-cardiac surgery after coronary stenting. Perioperative anti-platelet and anti-coagulation therapy was standardized. A total of 103 non-cardiac surgical patients who had undergone coronary stenting in the preceding 12 months were enrolled. Patients undergoing all types of elective or urgent non-cardiac surgery were included. Patients with a plasma cardiac troponin-T (cTnT) concentration above the detection limit (0.01 ng/ml) and those who had undergone prophylactic preoperative PCI as a cardioprotective strategy were excluded. Anti-platelet therapy (aspirin ± clopidogrel) was either continued throughout the perioperative period or discontinued for less than 3 days at the discretion of attending physician. All patients received subcutaneous unfractionated heparin (UFH; to maintain activated partial thromboplastin time > 1.5 times normal) or enoxaparin 1 mg/kg/day throughout the perioperative period. Patients were monitored for early complications for a minimum of 12 h on an intensive or intermediate care unit after surgery. The primary outcome measure was the combined (cardiac, haemorrhagic, surgical, septic) perioperative complication rate during hospitalization and 3 months after surgery.

INTERPRETATION. Forty-six patients (44.7%, 95% CI 34.9–54.8) had at least one perioperative complication in the follow-up period (median 399 days, range 93–912 days). The five deaths (4.9%, 95% CI 1.6–11.0) were all attributed to a major adverse cardiac event. Forty-four patients (42.7%) had cardiac complications (cardiac death, 5; MI, 12; redo-PCI, 8; myocardial ischaemia, 5; cardiac arrhythmia, 1; cTnT > 0.035 ng/ml without other evidence of MI, 22) and 4 patients (3.9%) had haemorrhagic complications. There were no surgical or septic complications. Patient characteristics, co-morbidities, concomitant medication, type of surgery (39.8% major surgery, 33.0% intermediate surgery, 27.7% minor surgery) and urgency of surgery (71.8% elective surgery, 28.2% urgent surgery) were similar in patients with and without adverse events. The median time from stent insertion to surgery was significantly shorter in patients with adverse events compared with patients without adverse events (60 days [range 2–348] vs. 123 days [range 20–350]; $P = 0.045$). Compared with patients with a PCI–surgery interval of > 90 days, the risk of perioperative complications was greater in patients with an interval of 35–90 days (OR 1.3, 95% CI 0.5–3.1) and in patients with a interval of <35 days (OR 2.1, 95% CI 1.1–4.3) (Fig. 3.3). Patients were much more likely to receive UFH than enoxaparin (84.5% vs. 14.5%), and multivariate analysis revealed that UFH was associated with more major adverse cardiac events than enoxaparin ($P<0.01$).

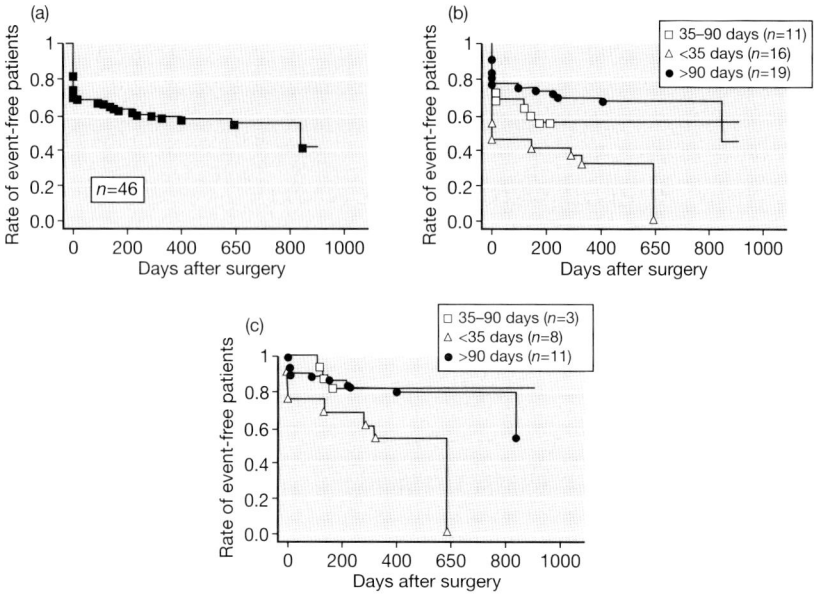

Fig. 3.3 (a) Kaplan–Meier event time curve. The x-axis is elapsed time in days after surgery, the y-axis is the cumulative rate of patients remaining free from any event. (b) Kaplan–Meier event time curves, separated by the time intervals between PCI and surgery. The x-axis is elapsed time in days after surgery, the y-axis is the cumulative rate of patients remaining free from any event. P<0.05 between the curves by log-rank tests. (c) Kaplan–Meier event time curves, separated by the time intervals between PCI and surgery. The x-axis is elapsed time in days after surgery, the y-axis is the cumulative rate of patients remaining free from any severe cardiac event (re-PCI, myocardial infarction or death). P<0.05 between the curves by log-rank tests. Source: Vicenzi et al. (2006).

Comment

Although this is the largest prospective study to date of the impact of PCI–surgery interval on outcome after non-cardiac surgery, the study population is small when compared with the cardiology literature. The results confirm that MACEs are the major cause of perioperative morbidity and mortality in patients undergoing non-cardiac surgery following PCI, and that despite continuation of anti-platelet therapy and heparin administration, haemorrhagic complications are both relatively uncommon and non-critical. The observation that a short PCI–surgery interval (<35 days) is associated with the highest risk of MACEs clearly has implications for patients requiring surgery soon after PCI, and confirms the findings of previous retrospective studies |**20,26**|. Whilst an interesting finding, the authors rightly advise extreme caution in interpreting the influence of the heparin regimen on outcome on the grounds that this factor was not subject to randomization and was unbalanced. Because no distinction was made between the type (i.e. bare metal vs. drug-eluting), number or length of stents present, it is not possible to draw any conclusions about the contribution of stent-related risk factors. Furthermore, it cannot be concluded that preoperative PCI is more effective than conventional therapy alone.

Pharmacological cardioprotection

Pharmacological interventions are likely to play a major role in perioperative cardioprotection as increasing evidence emerges for their efficacy and safety. Several pharmacological agents, including volatile anaesthetic agents, opioids, statins, α_2-blockers, beta-blockers and anti-platelet drugs have demonstrated the potential to reduce the incidence of both perioperative and long-term cardiac injury.

Volatile anaesthetic agents

A considerable body of experimental and clinical evidence suggests that volatile anaesthetic agents confer direct cardioprotection by the phenomenon of myocardial preconditioning. The mechanisms believed to underlie the phenomenon were discussed in the previous edition of this publication |28|. Exposure of the myocardium to a volatile anaesthetic agent before the onset of myocardial ischaemia reduces the impact of subsequent ischaemia–reperfusion injury – that is, myocardial infarction, myocardial stunning and ventricular dysrhythmias. Our understanding of the complex mechanisms underlying volatile anaesthetic preconditioning (APC) have largely been derived from laboratory investigations |29|. In contrast to the large volume of experimental work, there have been few clinical studies investigating the cardioprotective effects of volatile anaesthetic agents |30,31|. The requirement for a standardized 'ischaemic insult' means that all clinical studies to date have been undertaken in patients undergoing cardiac surgery |32–38|.

Myocardial damage prevented by volatile anaesthetics: a multicentre, randomized, controlled trial

Guarracino F, Landoni G, Tritapepe L, *et al. J Cardiothorac Vasc Anesth* 2006; **20**: 477–83

BACKGROUND. This randomized controlled trial, performed at three Italian centres, set out to compare the effects of volatile anaesthesia and total intravenous anaesthesia (TIVA) on the release of cardiac troponin-I (cTnI) in elective, isolated off-pump coronary artery bypass (OPCAB) surgery. All adult patients in whom OPCAB surgery was considered technically feasible were eligible. Patients with recent MI and acute decompensated heart failure were excluded. Fifty-seven patients were assigned to desflurane (0.5–2.0 end-tidal

minimum alveolar concentration) and 55 patients were assigned to propofol (2.0–3.0 µg/ml target-controlled infusion) administered throughout the duration of surgery. In addition to either desflurane or propofol, all patients received midazolam, fentanyl and pancuronium during surgery. All other aspects of perioperative care were standardized. The primary outcome measure was peak postoperative cTnI concentration. The secondary outcome measure was prolonged hospitalisation (≥7 days).

INTERPRETATION. The mean patient age was 69 years and 82% of patients were male. There were no significant differences between the preoperative and operative characteristics of the two groups. Patients in the volatile anaesthesia group had a significant reduction in peak postoperative median [interquartile range] cTnI concentration (1.2 ng/dl [0.9–1.9]) compared with patients in the TIVA group (2.7 ng/dl [2.1–4.0]; $P<0.001$; median difference 1.5 ng/dl, 95% CI, 1.9–1.0) (Fig. 3.4). A significantly smaller percentage of patients who received desflurane required prolonged hospitalization compared with patients who received TIVA (12.3% vs. 36.4%; $P = 0.005$; percentage difference 24.1%, 95% CI 38.6–8.1). Patients in the desflurane group had significantly less need for postoperative inotropic support.

Comment

This is the first multicentre randomized controlled trial to demonstrate reduction in postoperative myocardial injury and improved clinical outcome associated with volatile anaesthesia in patients undergoing OPCAB surgery. Previous studies of the putative cardioprotective effects of sevoflurane in OPCAB surgery have been small and have reached contradictory conclusions. In a study of 52 patients randomized to either propofol or sevoflurane anaesthesia for minimally invasive direct OPCAB, sevoflurane was associated with better preservation of myocardial performance

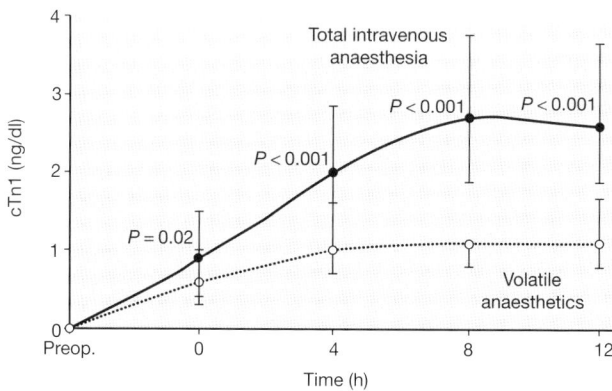

Fig. 3.4 Median (25th–75th percentiles) of troponin I after off-pump coronary artery bypass grafting in patients receiving either volatile anaesthetics or total intravenous anaesthesia. Source: Guarracino *et al.* (2006).

both during and after occlusion of the left anterior descending coronary artery |39|. The type of anaesthesia had no significant impact on postoperative cTnT concentrations. In a study of 20 OPCAB patients randomized to propofol or sevoflurane anaesthesia, patients in the propofol group had a significantly greater rise in cTnI concentrations in the first 24 h after surgery |32|. In contrast, a study of 18 OPCAB patients randomized to either sevoflurane-remifentanil or propofol-remifentanil anaesthesia to achieve a similar bispectral index level, revealed no significant difference in cumulative postoperative cTnI concentrations |40|.

The authors of the present study hypothesized that volatile anaesthesia improved myocardial protection, indicated by reduced postoperative peak cTnI, leading to a more rapid recovery, evidenced by the reduced need for prolonged hospitalization. Although the volatile anaesthesia group had a significantly shorter intensive care unit (ICU) and hospital length of stay, the differences were not clinically important.

The implications of this study are two-fold. First, volatile anaesthesia may be considered for OPCAB surgery to reduce perioperative myocardial injury and reduce the need for prolonged hospitalization. Second, because OPCAB surgery represents surgery on the beating heart, volatile anaesthesia may also be cardioprotective for patients at risk of myocardial ischaemia undergoing non-cardiac surgery – a hypothesis that, as yet, remains untested.

More recently, the same group published the results of a similar trial in 150 patients undergoing CABG surgery with cardiopulmonary bypass (CPB) |41|. In comparison with target-controlled propofol anaesthesia, desflurane anaesthesia was associated with significantly lower peak postoperative concentrations of cTnI and a reduced requirement for postoperative inotropic support. Further studies are required to confirm the clinical significance of anaesthetic preconditioning and to determine optimal administration protocols to improve perioperative outcomes.

Myocardial protection with volatile anaesthetic agents during coronary artery bypass surgery: a meta-analysis

Symons JA, Myles PS. *Br J Anaesth* 2006; **97**: 127–36

BACKGROUND. Previous studies investigating the use of volatile anaesthetic agents for cardioprotection during CABG surgery have been insufficiently powered to detect a significant effect on either perioperative MI or mortality. The aim of this Australian study was a systematic review and meta-analysis of all randomized controlled trials comparing volatile with non-volatile anaesthetic agents in adult patients undergoing isolated CABG surgery with or without CPB. A comprehensive systematic search was performed for all relevant trials published between January 1985 and March 2005. The outcome measures analysed included: myocardial ischaemia in the first 24 h after surgery, in-hospital MI, hospital mortality, post-CPB cardiac index, postoperative cTnI concentration, the requirement for postoperative inotropic support, duration of mechanical ventilation, and duration

of ICU and hospital stay. Odds ratios were estimated for dichotomous variables and weighted mean differences (WMDs) estimated for continuous variables. Subgroup analyses were carried out to assess the effect of the duration of volatile anaesthetic agent administration on outcome.

INTERPRETATION. Of the 43 studies identified, 27 with 2797 patients were analysed. No significant differences in MI, mortality, myocardial ischaemia or ICU length of stay were identified. Compared with non-volatile anaesthetics, volatile anaesthesia was associated with significantly higher cardiac indices (WMD 22%, 95% CI 6–38; $P<0.006$), lower cTnI concentration (WMD 1.44 ng/ml, 95% CI 2.34–0.55; $P<0.002$), less requirement for inotropic support (OR 0.50, 95% CI 0.31–0.80; $P<0.004$), shorter duration of mechanical ventilation (WMD 2.71 h, 95% CI 5.30–0.12; $P<0.04$) and shorter length of hospital stay (WMD 1.05 days, 95% CI 1.68–0.43 days; $P<0.001$). Subgroup analyses of the duration of volatile anaesthetic agent administration revealed no significant difference in MI or mortality between patients who received continuous administration and patients who received intermittent administration during surgery. No volatile agent was found to be superior to others in terms of myocardial protection (Table 3.2).

Comment

Despite the finding that volatile anaesthetic agents are associated with surrogate markers of improved clinical outcome, it was not possible to demonstrate any impact on MI or mortality. The study suffers from weaknesses associated with meta-analyses that limit the validity of the results: differences between trials in the outcome measures used, inconsistency in the definition of outcome measures and variation in clinical practice. There was evidence of statistical heterogeneity for the following endpoints: cardiac index, cTnI concentration, inotropic support, duration of mechanical ventilation, and ICU and hospital length of stay. Therefore, the results of these endpoints should be interpreted with caution. Although no difference in effects due to the duration of volatile anaesthetic agent administration was identified, an understanding of the mechanisms of anaesthetic preconditioning suggests that continuous administration throughout surgery should be beneficial |34|. A large, adequately powered, randomized controlled trial to definitively establish the benefits of volatile anaesthetic-mediated cardioprotection in CABG surgery is now required.

Opioids

Experimental evidence suggests that opioids induce myocardial preconditioning and enhance the protective effects of volatile anaesthetics |42|. Compared with other opioids, morphine is reported to produce a more potent cardioprotective effect |43|. There are few clinical studies investigating opioid preconditioning.

Table 3.2 Variables comparing volatile agent with a non-volatile agent anaesthetic regimen in coronary artery bypass graft surgery

Variable	Volatile no. (%)	Non-volatile no. (%)	OR or WMD (95% CI)	P-value
At specific times				
Mortality	12/782 (1.53)	7/320 (2.19)	0.73 (0.28–1.90)*	0.52
Myocardial infarction	41/1110 (3.69)	18/513 (3.51)	1.09 (0.61–1.93)*	0.77
Myocardial ischaemia	279/971 (28.73)	111/473 (2.33)	1.09 (0.84–1.43)*	0.51
Inotrope use	91/364 (25.00)	111/290 (38.28)	0.48 (0.25–0.90)*	0.02
ICU length of stay (h)			−1.60 (−9.91 to 6.71)†	0.71
Cardiac index			0.09 (−0.12 to 0.29)†	0.41
Troponin I (ng/ml)			−0.59 (−0.9 to −0.23)†	0.001
Mechanical ventilation time (h)			−1.60 (−10.01 to 6.80)†	0.71
Hospital length of stay (days)			26.69 (−1.98 to −0.62)†	0.0002
All times				
Mortality	4/426 (0.94)	4/293 (1.37)	0.6 (0.16–2.19)*	0.44
Myocardial infarction	10/459 (2.18)	10/327 (3.06)	0.77 (0.32–1.85)*	0.56
Myocardial ischaemia	5/24 (20.83)	8/26 (30.77)	0.59 (0.16–2.15)*	0.43
Inotrope use	203/529 (38.37)	198/402 (49.25)	0.54 (0.26–1.12)*	0.10
ICU length of stay (h)			−7.37 (−15.57 to 0.83)†	0.08
Cardiac index			0.35 (0.17–0.53)†	0.0001
Troponin I (ng/ml)			−2.29 (−4.57 to −0.01)†	0.05

Table 3.2 Variables comparing volatile agent with a non-volatile agent anaesthetic regimen in coronary artery bypass graft surgery (continued)

Variable	Volatile no. (%)	Non-volatile no. (%)	OR or WMD (95% CI)	P-value
Mechanical ventilation time (h)			−2.19 (−3.70 to −0.67)†	0.005
Hospital length of stay (days)			−0.86 (−1.89 to 0.16)†	0.10
Pooled studies				
Mortality	16/1208 (1.32)	11/613 (1.79)	0.68 (0.32–1.47)*	0.33
Myocardial infarction	51/1569 (3.25)	28/840 (3.33)	0.98 (0.61–1.58)*	0.94
Ischemia	284/995 (28.54)	119/499 (23.85)	1.07 (0.82–1.38)*	0.63
Inotrope use	294/893 (32.92)	309/692 (44.65)	0.50 (0.31–0.80)*	0.004
ICU length of stay (h)			−3.87 (−8.76 to 1.03)†	0.12
Cardiac index			0.22 (0.06–0.38)†	0.006
Troponin I (ng/ml)			−1.44 (−2.34 to −0.55)†	0.002
Mechanical ventilation time (h)			−2.71 (−5.30 to −0.12)†	0.04
Hospital length of stay (days)			−1.05 (−1.68 to −0.43)†	0.0009

*OR, odds ratio.
†WMD, weighted mean difference; CI, confidence interval.
Source: Symons et al. (2006).

Opioids and cardioprotection: the impact of morphine and fentanyl on recovery of ventricular function after cardiopulmonary bypass

Murphy GS, Szokol JW, Marymont JH, *et al. J Cardiothorac Vasc Anesth* 2006; **20**: 493–502

BACKGROUND. This single-centre study compared the effects of morphine and fentanyl on myocardial function and myocardial injury in patients undergoing elective isolated CABG surgery. Patients with valve disease or left ventricular ejection fraction <40% were excluded. Forty-six patients were randomized to receive an infusion of either morphine 40 mg ($n = 23$) or fentanyl 1 mg ($n = 23$) from induction of anaesthesia to application of the aortic cross-clamp. All patients received isoflurane before and after CPB and midazolam during CPB. All other aspects of perioperative care were standardized. The myocardial performance index (MPI) |44|, a relatively load-independent echocardiographic measure of combined systolic and diastolic ventricular function, was calculated at baseline after induction of anaesthesia, at 15-minute intervals after CPB and at the end of surgery (Fig. 3.5). Plasma BNP and cTnI concentrations were used to assess perioperative myocardial dysfunction and injury respectively.

INTERPRETATION. Preoperative, intraoperative and surgical characteristics, haemodynamic variables, and mean end-tidal isoflurane concentrations were similar in the two groups. MPI values did not differ between groups at baseline. Patients in the morphine group demonstrated a significant decrease in median [range] MPI following CPB, indicating an improvement in global ventricular function (0.44 [0.32–0.64] at baseline; 0.36 [0.24–0.45] at 15 minutes post-CPB; 0.34 [0.20–0.46] at end of surgery; $P<0.05$ post CPB compared with baseline). Patients in the fentanyl group

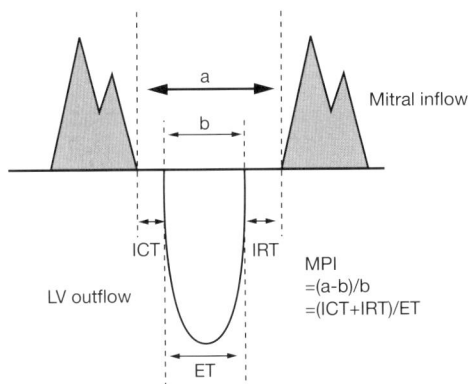

Fig. 3.5 The myocardial performance index (MPI). Interval 'a' represents the time (in ms) from cessation to onset of mitral inflow and is the sum of isovolumetric contraction time (ICT), isovolumetric relaxation time (IRT) and ejection time (ET). Ejection time (interval 'b') represents the duration of the left ventricular (LV) outflow velocity. The MPI was calculated by the formula MPI = $(a-b)/b$. Source: Murphy *et al.* (2006).

demonstrated a significant increase in MPI following CPB (0.43 [0.28–0.54] at baseline; 0.49 [0.32–0.64] at 15 min post CPB; 0.51 [0.36–0.63] at end of surgery; $P<0.05$ post CPB compared with baseline). There was a significant difference in MPI 15 min post CPB ($P<0.05$). Postoperative concentrations of both BNP and cTnI were significantly elevated in both groups, although there was no significant difference between groups.

Comment

This study provides clinical evidence for a cardioprotective effect of morphine, and the lack of such an effect of fentanyl, in patients undergoing on-pump CABG surgery. As patients in both groups had similar mean intraoperative end-tidal isoflurane concentrations, the beneficial effect appears to be morphine-mediated. The doses of opioids were not based on patient weight but chosen on the basis of an unpublished pilot study so as not to adversely prolong postoperative mechanical ventilation. Further studies need to address the appropriate opioid doses to achieve cardioprotection and minimise adverse effects. The discrepancy between the echocardiographic findings and the biomarker findings is noteworthy. The lack of effect of morphine on BNP and cTnI suggests that morphine-mediated cardioprotection is clinically insignificant and that echocardiography is, indeed, a very sensitive monitor of myocardial ischaemia. This study supports the need for a large trial to assess the effect of opioid preconditioning on clinically important outcome measures in CABG surgery.

Statins

Treatment with 3-hydroxy-3-methylglutaryl (HMG) coenzyme A inhibitors ('statins') has been shown to reduce low-density lipoprotein cholesterol in patients with hypercholesterolaemia and decrease cardiovascular morbidity and mortality in patients with known, or at risk of having, coronary artery disease. Statins also appear to have a wide range of pleiotropic effects, independent of their lipid-lowering action, which may contribute to the beneficial influence on cardiovascular outcomes |45|. Statins appear to stabilize vulnerable coronary atherosclerotic plaques by anti-inflammatory and anti-thrombotic actions. Coronary plaque rupture, leading to thrombus formation and vessel occlusion, is believed to play a key role in the pathophysiology of perioperative MI |13|. Hence, the cardioprotective effect of perioperative statin therapy for the prevention of perioperative MI has been extensively investigated. Perioperative use of statins in patients with cardiovascular disease has recently been recommended, but the evidence of benefit remains unclear |46|.

Strength of evidence for perioperative use of statins to reduce cardiovascular risk: systematic review of controlled studies

Kapoor AS, Kanji H, Buckingham J, *et al. BMJ* 2006; **333**: 1149

BACKGROUND. This group of Canadian authors set out to systematically review the existing evidence for the perioperative use of statins to reduce the risk of cardiovascular events. An extensive literature search was performed in September 2005 and repeated in February 2006 to identify studies that reported acute coronary syndromes or mortality in patients who were either receiving or not receiving perioperative statin treatment. Uncontrolled studies, studies published in abstract form, and studies in which statin treatment was started postoperatively were excluded. Intention-to-treat data were extracted on acute coronary syndrome or death in the 30-day postoperative period. Meta-analysis was performed on methodologically similar studies.

INTERPRETATION. Eighteen studies reporting data in 800 106 patients were eligible for analysis. The studies selected included two randomized controlled trials, one case–control study, three prospective cohort studies and 12 retrospective cohort studies. The use of statins was evaluated in patients undergoing vascular surgery (12 studies), cardiac surgery (four studies) and non-cardiovascular surgery (two studies). Perioperative statin use was associated with a reduction in acute coronary syndrome or death in the two pooled randomized trials (13 events in 177 patients, OR 0.26, 95% CI 0.07–0.99) and in the 13 pooled cohort studies (1004 events in 18 463 patients, OR 0.70, 95% CI 0.57–0.87, $P < 0.001$).

Comment

The findings of this systematic review must be interpreted with caution, as most of the included studies are observational studies. Even when pooled, the two randomized trials are too small for conclusions to be made based on these results. The results from the 13 pooled cohort studies revealed that perioperative statin therapy reduces the odds of acute coronary syndrome or death by 30% in patients undergoing surgery. The validity of these results is limited by significant statistical heterogeneity. The majority of the included studies were limited by a lack of data regarding the type, dosage and duration of preoperative statin therapy; treatment compliance; preoperative withdrawal and postoperative reintroduction of statin therapy; and adverse effects of statin treatment. The authors concluded that there is inadequate evidence to recommend the routine use of statins to reduce perioperative cardiovascular risk. Instead, they recommended that preoperative statin therapy be started in patients with known, or at risk of having, coronary artery disease, for whom statin therapy is currently indicated independent of the proposed surgery. Further large randomized controlled trials have been called for by this group and by the authors of another meta-analysis who reached similar conclusions |**47**|.

Beta-blockers

Beta-adrenoreceptor antagonists exert a range of antiarrhythmic, anti-inflammatory and genetic actions that may account for their ability to reduce mortality in patients with MI and stable cardiac failure. The rationale for the perioperative use of beta-blockers relates to the reduction in myocardial contractility and sympathetic tone mediated by these agents. Myocardial oxygen supply–demand mismatch, in addition to coronary plaque rupture, significantly contributes to the pathophysiology of perioperative MI |13|. Accordingly, the effects of perioperative beta-blockade have been subjected to intense scrutiny in the quest for effective cardioprotection for patients at risk of major adverse cardiac events. Although two systematic reviews have been performed to address the subject, there is relatively limited good evidence on which to base clinical guidelines for perioperative beta-blocker therapy |48,49|. The disproportionate influence of two studies |50,51| that have been heavily criticized |13| and the adoption of universal perioperative beta-blockade, as a measure of clinical performance, by patients and health maintenance organizations prompted the ACC and AHA to issue updated guidelines |52,53|.

Perioperative β-blockers for preventing surgery-related mortality and morbidity: a systematic review and meta-analysis

Wiesbauer F, Schlager O, Domanovits H, et al. Anesth Analg 2007; **104**: 27–41

BACKGROUND. Wiesbauer and his Austrian colleagues systematically reviewed the evidence supporting the use of perioperative beta-blockade for preventing major adverse cardiac events and improving outcome after cardiac and non-cardiac surgery. An expansive literature search identified randomized controlled trials published as full manuscripts or abstracts before October 2005 comparing beta-blocker treatment with either placebo or usual standard care in patients undergoing surgery. For studies to be included, beta-blockers had to be given preoperatively, intraoperatively or within 24 h postoperatively. The duration of treatment could be variable. The reviewers considered the following outcomes within 30 days postoperatively or prior to hospital discharge as study endpoints: mortality, MI, length of hospital stay, myocardial ischaemia, atrial fibrillation, other supraventricular arrhythmias, ventricular arrhythmias, stroke, cardiac failure, bradycardia and hypotension. Odds ratios were estimated for dichotomous variables and WMDs estimated for continuous variables.

INTERPRETATION. Sixty-nine studies were included for analysis. Beta-blockers were found not to reduce mortality (cardiac surgery: OR 0.55, 95% CI 0.17–1.83; non-cardiac surgery: OR 0.78, 95% CI 0.33–1.87), myocardial infarction (cardiac surgery: OR 0.89, 95% CI 0.53–1.5; non-cardiac surgery: OR 0.59, 95% CI 0.25–1.39) or length of hospital stay (cardiac surgery: WMD –0.35 days, 95% CI –0.77 to 0.07; non-cardiac surgery: WMD –5.59 days, 95% CI –12.22 to 1.04). Beta-blockers reduced the incidence of myocardial ischaemia in non-cardiac surgery (OR 0.38, 95% CI 0.21–0.69) but not in cardiac surgery (OR 0.49, 95% CI 0.17–1.4). Beta-blockers reduced the frequency of atrial fibrillation (OR 0.37, 95% CI 0.28–0.48), other supraventricular arrhythmias (OR 0.25, 95% CI 0.18–0.35) and ventricular arrhythmias (OR 0.28, 95% CI 0.13–0.57) in patients undergoing cardiac surgery but not in patients undergoing non-cardiac surgery (atrial fibrillation: OR 0.59, 95% CI 0.13–2.6; other supraventricular arrhythmias: OR 0.43, 95% CI 0.14–1.37; ventricular arrhythmias: OR 0.56, 95% CI 0.21–1.45). Beta-blockers significantly increased the risk of bradycardia and hypotension but had no effect on the risk of stroke or cardiac failure.

Comment

The authors of this systematic review did not identify a beneficial effect of perioperative beta-blockade on mortality or MI after either cardiac or non-cardiac surgery. The low mortality rates reported for cardiac surgery suggest that the lack of demonstrable mortality benefit may not be valid. The absence of an effect on mortality and MI in non-cardiac surgery is in stark contrast to previous reports |50,51,54|. The authors suggested that the adjustment for publication bias in their meta-analysis may have influenced the overall results. Beta-blockers were beneficial in preventing myocardial ischaemia in non-cardiac surgery and in preventing arrhythmias in cardiac surgery. The small number of patients in trials that assessed the frequency of arrhythmias during the non-cardiac surgery may have made it impossible to detect a significant effect of beta-blockade.

There are few adequately powered randomized trials of perioperative beta-blocker therapy. The current literature does not provide evidence to guide the choice of drug, dose, administration route, target heart rate, timing of treatment initiation, duration of therapy or target population. It is hoped that the results of a large randomized controlled trial will definitively ascertain the cardioprotective role of beta-blockers in non-cardiac surgery |55|.

At present, the approach to perioperative beta-blockade should follow recently revised consensus recommendations (Table 3.3) |52,53|. The recent finding that β_2-adrenergic receptor genotype may underlie the differential survival observed in patients prescribed a beta-blocker after acute coronary syndrome |56| reiterates the notion that low-risk patients undergoing non-cardiac surgery may derive no benefit from perioperative beta-blockade and might actually be harmed |54|.

Alpha-2-adrenoceptor agonists

Patients with asthma, cardiac conduction disorders or other adverse drug reactions who are at risk of perioperative major adverse cardiac events often cannot tolerate beta-blockers. For this group of patients, the α_2-agonist clonidine may offer an alternative means of providing perioperative cardioprotection |57|. Unlike beta-blockers, which block the end-organ effects of catecholamines, α_2-agonists reduce

Table 3.3 Recommendations for perioperative beta-blocker therapy based on published randomized trials

Type of surgery	Level of cardiac risk		
	Low	Intermediate	High or CHD[a]
Vascular	Class IIb Evidence level: C	Class IIb Evidence level: C	Class I[b] Evidence level: B Class IIa[c] Evidence level: B
High risk	Insufficient data	Class IIb Evidence level: C	Class IIa Evidence level: B
Intermediate risk	Insufficient data	Class IIb Evidence level: C	Class IIa Evidence level: B
Low risk	Insufficient data	Insufficient data	Insufficient data

[a]Patients found to have myocardial ischaemia on preoperative testing. [b]Applies to patients found to have coronary ischaemia on preoperative testing. [c]Applies to patients found to have coronary heart disease. Source: Fleisher et al. (2007).

catecholamine secretion via a central mechanism. The magnitude of the protective effects of clonidine on perioperative myocardial ischaemia and postoperative mortality are reported to be similar to those of atenolol |58|. Curiously, two studies of patients undergoing non-cardiac surgery have demonstrated that, while clonidine reduced the incidence of perioperative ischaemic episodes, it had no impact on either myocardial infarction or mortality |59,60|. To date, no study has assessed the effect of perioperative clonidine therapy on long-term outcome.

Discontinuing medication

Advances in pharmacotherapy and the introduction of new indications for existing agents means that a significant number of patients admitted for surgery may be taking four or more drugs unrelated to their surgery |61|. Accumulating evidence suggests that the acute withdrawal of certain types of drugs (e.g. beta-blockers, anti-platelet agents and statins) may be associated with adverse cardiac outcome. In a study of 1521 patients admitted with acute myocardial infarction, failure to comply with evidence-based medication 1 month after hospital discharge was shown to significantly reduce 12-month survival (88.5% vs. 97.7%; $P < 0.001$) |62|. While the temporary cessation of oral medication is frequently an unavoidable consequence of major surgery, failure to reinstitute medication after surgery in a timely fashion may have grave consequences. In a retrospective study of 140 consecutive vascular surgery patients receiving beta-blockers preoperatively, four of the eight patients who had beta-blockers discontinued postoperatively died |63|. Failure to reinstitute aspirin therapy after surgery has also been shown to be associated with adverse cardiac outcome. An analysis of three retrospective studies reporting the frequency of aspirin withdrawal preceding acute cardiovascular syndromes in 93 patients revealed that the interval to a major adverse cardiac event was 8.5 ± 3.6 (mean $\pm$ SD) days for acute coronary syndrome ($n=64$); 14.3 ± 11.3 days for cerebrovascular event ($n=14$); and 25.8 ± 18.1 days for acute peripheral vascular event ($n=12$) |64|. The implication is that delaying the reinstitution of aspirin for less than 1 week after surgery may be associated with adverse cardiac outcome.

The impact of postoperative discontinuation or continuation of chronic statin therapy on cardiac outcome after major vascular surgery

Le Manach Y, Godet G, Coriat P, *et al. Anesth Analg* 2007; **104**: 1326–33

BACKGROUND. A number of clinical and experimental studies have suggested that perioperative cessation of statin therapy is associated with adverse events. Prompted by an analysis of their vascular surgery register, which revealed a surprisingly high level of cardiac risk in patients chronically treated with statins, the investigators questioned their practice of withdrawing statin therapy for several days after major abdominal vascular surgery. The purpose of this retrospective analysis of prospectively collected data was to compare outcomes before and after the adoption of a modified approach to the reinstitution of statin therapy. All patients undergoing elective infrarenal aortic reconstructive surgery or endoprosthetic procedures between January 2001 and December 2004 were considered. Patient risk assessment and stratification was conducted in accordance with ACC/AHA guidelines using the Lee RCRI. Patients referred for PCI received only bare-metal stents and were treated with aspirin indefinitely and clopidogrel for 4 weeks before surgery. Blood was drawn from all patients for cTnI concentrations on admission to the recovery unit and on the first three postoperative days. From January to December 2004 (continuation group) all patients chronically treated with statins had their therapy restarted as soon as practicable after surgery – by mouth or nasogastric tube. The primary outcome variable was an elevation in cTnI concentration > 0.2 ng/ml.

INTERPRETATION. Data on 671 patients (discontinuation group, 491; continuation group, 178) were reviewed. During the 4-year preiod, 294 patients (44%) were chronically treated with statins. Statins were more frequently used in the second (continuation) cohort (51% vs. 41%, $P = 0.02$). The 29 patients for whom the delay between surgery and recommencement of statin therapy could not be determined were excluded from analysis. The median (95% CI) delay for resuming statin therapy was 4 (3.7–4.3) days in the discontinuation group and 1 (0.7–1.3) day in the continuation group ($P < 0.001$). Interruption of more than 4 days of chronic statin therapy was associated with a 2.9-fold increase in the rate of postoperative cTnI elevation.

Comment

This study confirms the findings of other studies of high-risk surgical patients. Poldermans and colleagues |65| reported that statin therapy was associated with a 4.5-fold reduction in perioperative mortality following vascular surgery. In a study of 780 591 patients, Lindenauer and colleagues |66| observed that perioperative statin therapy reduced the risk of postoperative death. While the present study undoubtedly supports the early recommencement of statin therapy after major vascular surgery, the strength of any inference must be tempered by the retrospective study design. Chronic statin therapy identified patients at greater cardiac risk in the discontinuation cohort than the continuation cohort. In addition, factors such as the perioperative use of angiotensin-converting enzyme inhibitors, anti-platelet drugs and beta-blockers were uncontrolled. Because plasma statin concentrations were not monitored in the continuation group, it cannot be said with any certainty that early reinstitution of statin therapy achieves therapeutic concentrations in patients recuperating from major abdominal surgery.

Pre-optimization

Since Shoemaker's observation |67| that 'goal-directed' therapy could reduce mortality and morbidity in high-risk surgical patients, a number of prospective studies have demonstrated that preoperative and intraoperative optimization of cardiovascular function can improve outcome after both cardiac and non-cardiac surgery |68–71|. Although a recent meta-analysis of 21 studies confirms the benefit of pre-optimization in high-risk patients |72|, it is unclear whether the improvement in outcomes observed is a manifestation of a global improvement in tissue oxygen delivery or direct myocardial protection. However, a recent small, single-centre study in cardiac surgical patients provides some evidence of cardioprotection |73|. In comparison with historical controls, patients managed using an algorithm-driven, goal-directed haemodynamic intervention (mean arterial pressure >70 mmHg, cardiac index >2.5 l/min/m², global end-diastolic volume index >640 ml/m²) had a shortened and reduced requirement for vasopressor and inotropic support and a shortened duration of mechanical ventilation.

General versus regional anaesthesia

When compared with general anaesthesia alone, regional or central neuraxial anaesthesia is known to have several potentially beneficial effects. Varying degrees of sympathetic blockade, a reduction in the metabolic stress associated with surgery, improved postoperative analgesia and respiratory function, and diminished hypercoagulability should – at least in theory – reduce the incidence of perioperative major adverse cardiac events, but convincing evidence has eluded the best efforts of researchers |74–76|. Most recently, in the largest study of its type, 423 patients undergoing peripheral vascular surgery were randomly assigned to undergo general ($n = 138$), epidural ($n = 149$) or spinal ($n = 136$) anaesthesia |77|. There was no significant difference in either mortality or cardiovascular morbidity between the groups, with a trend towards fewer postoperative events in patients who had general anaesthesia. The authors of the accompanying editorial |78| concluded that 'Additional ... trials ... are unlikely to be useful ... further trials are not needed'.

Conclusion

The evolution of perioperative cardioprotective strategies continues as consensus guidelines are tested in prospective, randomized studies. Recent evidence suggests that in certain groups of patients, routine non-invasive testing in the presence of one or two cardiac risk factors has no discernable impact on short- and long-term outcome. Preoperative PCI or CABG surgery should be reserved for patients who require coronary revascularization on symptomatic or prognostic grounds. There is no place for prophylactic revascularization in patients with stable but significant coronary disease. Emerging evidence supports the use of perioperative beta-blockade and the use of statins. Existing therapy with anti-platelet agents, beta-blockers and statins should not be stopped perioperatively and should be reinstituted as soon as possible after surgery.

References

1. Bursi F, Babuin L, Barbieri A, Politi L, Zennaro M, Grimaldi T, *et al*. Vascular surgery patients: perioperative and long-term risk according to the ACC/AHA guidelines, the additive role of post-operative troponin elevation. *Eur Heart J* 2005; **26**: 2448–56.

2. Eagle KA, Brundage BH, Chaitman BR, Ewy GA, Fleisher LA, Hertzer NR, *et al*. Guidelines for perioperative cardiovascular evaluation for noncardiac surgery. Report of the American College of Cardiology/American Heart Association Task Force on Practice Guidelines. Committee on Perioperative Cardiovascular Evaluation for Noncardiac Surgery. *Circulation* 1996; **93**: 1278–317.

3. Eagle KA, Berger PB, Calkins H, Chaitman BR, Ewy GA, Fleischmann KE, *et al*. ACC/AHA guideline update for perioperative cardiovascular evaluation for noncardiac surgery – executive summary. A report of the American College of Cardiology/American Heart Association Task Force on Practice Guidelines (Committee to Update the 1996 Guidelines on Perioperative Cardiovascular Evaluation for Noncardiac Surgery). *Circulation* 2002; **105**: 1257–67.

4. Auerbach A, Goldman L. Assessing and reducing the cardiac risk of noncardiac surgery. *Circulation* 2006; **113**: 1361–76.

5. Lee TH, Marcantonio ER, Mangione CM, Thomas EJ, Polanczyk CA, Cook EF, *et al*. Derivation and prospective validation of a simple index for prediction of cardiac risk of major noncardiac surgery. *Circulation* 1999; **100**: 1043–9.

6. Raux M, Godet G, Isnard R, Mergoni P, Goarin JP, Bertrand M, *et al.* Low negative predictive value of dobutamine stress echocardiography before abdominal aortic surgery. *Br J Anaesth* 2006; **97**: 770–6.

7. Wesorick DH, Eagle KA. The preoperative cardiovascular evaluation of the intermediate-risk patient: new data, changing strategies. *Am J Med* 2005; **118**: 1413.

8. Juul AB, Wetterslev J, Gluud C, Kofoed-Enevoldsen A, Jensen G, Callesen T, *et al.* Effect of perioperative beta blockade in patients with diabetes undergoing major non-cardiac surgery: randomised placebo controlled, blinded multicentre trial. *BMJ* 2006; **332**: 1482.

9. Brady AR, Gibbs JS, Greenhalgh RM, Powell JT, Sydes MR. Perioperative beta-blockade (POBBLE) for patients undergoing infrarenal vascular surgery: results of a randomized double-blind controlled trial. *J Vasc Surg* 2005; **41**: 602–9.

10. Feringa HH, Bax JJ, Elhendy A, de Jonge R, Lindemans J, Schouten O, *et al.* Association of plasma N-terminal pro-B-type natriuretic peptide with postoperative cardiac events in patients undergoing surgery for abdominal aortic aneurysm or leg bypass. *Am J Cardiol* 2006; **98**: 111–15.

11. Feringa HH, Schouten O, Dunkelgrun M, Bax JJ, Boersma E, Elhendy A, *et al.* Plasma N-terminal pro-B-type natriuretic peptide as long-term prognostic marker after major vascular surgery. *Heart* 2007; **93**: 226–31.

12. Augoustides J, Fleisher LA. Advancing perioperative prediction of cardiac risk after vascular surgery: does postoperative N-terminal pro-brain natriuretic peptide do the trick? *Anesthesiology* 2007; **106**: 1080–2.

13. Priebe HJ. Perioperative myocardial infarction – aetiology and prevention. *Br J Anaesth* 2005; **95**: 3–19.

14. Allen JR, Helling TS, Hartzler GO. Operative procedures not involving the heart after percutaneous transluminal coronary angioplasty. *Surg Gynecol Obstet* 1991; **173**: 285–8.

15. Huber KC, Evans MA, Bresnahan JF, Gibbons RJ, Holmes DR Jr. Outcome of noncardiac operations in patients with severe coronary artery disease successfully treated preoperatively with coronary angioplasty. *Mayo Clin Proc* 1992; **67**: 15–21.

16. Jones SE, Raymond RE, Simpfendorfer CC, Whitlow PL. Cardiac outcome of major noncardiac surgery in patients undergoing preoperative coronary angioplasty. *J Invasive Cardiol* 1993; **5**: 212–18.

17. Gottlieb A, Banoub M, Sprung J, Levy PJ, Beven M, Mascha EJ. Perioperative cardiovascular morbidity in patients with coronary artery disease undergoing vascular surgery after percutaneous transluminal coronary angioplasty. *J Cardiothorac Vasc Anesth* 1998; **12**: 501–6.

18. Posner KL, Van Norman GA, Chan V. Adverse cardiac outcomes after noncardiac surgery in patients with prior percutaneous transluminal coronary angioplasty. *Anesth Analg* 1999; **89**: 553–60.

19. Hassan SA, Hlatky MA, Boothroyd DB, Winston C, Mark DB, Brooks MM, *et al.* Outcomes of noncardiac surgery after coronary bypass surgery or coronary angioplasty in the Bypass Angioplasty Revascularization Investigation (BARI). *Am J Med* 2001; **110**: 260–6.

20. Kaluza GL, Joseph J, Lee JR, Raizner ME, Raizner AE. Catastrophic outcomes of noncardiac surgery soon after coronary stenting. *J Am Coll Cardiol* 2000; **35**: 1288–94.

21. McFalls EO, Ward HB, Moritz TE, Goldman S, Krupski WC, Littooy F, *et al.* Coronary-artery revascularization before elective major vascular surgery. *N Engl J Med* 2004; **351**: 2795–804.

22. Raghunathan A, Rapp JH, Littooy F, Santilli S, Krupski WC, Ward HB, *et al.* Postoperative outcomes for patients undergoing elective revascularization for critical limb ischemia and intermittent claudication: a subanalysis of the Coronary Artery Revascularization Prophylaxis (CARP) trial. *J Vasc Surg* 2006; **43**: 1175–82.

23. Ward HB, Kelly RF, Thottapurathu L, Moritz TE, Larsen GC, Pierpont G, *et al.* Coronary artery bypass grafting is superior to percutaneous coronary intervention in prevention of perioperative myocardial infarctions during subsequent vascular surgery. *Ann Thorac Surg* 2006; **82**: 795–800.

24. Eagle KA, Guyton RA, Davidoff R, Edwards FH, Ewy GA, Gardner TJ, *et al.* ACC/AHA 2004 guideline update for coronary artery bypass graft surgery: a report of the American College of Cardiology/American Heart Association Task Force on Practice Guidelines (Committee to Update the 1999 Guidelines for Coronary Artery Bypass Graft Surgery). *Circulation* 2004; **110**: e340–437.

25. Spahn DR, Howell SJ, Delabays A, Chassot PG. Coronary stents and perioperative anti-platelet regimen: dilemma of bleeding and stent thrombosis. *Br J Anaesth* 2006; **96**: 675–7.

26. Wilson SH, Fasseas P, Orford JL, Lennon RJ, Horlocker T, Charnoff NE, *et al.* Clinical outcome of patients undergoing non-cardiac surgery in the two months following coronary stenting. *J Am Coll Cardiol* 2003; **42**: 234–40.

27. Howard-Alpe GM, de Bono J, Hudsmith L, Orr WP, Foex P, Sear JW. Coronary artery stents and non-cardiac surgery. *Br J Anaesth* 2007; **98**: 560–74.

28. Howell S, Kimpson P. Protecting the heart in non-cardiac surgery. In: Hunter J, Cook T, Priebe HJ, Struys M, eds. *The Year in Anaesthesia and Critical Care.* 1st edn. Oxford: Clinical Publishing; 2005, pp. 103–108.

29. Tanaka K, Ludwig LM, Kersten JR, Pagel PS, Warltier DC. Mechanisms of cardioprotection by volatile anesthetics. *Anesthesiology* 2004; **100**: 707–21.

30. Zaugg M, Lucchinetti E, Uecker M, Pasch T, Schaub MC. Anaesthetics and cardiac preconditioning. Part I. Signalling and cytoprotective mechanisms. *Br J Anaesth* 2003; **91**: 551–65.

31. Zaugg M, Lucchinetti E, Garcia C, Pasch T, Spahn DR, Schaub MC. Anaesthetics and cardiac preconditioning. Part II. Clinical implications. *Br J Anaesth* 2003; **91**: 566–76.

32. Conzen PF, Fischer S, Detter C, Peter K. Sevoflurane provides greater protection of the myocardium than propofol in patients undergoing off-pump coronary artery bypass surgery. *Anesthesiology* 2003; **99**: 826–33.

33. De Hert SG, Van der Linden PJ, Cromheecke S, Meeus R, ten Broecke PW, De Blier IG, *et al.* Choice of primary anesthetic regimen can influence intensive care unit length of stay after coronary surgery with cardiopulmonary bypass. *Anesthesiology* 2004; **101**: 9–20.

34. De Hert SG, Van der Linden PJ, Cromheecke S, Meeus R, Nelis A, Van Reeth V, *et al.* Cardioprotective properties of sevoflurane in patients undergoing coronary surgery with cardiopulmonary bypass are related to the modalities of its administration. *Anesthesiology* 2004; **101**: 299–310.

35. De Hert SG, Turani F, Mathur S, Stowe DF. Cardioprotection with volatile anesthetics: mechanisms and clinical implications. *Anesth Analg* 2005; **100**: 1584–93.

36. De Hert SG. The concept of anaesthetic-induced cardioprotection: clinical relevance. *Best Pract Res Clin Anaesthesiol* 2005; **19**: 445–59.

37. Cromheecke S, Pepermans V, Hendrickx E, Lorsomradee S, ten Broecke PW, Stockman BA, *et al.* Cardioprotective properties of sevoflurane in patients undergoing aortic valve replacement with cardiopulmonary bypass. *Anesth Analg* 2006; **103**: 289–96.

38. Lee MC, Chen CH, Kuo MC, Kang PL, Lo A, Liu K. Isoflurane preconditioning-induced cardio-protection in patients undergoing coronary artery bypass grafting. *Eur J Anaesthesiol* 2006; **23**: 841–7.

39. Bein B, Renner J, Caliebe D, Scholz J, Paris A, Fraund S, Zaehle W, Tonner PH. Sevoflurane but not propofol preserves myocardial function during minimally invasive direct coronary artery bypass surgery. *Anesth Analg* 2005; **100**: 610–16.

40. Law-Koune JD, Raynaud C, Liu N, Dubois C, Romano M, Fischler M. Sevoflurane-remifentanil vs. propofol-remifentanil anesthesia at a similar bispectral level for off-pump coronary artery surgery: no evidence of reduced myocardial ischemia. *J Cardiothorac Vasc Anesth* 2006; **20**: 484–92.

41. Tritapepe L, Landoni G, Guarracino F, Pompei F, Crivellari M, Maselli D, De Luca M, Fochi O, D'Avolio S, Bignami E, Calabrò MG, Zangrillo A. Cardiac protection by volatile anaesthetics: a multicentre randomized controlled study in patients undergoing coronary artery bypass grafting with cardiopulmonary bypass. *Eur J Anaesthesiol* 2007; **24**: 323–31.

42. Ludwig LM, Patel HH, Gross GJ, Kersten JR, Pagel PS, Warltier DC. Morphine enhances pharmacological preconditioning by isoflurane: role of mitochondrial K(ATP) channels and opioid receptors. *Anesthesiology* 2003; **98**: 705–11.

43. Benedict PE, Benedict MB, Su TP, Bolling SF. Opiate drugs and delta-receptor-mediated myocardial protection. *Circulation* 1999; 100 (Suppl.): II357–60.

44. Tei C, Ling LH, Hodge DO, Bailey KR, Oh JK, Rodeheffer RJ, *et al.* New index of combined systolic and diastolic myocardial performance: a simple and reproducible measure of cardiac function – a study in normals and dilated cardiomyopathy. *J Cardiol* 1995; **26**: 357–66.

45. Liao JK. Clinical implications for statin pleiotropy. *Curr Opin Lipidol* 2005; **16**: 624–9.

46. Biccard BM, Sear JW, Foex P. Statin therapy: a potentially useful peri-operative intervention in patients with cardiovascular disease. *Anaesthesia* 2005; **60**: 1106–14.

47. Hindler K, Shaw AD, Samuels J, Fulton S, Collard CD, Riedel B. Improved postoperative outcomes associated with preoperative statin therapy. *Anesthesiology* 2006; **105**: 1260–72.

48. Stevens RD, Burri H, Tramer MR. Pharmacologic myocardial protection in patients undergoing noncardiac surgery: a quantitative systematic review. *Anesth Analg* 2003; **97**: 623–33.

49. Devereaux PJ, Beattie WS, Choi PT, Badner NH, Guyatt GH, Villar JC, Cinà CS, Leslie K, Jacka MJ, Montori VM, Bhandari M, Avezum A, Cavalcanti AB, Giles JW, Schricker T, Yang H, Jakobsen CJ, Yusuf S. How strong is the evidence for the use of perioperative beta blockers in non-cardiac surgery? Systematic review and meta-analysis of randomised controlled trials. *BMJ* 2005; **331**: 313–21.

50. Mangano DT, Layug EL, Wallace A, Tateo I. Effect of atenolol on mortality and cardiovascular morbidity after noncardiac surgery. Multicenter Study of Perioperative Ischemia Research Group. *N Engl J Med* 1996; **335**: 1713–20.

51. Poldermans D, Boersma E, Bax JJ, Thomson IR, van de Ven LL, Blankensteijn JD, Baars HF, Yo TI, Trocino G, Vigna C, Roelandt JR, van Urk H. The effect of bisoprolol on perioperative mortality and myocardial infarction in high-risk patients undergoing vascular surgery. Dutch Echocardiographic Cardiac Risk Evaluation Applying Stress Echocardiography Study Group. *N Engl J Med* 1999; **341**: 1789–94.

52. Fleisher LA, Beckman JA, Brown KA, Calkins H, Chaikof E, Fleischmann KE, *et al.* ACC/AHA 2006 guideline update on perioperative cardiovascular evaluation for noncardiac surgery: focused update on perioperative beta-blocker therapy: a report of the American College of Cardiology/American Heart Association Task Force on Practice Guidelines (Writing Committee to Update the 2002 Guidelines on Perioperative Cardiovascular Evaluation for Noncardiac Surgery) developed in collaboration with the American Society of Echocardiography, American Society of Nuclear Cardiology, Heart Rhythm Society, Society of Cardiovascular Anesthesiologists, Society for Cardiovascular Angiography and Interventions, and Society for Vascular Medicine and Biology. *J Am Coll Cardiol* 2006; **47**: 2343–55.

53. Fleisher LA, Beckman JA, Brown KA, Calkins H, Chaikof EL, Fleischmann KE, *et al.* ACC/AHA 2006 guideline update on perioperative cardiovascular evaluation for noncardiac surgery: focused update on perioperative beta-blocker therapy – a report of the American College of Cardiology/American Heart Association Task Force on Practice Guidelines (Writing Committee to Update the 2002 Guidelines on Perioperative Cardiovascular Evaluation for Noncardiac Surgery). *Anesth Analg* 2007; **104**: 15–26.

54. Lindenauer PK, Pekow P, Wang K, Mamidi DK, Gutierrez B, Benjamin EM. Perioperative beta-blocker therapy and mortality after major noncardiac surgery. *N Engl J Med* 2005; **353**: 349–61.

55. Devereaux PJ, Yang H, Guyatt GH, Leslie K, Villar JC, Monteri VM, Choi P, Giles JW, Yusuf S. Rationale, design, and organization of the PeriOperative ISchemic Evaluation (POISE) trial: a randomized controlled trial of metoprolol vs. placebo in patients undergoing noncardiac surgery. *Am Heart J* 2006; **152**: 223–30.

56. Lanfear DE, Jones PG, Marsh S, Cresci S, McLeod HL, Spertus JA. Beta2-adrenergic receptor genotype and survival among patients receiving beta-blocker therapy after an acute coronary syndrome. *JAMA* 2005; **294**: 1526–33.

57. Wallace AW, Galindez D, Salahieh A, Layug EL, Lazo EA, Haratonik KA, Boisvert DM, Kardatzke D. Effect of clonidine on cardiovascular morbidity and mortality after noncardiac surgery. *Anesthesiology* 2004; **101**: 284–93.

58. Wallace AW. Clonidine and modification of perioperative outcome. *Curr Opin Anaesthesiol* 2006; **19**: 411–17.

59. Ellis JE, Drijvers G, Pedlow S, Laff SP, Sorrentino MJ, Foss JF, Shah M, Busse JR, Mantha S, McKinsey JF. Premedication with oral and transdermal clonidine provides safe and efficacious postoperative sympatholysis. *Anesth Analg* 1994; **79**: 1133–40.

60. Stuhmeier KD, Mainzer B, Cierpka J, Sandmann W, Tarnow J. Small, oral dose of clonidine reduces the incidence of intraoperative myocardial ischemia in patients having vascular surgery. *Anesthesiology* 1996; **85**: 706–12.

61. Kennedy JM, van Rij AM, Spears GF, Pettigrew RA, Tucker IG. Polypharmacy in a general surgical unit and consequences of drug withdrawal. *Br J Clin Pharmacol* 2000; **49**: 353–62.

62. Ho PM, Spertus JA, Masoudi FA, Reid KJ, Peterson ED, Magid DJ, Krumholz HM, Rumsfeld JS. Impact of medication therapy discontinuation on mortality after myocardial infarction. *Arch Intern Med* 2006; **166**: 1842–7.

63. Shammash JB, Trost JC, Gold JM, Berlin JA, Golden MA, Kimmel SE. Perioperative beta-blocker withdrawal and mortality in vascular surgical patients. *Am Heart J* 2001; **141**: 148–53.

64. Burger W, Chemnitius JM, Kneissl GD, Rucker G. Low-dose aspirin for secondary cardiovascular prevention – cardiovascular risks after its perioperative withdrawal vs. bleeding risks with its continuation – review and meta-analysis. *J Intern Med* 2005; **257**: 399–414.

65. Poldermans D, Bax JJ, Kertai MD, Krenning B, Westerhout CM, Schinkel AF, Thomson IR, Lansberg PJ, Fleisher LA, Klein J, van Urk H, Roelandt JR, Boersma E. Statins are associated with a reduced incidence of perioperative mortality in patients undergoing major noncardiac vascular surgery. *Circulation* 2003; **107**: 1848–51.

66. Lindenauer PK, Pekow P, Wang K, Gutierrez B, Benjamin EM. Lipid-lowering therapy and in-hospital mortality following major noncardiac surgery. *JAMA* 2004; **291**: 2092–9.

67. Shoemaker WC, Appel PL, Kram HB, Waxman K, Lee TS. Prospective trial of supranormal values of survivors as therapeutic goals in high-risk surgical patients. *Chest* 1988; **94**: 1176–86.

68. Boyd O, Grounds RM, Bennett ED. A randomized clinical trial of the effect of deliberate perioperative increase of oxygen delivery on mortality in high-risk surgical patients. *JAMA* 1993; **270**: 2699–707.

69. Mythen MG, Webb AR. Perioperative plasma volume expansion reduces the incidence of gut mucosal hypoperfusion during cardiac surgery. *Arch Surg* 1995; **130**: 423–9.

70. Sinclair S, James S, Singer M. Intraoperative intravascular volume optimisation and length of hospital stay after repair of proximal femoral fracture: randomised controlled trial. *BMJ* 1997; **315**: 909–12.

71. Gan TJ, Soppitt A, Maroof M, el-Moalem H, Robertson KM, Moretti E, Dwane P, Glass PS. Goal-directed intraoperative fluid administration reduces length of hospital stay after major surgery. *Anesthesiology* 2002; **97**: 820–6.

72. Kern JW, Shoemaker WC. Meta-analysis of hemodynamic optimization in high-risk patients. *Crit Care Med* 2002; **30**: 1686–92.

73. Goepfert MS, Reuter DA, Akyol D, Lamm P, Kilger E, Goetz AE. Goal-directed fluid management reduces vasopressor and catecholamine use in cardiac surgery patients. *Intensive Care Med* 2007; **33**: 96–103.

74. Cook PT, Davies MJ, Cronin KD, Moran P. A prospective randomised trial comparing spinal anaesthesia using hyperbaric cinchocaine with general anaesthesia for lower limb vascular surgery. *Anaesth Intensive Care* 1986; **14**: 373–80.

75. Damask MC, Weissman C, Todd G. General versus epidural anesthesia for femoral-popliteal bypass surgery. *J Clin Anesth* 1990; **2**: 71–5.

76. Christopherson R, Beattie C, Frank SM, Norris EJ, Meinert CL, Gottlieb SO, Yates H, Rock P, Parker SD, Perler BA, *et al*. Perioperative morbidity in patients randomized to epidural or general anesthesia for lower extremity vascular surgery. Perioperative Ischemia Randomized Anesthesia Trial Study Group. *Anesthesiology* 1993; **79**: 422–34.

77. Bode RH Jr, Lewis KP, Zarich SW, Pierce ET, Roberts M, Kowalchuk GJ, Satwicz PR, Gibbons GW, Hunter JA, Espanola CC. Cardiac outcome after peripheral vascular surgery. Comparison of general and regional anesthesia. *Anesthesiology* 1996; **84**: 3–13.

78. Go AS, Browner WS. Cardiac outcomes after regional or general anesthesia. Do we have the answer? *Anesthesiology* 1996; **84**: 1–2.

4

Ambulatory and outpatient anaesthesia

GABRIELLA IOHOM, GIRISH JOSHI

Introduction

The advantages of surgery performed on a day-care basis (also known as outpatient or ambulatory surgery) include recovery in familiar environment, reduced separation from home and family, minimal disruption to daily life, greater convenience and greater cost-effectiveness. It has been estimated that approximately 60–70% of all surgical procedures performed in the USA are outpatient procedures [1].

Initially, less complex ambulatory surgical procedures were performed in relatively healthy patients. However, recent advances in surgical techniques and availability of anaesthetic agents that facilitate rapid recovery with fewer adverse effects have resulted in further increase in the scope and extent of surgical procedures that can be performed on an outpatient basis. A wide range of increasingly invasive surgical procedures are now being performed on medically complex patients in ambulatory facilities. Furthermore, there has been a growth of office-based procedures, which now approach 25% of outpatient surgery. Office-based anaesthesia is presently the most rapidly expanding area, but as yet inadequately taught in most anaesthesia residency programmes [2]. In addition, anaesthetists are increasingly required to anaesthetize outpatients in locations other than the operating room, such as the gastrointestinal suite, cardiac catheterization laboratory and interventional radiology.

Ambulatory anaesthetists are perioperative physicians who ensure optimal management of the patient's coexisting medical condition throughout the operative course. This includes preoperative evaluation and optimization, intraoperative management and postoperative care with the aim of facilitating early discharge home and rapid resumption of normal daily activities. The determination of suitability of a patient for ambulatory surgery is complex, and includes the nature of the surgical procedure (e.g. reduced risk of intraoperative and postoperative blood loss and ability to control pain after discharge home), patient's preoperative health, proposed anaesthetic technique, as well as suitability and location of surgical facility (e.g. free-standing surgery centre vs. physician's office) and social considerations such as home conditions, caregiver availability and access to a medical centre.

Fast-track anaesthesia techniques that provide excellent operative conditions and allow rapid emergence from anaesthesia as well as prevent common complications such as pain, nausea and vomiting should be utilized for ambulatory surgical procedures. Unnecessary delay in recovery after ambulatory surgery reduces the effectiveness and efficiency of an outpatient setting. Therefore, the time spent in the hospital is becoming an increasingly relevant issue from both a clinical and cost standpoint. A clear and coordinated postoperative plan, which is implemented as a clinical pathway, is necessary to achieve rapid discharge. The potential benefits of ambulatory surgery may cease to exist if patients require emergency care or unplanned hospital admission, which occurs in approximately 1% of cases |3|. The factors that might influence outcome after ambulatory surgery include general anaesthesia, duration of surgical procedure, uncontrolled pain and bleeding.

Overall, there is a general belief that surgical procedures performed on an outpatient basis are easy; however, in actual fact, these procedures can be some of the most challenging for the anaesthetist, given the increasing co-morbidities and complexity of the surgical procedures. In addition, an anaesthetist-led multidisciplinary management team can improve patient throughput and, thus, improve the efficiency of the outpatient centre. Furthermore, the demand for highly efficient and streamlined care, as well as expectations for improved patient satisfaction, has increased production pressures in the ambulatory surgical setting. Undoubtedly, delivery of safe and efficient anaesthetic care in these circumstances requires unique skills.

Practice guidelines for the perioperative management of patients with obstructive sleep apnea: a report by the American Society of Anesthesiologists Task Force on perioperative management of patients with obstructive sleep apnoea

Gross JB, Bachenberg KL, Benumof JL, et al. Anesthesiology 2006; **104**: 1081–93

BACKGROUND. Obstructive sleep apnoea (OSA) is a common sleep disorder that is associated with increased perioperative morbidity and mortality primarily due to difficulty in securing and maintaining the upper airway, postoperative airway obstruction and postoperative respiratory depression |4|. With the incidence of obesity increasing across the world, it is expected that the incidence of OSA will also increase. Inevitably, there will be an increase in OSA patients scheduled for ambulatory surgery. The American Society of Anesthesiologists (ASA) published Practice Guidelines for the Perioperative Management of Patients with Obstructive Sleep Apnea, which include recommendations for management of ambulatory surgery patients.

INTERPRETATION. The summary of the ASA–OSA practice guidelines is included in Table 4.1. These guidelines emphasize the need to identify OSA patients during preoperative evaluation (Table 4.2). If history and physical examination suggest the presence of

Table 4.1 Summary of ASA practice guidelines on obstructive sleep apnoea (OSA)

1 Preoperative evaluation
  a Medical records review
  b Patient and family interview
  c Screening questionnaire
  d Focused physical examination
  e Sleep study

2 Preoperative preparation
  a Preoperative treatment/optimization for OSA (e.g. continuous positive airway pressure [CPAP], non-invasive positive-pressure ventilation [NIPPV], mandibular appliances, surgical treatment)
  b Consult the ASA's *Practice Guidelines for Management of the Difficult Airway*
  c Limit procedures to facilities with full hospital services

3 Intraoperative management (no good data; avoid opioids and use regional, if possible)
  a Anaesthetic technique
    (i) Local or regional anaesthesia vs. general anaesthesia
    (ii) Combined regional and general anaesthesia vs. general anaesthesia
    (iii) Sedation vs. general anaesthesia
  b Monitoring
    (i) Continuously monitor the respiratory depressant effects of sedatives and/or opioids (e.g. level of consciousness, pulmonary ventilation, oxygenation, automated apnoea monitoring)
    (ii) Special intraoperative monitoring techniques (arterial line, pulmonary artery catheter)
  c Extubation
    (i) Verify the full reversal of neuromuscular block before extubation
    (ii) Extubate patients after they are fully awake (vs. asleep or partially awake)
    (iii) Extubate patients in the semi-upright, lateral or prone positions (vs. supine)

Table 4.1 Summary of ASA practice guidelines on obstructive sleep apnoea (OSA)   (continued)

4 Postoperative management
  a Analgesic use
    (i) Regional analgesic techniques without neuraxial opioids vs. systemic opioids
    (ii) Neuraxial opioids vs. systemic opioids
    (iii) Oral analgesics vs. parenteral opioids
    (iv) Patient-controlled analgesia (PCA) without a background infusion vs. PCA with a background infusion
    (v) Titration or lower dosage levels of systemic opioids
  b Oxygenation
    (i) Supplemental oxygen vs. no supplemental oxygen
    (ii) CPAP vs. no CPAP (oxygen or room air)
    (iii) CPAP for patients who had previously been on CPAP vs. CPAP for patients not previously on CPAP
    (iv) NIPPV vs. no NIPPV (CPAP, oxygen or room air)
  c Positioning patients in the lateral, prone or tonsil position vs. the supine position
  d Monitoring
    (i) Telemetry monitoring systems vs. no telemetry monitoring systems
    (ii) Monitored settings vs. routine hospital wards
  e Duration of stay
    (i) Extended stay in post-anaesthesia care unit (PACU) vs. no extended stay in PACU
    (ii) Hospital admission vs. discharge home

Source: American Society of Anesthesiologists Task Force on Perioperative Management of Patients with Obstructive Sleep Apnea (2006).

Table 4.2 Identification and assessment of OSA (modified from ASA Practice Guidelines)

A Clinical signs and symptoms suggesting the possibility of OSA

1   Predisposing physical characteristics

   a BMI $35 kg/m^2$ (95 percentile for age and gender)
   b Neck circumference 17 inches (men) or 16 inches (women)
   c Craniofacial abnormalities affecting the airway
   d Anatomical nasal obstruction
   e Tonsils nearly touching or touching in the midline

2   History of apparent airway obstruction during sleep (two or more the following are present; if patient lives alone or sleep is not observed by another person, then only one of the following needs to be present)

   a Snoring (loud enough to be heard through closed doors)
   b Frequent snoring
   c Observed pauses in breathing during sleep
   d Awakens from sleep with choking sensation
   e Frequent arousals from sleep
   f Intermittent vocalization during sleep*
   g Parental report of restless sleep, difficulty breathing or struggling respiratory efforts during sleep*

3 Somnolence (one or more of the following is present)

   a Frequent somnolence or fatigue despite adequate 'sleep'
   b Falls asleep easily in a non-stimulating environment (e.g. watching TV, reading, riding in or driving a car) despite adequate 'sleep'
   c Parent or teacher comments that child appears sleepy during the day, is easily distracted, is overly aggressive or has difficulty concentrating*
   d Child often difficult to arouse at usual awakening time*

If a patient has signs and symptoms in two or more categories of the above, there is a significant probability of OSA.

B If a sleep study has been done, it should be used to determine the perioperative management†

Severity of OSA	Adult AHI	Paediatric AHI
None	0–5	0
Mild OSA	6–20	1–5
Moderate OSA	21–40	6–10
Severe OSA	> 40	> 10

*Items in brackets refer to paediatric patients.
†Note that sleep laboratories' assessment of severity should take precedence over the actual apnoea–hypopnoea index (AHI).
Source: American Society of Anesthesiologists Task Force on Perioperative Management of Patients with Obstructive Sleep Apnea (2006).

OSA, the anaesthetist and surgeon should together determine if a sleep study should be obtained or to proceed with the surgery based on clinical criteria. Patients on preoperative continuous positive airway pressure (CPAP) should be asked to bring their CPAP equipment with them for use in the postoperative period. The ASA–OSA guidelines propose a scoring system (based on severity of OSA, invasiveness of diagnostic or surgical procedure and anaesthetic technique, and anticipated postoperative opioid requirements) that may be used to estimate the perioperative risk (Table 4.3). Although the type and extent of surgery and the need for postoperative opioids, rather than the choice of anaesthetic technique appear to be more important determinants of postoperative complications in patients with OSA, local or regional anaesthesia should be preferred whenever possible. During sedation, ventilation should be continuously monitored by capnography. Of note, general anaesthesia is preferred to unprotected airway during deep sedation. For patients requiring general anaesthesia, there is potential for difficult tracheal intubation and extubation. Most importantly, perioperative pain should be managed by non-opioids if possible, and opioids should be used judiciously. It is recommended that the OSA patients be monitored for a median of 3 h longer than their non-OSA counterparts before discharge from the ambulatory facility. In addition, the monitoring should continue for a median of 7 h after the last episode of airway obstruction

Table 4.3 Scoring system to estimate perioperative complications

(A) Severity of sleep apnoea based on sleep study (i.e. AHI) or clinical indicators if sleep study not available
- None = 0; mild OSA = 1; moderate OSA = 2; severe OSA = 3
- Subtract a point in patients using CPAP or NIPPV preoperatively and postoperatively, and add a point in a patient with $Paco_2 > 50$ mmHg

(B) Invasiveness of surgery and anaesthesia
- Superficial surgery under local or peripheral nerve block anaesthesia without sedation = 0
- Superficial surgery with moderate sedation or general anaesthesia or peripheral surgery under spinal or epidural anaesthesia (with no more than moderate sedation) = 1
- Peripheral surgery with general anaesthesia or airway surgery with moderate sedation = 2
- Major surgery or airway surgery under general anaesthesia = 3

(C) Requirement for postoperative opioid
- None = 0
- Low-dose oral opioids = 1
- High-dose oral or parenteral or neuraxial opioids = 3

(D) Estimation of perioperative risk
- Overall score = score of A + greater score of either B or C
- Patients with overall score of 4 or greater may be at increased perioperative risk from OSA
- Patients with a score of 5 or greater may be at significantly increased perioperative risk from OSA

Source: American Society of Anesthesiologists Task Force on Perioperative Management of Patients with Obstructive Sleep Apnea (2006).

or hypoxaemia while breathing room air in an unstimulated environment. These recommendations for longer postoperative stay may be the major limitation of performing ambulatory surgery in a free-standing ambulatory surgery centre or office setting as they may reduce the efficiency of the facility.

Comment

Although the ASA–OSA guidelines assist anaesthetists in the management of this challenging patient population, they are primarily based upon expert opinions rather than scientific evidence, which is lacking. Ambulatory surgery in OSA patients remains controversial because the literature regarding its safety is sparse and of limited quality. Because OSA is undiagnosed in approximately 60–70% of patients, it is imperative that anaesthetists identify patients with OSA at the time of preoperative evaluation. Although the criteria proposed by the ASA–OSA guidelines for identification of OSA are comprehensive (see Table 4.2), they are time-consuming. Recently, a simple and quick OSA screening tool has been shown to have the same sensitivity and specificity as the ASA–OSA criteria and the Berlin questionnaire |5|. The questions included in this new OSA screening tool are: Do you snore loudly (heard through closed doors)?; Do you often feel tired, fatigued or sleepy during daytime despite adequate sleep?; Has anyone observed that you stop breathing during sleep?; and Do you have or are treated for high blood pressure?

It is recommended that patients who are at significantly increased risk of perioperative complications (i.e. score ≥5, Table 4.3) are generally not good candidates for ambulatory surgery. It must be emphasized that this scoring system is not yet validated and clinical judgement should be used to assess the risk of an individual patient. In addition, the ability of the facility to manage OSA patients should be taken into consideration.

Finally, patients, their family members and surgeons should be informed of the potential perioperative concerns associated with OSA. Anaesthetists and surgeons should collaborate to develop protocols for preoperative identification and preparation, intraoperative management, and postoperative (including post-discharge) care, which is critical in the prevention of perioperative complications in OSA patients.

A novel index of elevated risk of inpatient hospital admission immediately following outpatient surgery

Fleisher LA, Pasternak LR, Lyles A. *Arch Surg* 2007; **142**: 263–8

BACKGROUND. Although the absolute rate of adverse effects following ambulatory surgery has been low, the increasing number and complexity of cases performed in a variety of outpatient settings (free-standing, hospital-affiliated facilities and physicians' offices) make the identification of factors associated with elevated relative risk critical. Using outpatient surgical encounter data from the Agency for

Healthcare Research and Quality, the authors report (i) rates of direct admission to a short-term hospital facility; (ii) death rates during ambulatory procedure; and (iii) a novel index to identify individuals at highest risk for hospital admission immediately following ambulatory surgery.

INTERPRETATION. After excluding cardiac catheterizations, endoscopies, cataract operations and discharges other than routine or short-term hospitalization, 783 558 patients were included in the study. Of these, 4351 were discharged directly for short-term hospitalization (1:180), and 19 died (1:41 240). The modified Deyo co-morbidity score |6| ranged from 0 to 5 and was substantially less for free-standing (0.040) than for hospital-affiliated (0.154) surgical centres. The data set was subsequently randomized into the following two subsets: the *analysis* data set (*n* = 392 107) was used for analysis and model development; the *holdout* data set (*n* = 391 415) was used for validation. An outpatient surgery admission index (OSAI) was developed from independent predictors of immediate hospital admission using the following point values: 65 years or older (1), operating time longer than 120 min (1), cardiac diagnoses (1), peripheral vascular disease (1), cerebrovascular disease (1), malignancy (1), seropositive findings for human immunodeficiency virus (1) and regional (1) or general anaesthesia (2). Increasing scores were associated with higher odds of admission relative to scores of 0 or 1. For scores of 4 or higher, the odds ratio was 31.96 (95% CI 26.29–38.86), and 2.8% of these patients were discharged to the hospital. For the holdout half of the data set, scores of 4 or higher had an odds ratio of 34.62 (95% CI 28.55–41.97).

Comment

Shortcomings include the retrospective nature of the study design, limited specificity of the OSAI, possibility of false-positive findings, and data obtained from facilities predominantly associated with outpatient hospital settings. Most importantly, it is not clear whether these admissions were planned or unplanned. This, for example, may explain the inclusion of HIV-positive status as a risk factor, because the surgery may be part of a planned admission. Subsequent prospective studies using this index will have to address some of these issues. However, the proposed OSAI provides an evidence-based guide to assist clinicians in identifying patients at higher risk of immediate hospital admission. This is not to suggest that patients with an OSAI of 4 or higher should universally undergo inpatient surgery; rather, clinicians should consider performing surgery on these patients in a setting where there is additional medical support to treat acute adverse events and to permit rapid transfer to an inpatient hospital. Including this information in physician and patient decisions regarding the surgical setting may lead to enhanced patient safety and high-quality care. The findings of this study point to the importance of a structured preoperative evaluation system that provides this information in a complete form and on a timely basis for review |7|.

Nitrous oxide in ambulatory anaesthesia: does it have a place in day surgical anaesthesia or is it just a threat for personnel and the global environment?

Smith I. *Curr Opin Anaesthesiol* 2006; **19**: 592–6

BACKGROUND. Being by far the oldest anaesthetic in current use, the question is legitimate. Therefore, the above review is undoubtedly timely and justified. The author gives a balanced perspective based on both historical and more recent research.

INTERPRETATION. *Drawbacks* of nitrous oxide include negative effect on the environment; toxicity with prolonged exposure to both patients and operating room personnel; pressure effects through expansion of closed air-filled spaces; and potentiation of postoperative nausea and vomiting (PONV). *Potential benefits* include the fact that, as an analgesic and a weak anaesthetic, nitrous oxide acts as an adjunct to other anaesthetics during the induction and maintenance phases improving the quality and safety of anaesthesia and facilitating faster recovery with minimal adverse effects. *Alternatives* suggested include remifentanil and xenon, with similar kinetics but substantially higher costs.

Comment

Drawbacks and harmful effects of nitrous oxide are realistic, but they are well recognized and can therefore be minimized or eliminated by judicious use. Although it is a greenhouse gas and contributes to depletion of the ozone layer, of all the nitrous oxide reaching the upper atmosphere, only about 1% originates from anaesthetic use |8|, the vast majority coming from denitrification of agricultural fertilizer and fossil fuels. The bone marrow depression through inhibition of methionine synthesis caused by nitrous oxide precludes its prolonged administration to critically ill patients, but poses a negligible risk to ambulatory patients. With modern scavenging systems – required for other inhalational agents, too – there is no convincing evidence of any adverse health effects on staff. While intraocular or intracranial air represents an absolute contraindication to nitrous oxide, bowel distension during laparoscopic surgery is not as clear-cut. The question was addressed in a blinded study, which concluded that intraoperative conditions and PONV were identical, irrespective of whether or not nitrous oxide was used in this 'at-risk' population |9|. In fact, the authors of a meta-analysis of randomized controlled trials stated that the 'clinically-important risk of major harm [intraoperative awareness] reduces the usefulness of omitting nitrous oxide to prevent postoperative nausea and vomiting' |10|.

Potential benefits can be observed throughout induction, maintenance and recovery. In addition to reducing the induction time or dose of the inducing agent, the use of nitrous oxide results in smoother induction, with fewer adverse airway events and a greater first-time successful insertion of the laryngeal mask |11|. Besides the well-known second-gas effect on inhalation agents, a persisting second-gas effect on oxygen uptake has recently been observed |12|, resulting in higher arterial oxygen partial pressures throughout anaesthesia supplemented with nitrous oxide, despite identical inspired oxygen concentrations. This advantage would translate into a greater margin of safety, especially desirable in frail elderly patients presenting now for ambulatory anaesthesia. An interesting finding is that bispectral index (as well as other brain function monitors, e.g. entropy) is 'blind' to nitrous oxide, with the unfortunate consequence of an unanticipated overdose of the primary anaesthetic agent when it is titrated solely against the bispectral index (BIS) value |13|. Nitrous oxide is rapidly eliminated, resulting in a faster recovery than when anaesthesia is maintained by higher concentrations of the primary anaesthetic agent. Diffusion hypoxia is well recognized, but perhaps overrated.

Alternatives considered could be total omission of nitrous oxide, its replacement with nitrogen, opioid supplementation (remifentanil in particular, with advantageous pharmacokinetics) or xenon. The last is undoubtedly an excellent anaesthetic, and as an environmental constituent it is promising in many respects. At present, the most likely application for xenon appears to be the high-risk cardiac surgery patient |14|. The author concludes that 'whereas potential alternatives to nitrous oxide exist, their use is usually more complex, more costly and less effective than nitrous oxide. In addition, the long-term effects of remifentanil and xenon on outcome are relatively unknown compared with the 162-year-long track record of nitrous oxide, which should retain a place in ambulatory anaesthesia for many years to come.'

Intraoperative awareness in a regional medical system: a review of 3 years' data

Pollard RJ, Coyle JP, Gilbert RL, *et al. Anesthesiology* 2007; **106**: 269–74

BACKGROUND. In an effort to achieve an expeditious recovery and discharge after ambulatory surgery, there is a tendency to maintain a 'lighter' plane of anaesthesia (i.e. fast-track anaesthesia technique) |15|. This increases the concerns of intraoperative awareness (or postoperative recall of intraoperative events) and justifies the focus on evaluation of the incidence of intraoperative awareness. Although intraoperative awareness is an infrequent complication, it may be associated with significant psychological consequences |16,17|. The overall incidence of intraoperative awareness varies between 0.1% and 0.9%, with a higher incidence in sicker patients undergoing major surgery than with surgical procedures that are commonly performed on an outpatient basis |16–19|. This large, prospective, observational study assessed the occurrence of intraoperative awareness. As part of the quality assurance process, 87 621 patients undergoing general anaesthesia were interviewed within 1–2 days after their anaesthetic. The interview consisted of a structured questionnaire (i.e. what was the last thing you remember before surgery; what was the first thing you remember once you woke up: did you have any dreams while you were asleep for surgery; were you put to sleep gently; did you have any problems going to sleep?).

INTERPRETATION. Of the 87621 patients considered at risk of awareness, six patients were determined to have intraoperative awareness, for an incidence of 0.0068%. Of these six patients, four had undergone cardiac surgery, for an incidence of 0.12% (4 in 3208 cases). None of the patients with awareness had undergone ambulatory surgery. All patients with awareness had received neuromuscular blockade and none of the patients had received nitrous oxide. Interestingly, the incidence of awareness in the academic centre was higher (5 of 52751 cases, 0.0095%) as compared with community centres (1 of 34610 cases, 0.003%), but this difference was not statistically significant.

Comment

In contrast to previous studies that have reported an incidence of awareness of 1–2 cases per 1000 patients, this study found a significantly lower incidence of awareness (one case per 14560 patients). The discrepancy between studies could not be explained by differences in the timing of the interview or differences in the questionnaires.

The possible causes of awareness include light general anaesthesia, increased anaesthetic requirements and anaesthetic machine malfunction or misuse |**17**|. Of note, the anaesthetic technique also influences the incidence of awareness. For example, use of neuromuscular blockade or omitting nitrous oxide may increase the incidence of awareness |**10,19**|. Because clinical signs of inadequate anaesthesia are unreliable, a number of brain function monitors have been developed. However, the brain function monitors do not have uniform sensitivity across all anaesthetic drugs and patients. Intrapatient variations have also been reported |**20**|. Awareness can still occur in patients receiving brain function monitoring |**17**|. Therefore, their ability to consistently reflect the state of hypnosis and prevent intraoperative awareness remains controversial |**17**|. A recent American Society of Anesthesiologists Task Force for the Practice Advisory for Intraoperative Awareness and Brain Function Monitoring concluded that brain function monitoring is not routinely indicated for patients undergoing general anaesthesia, either to reduce the frequency of intraoperative awareness or to monitor depth of hypnosis. Nevertheless, it is suggested that brain function monitors may be beneficial in patients at higher risk of awareness.

The brain function monitors have also been reported to improve titration of inhaled and intravenous sedative–hypnotic drugs, and allow faster emergence, as well as improve quality of recovery (reduced drowsiness, dizziness, fatigue, nausea and vomiting). However, these monitors may have limited benefits in patients breathing spontaneously or undergoing shorter surgical procedures with newer inhaled anaesthetics |**21**|. In addition, although these monitors hasten emergence from general anaesthesia, they do not influence phase II recovery and discharge to home. Furthermore, the cerebral function monitors might not be cost-effective, particularly if the policy of the recovery facility mandates a minimum length of stay.

Early reversal of profound rocuronium-induced neuromuscular blockade by sugammadex in a randomized multicentre study: efficacy, safety, and pharmacokinetics

Sparr HJ, Vermeyen KM, Beaufort AM, *et al. Anesthesiology* 2007; **106**: 935–43

BACKGROUND. It is well accepted that even a minor degree of residual blockade (train-of-four [TOF] ratio of 0.9), which is usually not appreciated clinically |22|, can increase postoperative morbidity, including inadequate ventilation, hypoxia, the need for reintubation and delayed discharge from the operating room and the recovery room |23–25|. In addition, a TOF ratio of > 0.9 is necessary to ensure return of adequate voluntary muscle strength and the ability to ambulate, both of which are of critical importance in outpatients |25|. Residual paralysis may be even more critical in the high-risk patients (e.g. obese, sleep apnoeic and elderly patients) who are increasingly undergoing surgical procedures on an outpatient basis. Clinically unrecognized residual paralysis is common despite routine neuromuscular monitoring |26| and the use of cholinesterase inhibitors (e.g. neostigmine) |22|. Furthermore, cholinesterase inhibitors are not effective if used in profound neuromuscular blockade. Sugammadex (Org 25969), a synthetic cyclodextrin derivative, is a selective relaxant-binding agent designed to reverse a rocuronium-induced neuromuscular block through chemical encapsulation |26|. The binding of sugammadex and rocuronium results in a rapid decrease in plasma concentration of rocuronium, and subsequently decreased concentration at the motor endplate. With decrease in the availability of rocuronium to block acetylcholine receptors in the neuromuscular junction, muscle activity should reappear |26|. In this multicentre, dose-finding study, 98 male patients were randomized to receive placebo or one of five sugammadex doses (1, 2, 4, 6 and 8 mg/kg) administered 3, 5 or 15 min after rocuronium 0.6 mg/kg. Pharmacokinetic evaluations were also performed to determine the effect of sugammadex on plasma concentrations of rocuronium. In addition, urinary excretion of rocuronium and sugammadex were measured.

INTERPRETATION. The times to recovery of TOF ratio to 0.9, measured using acceleromyography, were significantly shorter after sugammadex than that after placebo (Table 4.4). Sugammadex was found to be safe and well tolerated, and no signs of re-paralysis were observed during the postoperative period. The 24-h urinary rocuronium excretion was higher in the sugammadex group (30% for 1 mg/kg, 33% for 2 mg/kg, and 58–74% after ≥ 4 mg/kg) than in the placebo group (26%). There was no relationship between the sugammadex dose and percentage of the dose excreted in the urine. Interestingly, after administration of sugammadex, 20% of patients showed signs of inadequate anaesthesia, such as increase in BIS values, sucking, grimacing, moving and coughing on the tube.

Table 4.4 Time interval (min) from administration of placebo or sugammadex to a train-of-four ratio of 0.9

Time of administration of placebo or sugammadex (min)	Placebo (n = 3)	Sugammadex (mg/kg)				
		1.0 (n = 6)	2.0 (n = 6)	4.0 (n = 6)	6.0 (n = 6)	8.0 (n = 6)
3	52.1 (8.8)	22.7 (11.6)	4.9 (1.3)	6.3 (9.0)	1.9 (0.6)	1.8 (0.9)
5	51.7 (13.1)	27.4 (6.4)	8.9 (7.8)	2.3 (0.7)	2.1 (0.9)	1.5 (0.6)
15	35.6 (9.1)	6.5 (1.7)	2.7 (0.7)	2.1 (1.2)	2.1 (2.0)	1.4 (0.2)

Values are mean (SD).
Source: Sparr et al. (2007).

Comment

Sugammadex reversed profound neuromuscular blockade and the speed of recovery was dose dependent. Although this study included only a small number of patients, there was a narrow inter-individual variability in recovery times after sugammadex administration. A TOF ratio of 0.9 was achieved within 3 min at $\geq 6\,mg/kg$ sugammadex administered 3 min after rocuronium, at $4\,mg/kg$ sugammadex administered 5 min after rocuronium, and at $2\,mg/kg$ sugammadex administered 15 min after rocuronium. This suggests that the sugammadex dose would depend upon the time interval between administration of rocuronium and reversal. Unfortunately, the authors did not recommend an appropriate sugammadex dose for clinical use. The clinical significance of signs of inadequate anaesthesia in 20% of patients is unknown.

Sugammadex was designed to reverse rocuronium-induced neuromuscular blockade |27,28|. However, a recent study reported that it was also effective in reversing vecuronium-induced neuromuscular blockade |29|. By contrast, sugammadex was not effective in reversing atracurium or mivacurium-induced neuromuscular blockade |30|. Thus, if there is a need for re-paralysis after administration of sugammadex, benzylisoquinolonium muscle relaxants might still be effective.

It is to be expected that sugammadex would eliminate the limitations of neuro-muscular function monitoring and neostigmine, as well as reduce the concerns of residual neuromuscular blockade and, thus, improve patient safety. However, there is no such clinical evidence as of yet. The rapid reversal of profound rocuronium-induced neuromuscular blockade might eliminate the need for succinylcholine for rapid tracheal intubation or in patients with suspected difficult tracheal intubation. Future studies need to compare the recovery after succinylcholine and rocuronium–sugammadex.

Spinal anesthesia with lidocaine or preservative-free 2-chloroprocaine for outpatient knee arthroscopy: a prospective, randomized, double-blind comparison

Casati A, Fanelli G, Danelli G, *et al. Anesth Analg* 2007; **104**: 959–64

BACKGROUND. Lidocaine had been the agent of choice for short-acting spinal anaesthesia in the outpatient setting until transient neurological symptoms (TNS) were consistently reported |31|. A preservative-free solution of 2-chloroprocaine has recently been reintroduced and is available for off-label use. Its short half life and potentially favourable evolution of subarachnoid block make it attractive for short outpatient procedures |32|. The hypothesis tested by the authors in this prospective, randomized, double-blind study was that 50 mg of 1% 2-chloroprocaine would provide similarly effective spinal block with a faster recovery of sensory and motor function than an equivalent dose of 1% plain lidocaine.

INTERPRETATION. Thirty outpatients undergoing knee arthroscopy were randomly allocated to receive 50 mg of either 1% plain lidocaine ($n = 15$) or 1% preservative-free plain chloroprocaine ($n = 15$). Spinal anaesthesia was successful in all patients. No differences in the maximum level of sensory block and degree of motor blockade were noted between the groups. Recovery of sensory and motor function and unassisted ambulation was faster in patients receiving chloroprocaine than in those receiving lidocaine. No difference in first voiding was reported between the two groups (Table 4.5). TNS were reported in five patients in the lidocaine group compared with none in the 2-chloroprocaine group ($P = 0.042$).

Comment

The authors of this study confirmed previous observations in volunteers |**32,33**|, that intrathecal injection of 50 mg of 1% preservative-free 2-chloroprocaine produced a reliable subarachnoid block for outpatient knee arthroscopy, with quicker recovery of sensory and motor function and earlier unassisted ambulation than with the same dose of 1% lidocaine. The implication of this is that faster resolution of the spinal block may accelerate home discharge in patients undergoing procedures at low risk of urinary retention, in whom presence of first voiding can be excluded from standard discharge criteria. In a previous dose-finding study, the same group demonstrated that while 40 and 50 mg of 2-chloroprocaine provide adequate spinal anaesthesia for outpatient procedures lasting 45–60 min, 30 mg produces a spinal block of insufficient duration |**34**|. The 4-min difference in the onset time of spinal block between the two groups in the present study, though statistically significant, may arguably be clinically irrelevant. This study was not powered to assess the safety of the two drugs. However, the 33% incidence of TNS in the lidocaine group and none in the 2-chloroprocaine group is consistent with previous findings in healthy volunteers (seven out of eight subjects after spinal lidocaine and none after chloroprocaine) |**32**|. All of these advantages make 2-chloroprocaine a suitable drug

Table 4.5 Times from spinal injection to complete recovery of motor and sensory function, unassisted ambulation, and first voiding in patients receiving intrathecal injection of 50 mg of either 1% lidocaine or 1% plain chloroprocaine

	Lidocaine (n = 15)	Chloroprocaine (n = 15)	P-value
Duration of motor block (min)	100 (60–140)	60 (45–120)	0.0005
Duration of sensory block (min)	120 (80–175)	95 (68–170)	0.019
Recovery of ambulation (min)	152 (100–185)	103 (70–191)	0.003
First voiding (min)	190 (148–340)	180 (100–354)	0.191

Data are median (range).
Source: Casati et al. (2007).

for providing spinal anaesthesia in the ambulatory setting, but more data are needed before it can be safely incorporated into clinical practice. It is of note that neither clinical reports on its off-label intrathecal use in more than 1000 patients, nor rigorous investigations in more than 100 volunteers and outpatients have reported any cases of neurological toxicity to date |34|.

Effect of patient-controlled perineural analgesia on rehabilitation and pain after ambulatory orthopaedic surgery

Capdevila X, Dadure C, Bringuier S, *et al. Anesthesiology* 2006; **105**: 566–73

BACKGROUND. Postoperative analgesia and rapid recovery may be challenging in the clinical setting of ambulatory orthopaedic surgery. Peripheral nerve blocks provide superior same-day recovery and decrease hospital readmission compared with general anaesthesia. Single-injection regional anaesthesia, despite using long-acting local anaesthetics, provides early but not long-term benefits compared with general anaesthesia. In addition, continuous peripheral nerve blocks have been shown to facilitate early rehabilitation after inpatient orthopaedic surgery. Furthermore, continuous infusion of local anaesthetic combined with patient-controlled bolus doses optimizes analgesia and increases the duration of infusion in comparison with continuous infusion or bolus alone. The primary objective of this study was to determine whether patient-controlled perineural analgesia provides optimal postoperative patient functional exercise capacity and daily activity at home. Secondary outcomes investigated postoperative analgesia, opioid-related side-effects and overall satisfaction.

INTERPRETATION. In this multicentre randomized prospective trial, 83 patients scheduled to undergo acromioplasty or hallux valgus surgery received an interscalene ($n = 40$) or popliteal ($n = 43$) peripheral nerve block with 30 ml of ropivacaine 0.5%. After randomization, patients were discharged home 24 h following surgery with a disposable infusion pump delivering either patient-controlled intravenous morphine ($n = 23$) or perineural ropivacaine 0.2%, either as continuous infusion without bolus ($n = 30$) or as basal infusion plus bolus ($n = 30$). Basal infusion plus bolus ropivacaine decreased the time to 10 min walk, optimized daily activities ($P<0.05$) (Fig. 4.1) and decreased the amount of ropivacaine used. Higher pain scores and rescue analgesic consumption, higher incidences of nausea/vomiting, sleep disturbance and dizziness, and less patient satisfaction scores were recorded in the morphine group ($P<0.05$).

Comment

The novelty of this study lies with the 72 h post-surgery analysis of the impact of the postoperative analgesic technique on the quality of patients' daily activities and functional exercise capacity. After ambulatory orthopaedic surgery, ropivacaine 0.2% delivered as a perineural infusion via a disposable elastomeric pump with

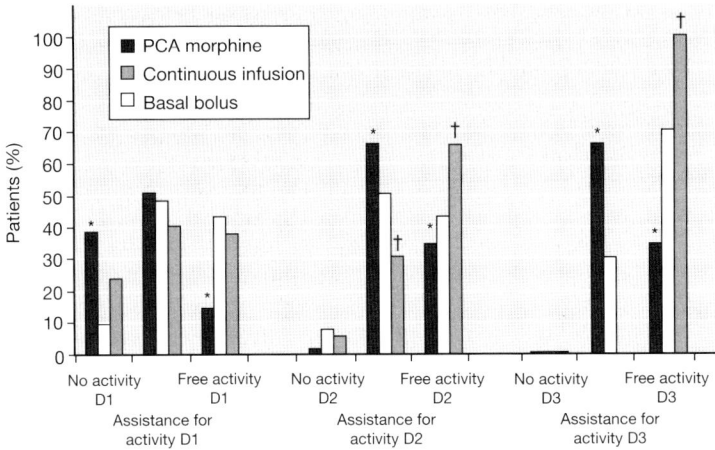

Fig. 4.1 Percentages of patients without daily activity, with assistance for daily activity, or with complete free activity at home in the three groups of patients. D1, D2, D3 = postoperative days 1, 2 and 3. *$P<0.05$ vs. both regional anaesthesia groups. †$P<0.05$ vs. the other two groups. PCA, patient-controlled anaesthesia. Source: Capdevila et al. (2006).

patient-controlled anaesthesia bolus doses optimized functional recovery and analgesia while decreasing the consumption of rescue analgesics and ropivacaine and the number of adverse events. Of the patients in the basal infusion plus bolus group, 70% and 100% had no limitation in their activity level including walking at 48 and 72 h, respectively. The main reasons for lack of activity or need for assistance during home activities were essentially pain and fatigue in the patient-controlled intravenous morphine group. One might infer from the current study that excellent pain relief coupled with a reduction in side-effects would facilitate postoperative mobilization at home. Probably the most important conclusion to be drawn from this study is that future investigations should focus on improvements in quality of functional outcome. Continuous peripheral nerve blocks appear to be one of the key elements.

PROSPECT: evidence-based, procedure-specific postoperative pain management

Kehlet H, Wilkinson RC, Fischer HBJ, et al., on behalf of the PROSPECT Working Group. Best Prac Res Clin Anaesthesiol 2007; **21**: 149–59

BACKGROUND. Inadequate pain management after ambulatory surgery continues to be a major concern |35,36|. One of the reasons for this is inadequate or improper application of available analgesic therapies, which may partly be due to the significant amount of conflicting information that is being made increasingly available. The currently available evidence-based pain management guidelines

may influence clinical practice |37–39|. However, they are derived from multiple
surgical procedures that have different pain characteristics (e.g. location,
intensity, type and duration). In addition, the risks and benefits of different
analgesic techniques differ between surgical procedures. Furthermore, some
analgesic techniques are applicable to specific surgical procedures (e.g. intra-
articular and intraperitoneal techniques for joint surgery and abdominal surgery,
respectively). Also, some pain management guidelines use the number needed
to treat (NNT) values (e.g. number of patients who achieve at least a 50% pain
relief compared with placebo), which are derived from a variety of surgical
procedures. However, efficacy of an analgesic may vary depending upon the type
of surgical procedure as well as on the combination of analgesics |40|. Therefore,
it is clear that the NNT may not necessarily be valid in all types of surgery and
for all intensities of pain. The PROSPECT (procedure-specific postoperative
pain management) initiative was developed to overcome the limitations of
generalized pain management guidelines. It provides comprehensive web-based
recommendations derived from systematic reviews of the literature (using the
Cochrane Collaboration of randomized controlled trials of analgesic, anaesthetic
and surgical interventions affecting postoperative pain) for the specific type of
surgery. These procedure-specific systematic reviews are supplemented with
evidence from other surgical procedures with similar pain profile (e.g. transferable
evidence) and clinical practice information (e.g. practical guidelines from
the PROSPECT Working Group that consists of an international panel of both
anaesthetists and surgeons) is taken into consideration (Fig. 4.2) |41|.

INTERPRETATION. The recommendations available online (www.postoppain.org) are
presented in the form of a flow diagram arranged into folders labelled as preoperative,
intraoperative and postoperative interventions. Within the folders, evidence and clinical
practice are presented as argument for and against an analgesic, anaesthetic or surgical

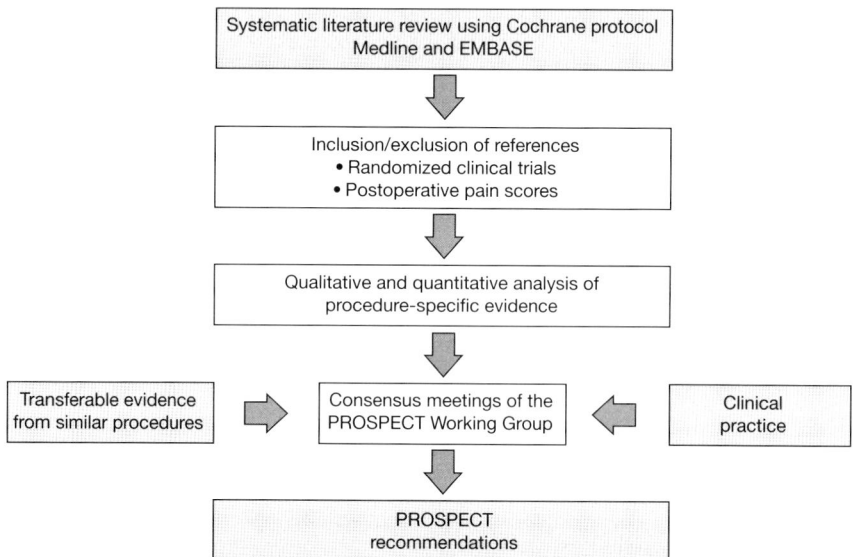

Fig. 4.2 Formulation of PROSPECT recommendations. Source: Kehlet *et al.* (2007).

intervention, together with links to abstracts. The detailed information, including level of evidence and grade of recommendation, allows the readers to make their own decisions based on the strength of the recommendation (Table 4.6). Most importantly, the user can assess the references as well as the quantitative meta-analyses that form the basis of the recommendations.

Table 4.6 The use of local anaesthetic in herniorraphy, laparoscopic cholecystectomy and abdominal hysterectomy

(A) Herniorraphy
- Local anaesthetic injection techniques (inguinal nerve block/field block/infiltration), administered preoperatively or intraoperatively, or both, are recommended (grade A) because they reduce early postoperative pain and supplementary analgesic use compared with placebo. The effect of preoperative administration is similar to that of post-incisional administration
- There are insufficient data to recommend (grade D) one injection technique (inguinal nerve block/field block/infiltration), or combination, in preference to another
- Local anaesthetic instillation administered at closure cannot be recommended at this time despite evidence for its analgesic efficacy, because of limited data (grade D)
- Long-acting local anaesthetics are recommended in preference to short-acting local anaesthetics (grade D)
- Addition of adrenaline to local anaesthetic solution is not recommended because of lack of additional or prolonged analgesic effect from limited procedure-specific data (grade A)
- Postoperative continuous wound infusion with local anaesthetic cannot be recommended at this time, despite evidence for its analgesic efficacy, because of limited data (grade D)
- Postoperative single/repeat dose of local anaesthetic by catheter in the wound is not recommended because of lack of analgesic effect (grade A)
- Subfascial infiltration with local anaesthetic cannot be recommended in preference to subcutaneous infiltration at this time because of limited data (grade D)

(B) Laparoscopic cholecystectomy
- Incisional local anaesthetic infiltration is recommended at the end of surgery (grade A). Combined incisional/intraperitoneal local anaesthetic is recommended (grade C) provided dose is monitored to prevent toxicity
- Despite analgesic effects (grade C), interpleural local anaesthetics are not recommended due to the invasive nature of the technique
- Intraperitoneal local anaesthetics are recommended, although the effects are of limited duration (grade A)

(C) Abdominal hysterectomy
- Intraoperative wound infiltration is recommended based on specific evidence that it reduces pain following hysterectomy at 8h (grade A). Although this outcome did not reach clinical significance, this method of analgesia is convenient and has a favourable safety profile
- Intraperitoneal analgesia is not recommended based on its lack of benefit in reducing pain scores and supplementary analgesic consumption following abdominal hysterectomy (grade A)
- Postoperative wound infiltration administered by PCA may have a benefit in controlling postoperative pain, but there is not currently enough evidence to recommend it

Source: Kehlet *et al.* (2007).

Comment

With more extensive and potentially more painful surgical procedures being performed on an outpatient basis, there is an increased need for prolonged dynamic postoperative pain relief, particularly after discharge home |42|. Procedure-specific pain management protocols should facilitate postoperative pain therapy. These protocols consider all aspects of perioperative period, including surgical techniques, and provide an optimal multimodal approach to perioperative pain management.

Ondansetron and dexamethasone dose combinations for prophylaxis against postoperative nausea and vomiting

Paech MJ, Rucklidge MW, Lain J, *et al*. *Anesth Analg* 2007; **104**: 808–14

BACKGROUND. Postoperative nausea and vomiting (PONV) is one of the common complications that can delay recovery after ambulatory surgery. The incidence of PONV can be minimized by using prophylactic anti-emetics in patients 'at risk' for developing this complication |43|. Limited efficacy of a single anti-emetic has prompted the use of combinations of anti-emetics with different mechanism of action (e.g. 5-HT$_3$-receptor antagonists, droperidol, dexamethasone, scopolamine patch and neurokinin (NK$_1$)-receptor antagonist, aprepitant). The potential combinations include a 5HT$_3$ antagonist (particularly ondansetron because it is now generic) and droperidol or dexamethasone. Droperidol (0.625–1.25 mg) is an excellent anti-emetic, but it has fallen out of favour because of the 'boxed' warning for arrhythmias, although this warning is unfounded. Dexamethasone is becoming popular because in addition to its anti-emetic effects |44| it also has analgesic properties that could be highly beneficial in the ambulatory setting. Furthermore, steroids may attenuate postoperative fatigue and improve outcome |45–47|. The combination of ondansetron and dexamethasone appears to be most appealing. However, the optimal doses of these anti-emetic combinations remain unclear. This double-blind study was designed to determine the efficacy of combinations of ondansetron and dexamethasone in preventing postoperative nausea and vomiting. Women undergoing ambulatory gynaecological laparoscopic procedures were randomized to receive combinations of dexamethasone 4 mg and ondansetron 4 mg; dexamethasone 4 mg and ondansetron 2 mg; dexamethasone 2 mg and ondansetron 4 mg; or dexamethasone 2 mg and ondansetron 2 mg.

INTERPRETATION. There were no differences between the groups with respect to incidence of vomiting, no nausea and no vomiting, need for anti-emetic therapy until 24 h postoperatively (Table 4.7, Fig. 4.3). In addition, there were no differences in the recovery scores, time to discharge or patient satisfaction. However, the 24-h incidence of nausea in patients receiving dexamethasone 2 mg and ondansetron 2 mg was higher than the other groups.

Table 4.7 Incidence of nausea, vomiting and need for rescue anti-emetics in the four groups

	D4/04	D4/02	D2/04	D2/02
PACU data (n)	154	151	154	155
24-h data (n)	141	140	149	149
Nausea				
PACU	17 (11)	12 (8)	18 (12)	19 (13)
Until discharge	48 (31)	38 (25)	59 (38)	56 (37)
From discharge to 24 h	38 (25)	28 (20)	42 (28)	45 (31)
Any time	65 (43)	52 (36)	77 (51)	76 (51)*
No nausea and no vomiting				
Until discharge	106 (69)	116 (77)	108 (70)	105 (68)
Until 24 h	79 (53)	94 (65)	90 (59)	82 (54)
Rescue anti-emetics				
PACU	6 (4)	7 (5)	12 (8)	10 (7)
Until discharge	23 (15)	24 (16)	28 (18)	30 (19)
From discharge to 24 h	6 (4)	2 (1)	4 (3)	1 (0.7)
Any time	25 (17)	24 (17)	29 (19)	31 (20)
Complete response	127 (82)	125 (83)	124 (81)	124 (80)

Values are number (%); *$P = 0.03$. D4/04 = dexamethasone 4 mg/ondansetron 4 mg, D4/02 = dexamethasone 4 mg/ondansetron 2 mg, D2/04 = dexamethasone 2 mg/ondansetron 4 mg, D2/02 = dexamethasone 2 mg/ondansetron 2 mg.
Source: Paech et al. (2007).

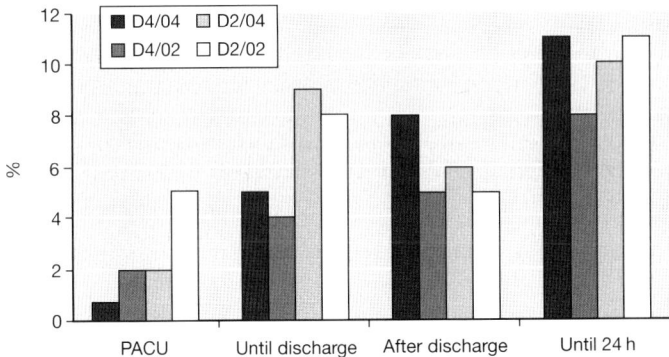

Fig. 4.3 The incidence of vomiting. PACU, post-anaesthesia care unit; D4/04, dexamethasone 4 mg/ondansetron 4 mg; D4/02, dexamethasone 4 mg/ondansetron 2 mg; D2/04, dexamethasone 2 mg/ondansetron 4 mg; D2/02, dexamethasone 2 mg/ondansetron 2 mg. Source: Paech et al. (2007).

Comment

This study provides the optimal doses for ondansetron and dexamethasone combinations. However, the study was limited by the small sample size. Although some might criticize the lack of a placebo group, it may not be considered ethical to omit prophylactic anti-emetics in patients at high PONV risk. Although steroids appear to be optimal for ambulatory surgery, there are concerns regarding the potential adverse effects, which include increased infection rate, gastrointestinal side-effects and delayed wound healing. However, single doses of steroids have not been found to cause any significant adverse effects |47|. Of note, the studies have been small and have not included patients at risk.

It is recommended that the number of prophylactic anti-emetics should be based on the patient's level of risk. The risk factors for PONV include female gender, non-smoker status, history of motion sickness or previous PONV, use of inhalation anaesthesia, postoperative use of opioids and duration of surgery. A large, multicentre, randomized trial found that ondansetron, droperidol, dexamethasone and total intravenous anaesthesia (TIVA) with propofol all reduced the relative PONV incidence by approximately 25–30%. Combining any of these anti-emetics leads to additive (not synergistic) effects. Thus, the first anti-emetic leads to the largest absolute reduction; each subsequent anti-emetic results in a smaller absolute additional effect.

Finally, anti-emetic prophylaxis with $5HT_3$ antagonist has become standard of care in ambulatory anaesthesia. In patients at moderate-to-severe PONV risk, a $5HT_3$ antagonist is usually combined with other anti-emetics (e.g. dexamethasone and/or droperidol). In addition, scopolamine patch and/or aprepitant may be used in patients at very high PONV risk.

An analysis of factors influencing post-anaesthesia recovery after paediatric ambulatory tonsillectomy and adenoidectomy

Edler AA, Mariano ER, Golianu B, et al. Anesth Analg 2007; **104**: 784–9

BACKGROUND. There are several unique aspects to the post-anaesthesia care of the paediatric patient, such as emergence agitation, post-intubation croup, apnoea of prematurity and parental presence, that can contribute to prolonged length of stay (LOS) for paediatric patients in the PACU |48,49|. So far, studies have identified individual preoperative risk factors or adverse effects which can prolong LOS. No study to date has explored the interaction between these independent factors or identified their composite impact on prolonging LOS. The authors set out to identify in a prospective manner the pre- and postoperative factors that prolong LOS for paediatric patients in the PACU following tonsillectomy and adenoidectomy, and bilateral myringotomy with tube insertion under general anaesthesia.

INTERPRETATION. Of the 169 patients aged 1–18 years enrolled in the study over a period of 13 months, three required unplanned hospital admission (two due to postoperative bleeding, the third due to lack of transportation). The primary outcome measure was LOS in the PACU, defined as the time interval from time of arrival in the PACU until the patient was deemed 'home-ready', based on a standard Aldrete score modified for paediatric patients. Mean LOS was 106 ± 52 min. The authors found significant associations ($P<0.05$) between increasing age, number of episodes of PONV or retching (accounting for anti-emetic treatment), and number of oxygen desaturations when supplemental opioid was administered in the PACU. Each episode of postoperative nausea and vomiting or oxygen desaturation to <95% increased the patient's LOS by 0.5 h. For each year of age above 1, the chances of prolonged LOS decreased by 2.2% (Table 4.8).

Comment

Surprisingly, history of upper respiratory tract infection, emergence agitation and parental anxiety did not significantly predict increased LOS. However, the statistical model used was able to account for only 43% of the variability in LOS. Although this was significantly more than in past investigations, this finding confirms the presence and importance of individual variability in post-anaesthetic recovery (e.g. emergence agitation may affect LOS in the PACU in one patient but not another). The strength of this study lies with the fact that it provides the first composite view of LOS in paediatric patients after ambulatory surgery. The authors identified PONV and desaturation as the two major factors contributing to prolonged LOS in paediatric patients undergoing tonsillectomy and adenoidectomy, with the overall risk of prolonged LOS decreasing with age. Patients who did not experience PONV had up to 80% shorter recovery times in the PACU. Similarly, patients who did not experience oxygen desaturation required 50% less recovery time in the PACU. The implication of this is that aggressive prophylaxis of PONV, careful airway management and pain strategies not requiring supplemental opioids in PACU can potentially reduce LOS and thus improve outcome and cost-effectiveness of care in paediatric surgical outpatients.

Table 4.8 Final linear regression model

	B coefficient (min)	95% CI (min)	P-value
Age	0.022	0.01–0.05	<0.05
Episodes of PONV, complaints of nausea or episodes of retching	31*	7–54	<0.05
Episodes of oxygen desaturation <95%	28†	10–47	<0.05

PONV, postoperative nausea and vomiting.
*Adjusted for the use of varied and/or multiple intraoperative anti-emetic regimes.
†Adjusted for supplemental doses of opioid in the post-anaesthesia care unit.
Source: Edler et al. (2007)

Conclusion

Ambulatory anaesthesia has a secure place in our current clinical practice. The focus is now on quality assurance and patient satisfaction throughout the perioperative patient care. Practice guidelines for the perioperative management of patients (e.g. for patients with obstructive sleep apnoea) are intended to enhance patient safety. Similarly, using a reliable index of elevated risk of inpatient hospital admission immediately following outpatient surgery may lead to improved patient safety and high-quality care. Although the controversy around the use of nitrous oxide may not seem to affect the ambulatory setting, its use may reduce the incidence of awareness. The incidence of intraoperative awareness in ambulatory anaesthesia, although very low, is of major concern to patients. Similar to the introduction of propofol that revolutionized anaesthesia practice, it is expected that sugammadex has the potential to revolutionize reversal of neuromuscular blockade and improve patient safety.

Regional anaesthesia proves to be the cornerstone of multimodal analgesia in the ambulatory setting. Spinal anaesthesia is not only feasible but advocated with certain modifications of the technique and reintroduction of local anaesthetic agents such as 2-chloroprocaine |34,50–51| and articaine |52|. The duration of analgesia obtained with peripheral nerve blocks could be extended beyond the effect of a single bolus using perineural continuous infusions. They provide excellent analgesia, facilitate early discharge, optimal functional exercise capacity and daily activity at home. In addition, ambulatory perineural catheters may be a rare instance of a new technology holding the promise of both improving outcomes and reducing societal costs |53|. Implementation of PROSPECT evidence-based procedure-specific postoperative pain management protocols should improve postoperative pain relief and facilitate recovery and return to daily living. A multimodal approach to the prophylaxis and treatment of PONV will increase patient satisfaction. It should extend beyond the immediate postoperative period in order to minimize PONV after discharge home.

Children benefit particularly from day-care surgery, and recent years have seen a huge expansion of this modality of care. Attitudes are changing with regard to the management of children undergoing tonsillectomy and adenoidectomy. More units in Europe are moving towards North American-style same-day care. Improvements in anaesthetic techniques, pain control, PONV prophylaxis and surgical techniques have all contributed to this trend |54|.

References

1. National Center for Health Statistics. Hospital admissions, average length of stay, and outpatient visits, according to type of ownership and size of hospital, and percent outpatient surgery; United States, selected years 1975–2000 [Table 96]. I: Health, United States, 2002, With Chartbook on Trends in the Health of Americans. Hyattsville, MD; NCHS; 2002.

2. Hausman LM, Levine AI, Rosenblatt MA. A survey evaluating the training of anesthesiology residents in office-based anesthesia. *J Clin Anesth* 2006; **18**: 499–503.

3. Mezei G, Chung F. Return hospital visits and hospital readmissions after ambulatory surgery. *Ann Surg* 1999; **230**: 721–7.

4. Joshi GP. Ambulatory surgery for the patient with obstructive sleep apnea syndrome. *American Society of Anesthesiologists Refresher Course lectures* 2007; **35**: 97–106.

5. Yogneswaran B, Yuan H, Chung S, Shapiro C, Chung F. OSA questionnaire: a new short-form screening tool for obstructive sleep apnea (OSA) patients. *Anesthesiology* 2006; **105**: A993.

6. Deyo RA, Cherkin DC, Ciol MA. Adapting a clinical comorbidity index for use with *ICD-9-CM* administrative databases. *J Clin Epidemiol* 1992; **45**: 613–19.

7. Correll DJ, Bader AM, Hull MW, Hsu C, Tsen LC, Hepner DL. Value of preoperative clinic visits in identifying issues with potential impact on operating room efficiency. economics. *Anesthesiology* 2006; **105**: 1254–9.

8. Sherman SJ, Cullen BF. Nitrous oxide and the greenhouse effect (editorial). *Anesthesiology* 1988; **68**: 816–17.

9. Taylor E, Feinstein R, White PF, Soper N. Anesthesia for laparoscopic cholecystectomy. Is nitrous oxide contraindicated? *Anesthesiology* 1992; **76**: 541–3.

10. Tramér M, Moore A, McQuay H. Omitting nitrous oxide in general anaesthesia: meta-analysis of intraoperative awareness and postoperative emesis in randomized controlled trials. *Br J Anaesth* 1996; **76**: 186–93.

11. Hall JE, Stewart JIM, Harmer M. Single-breath inhalation induction of sevoflurane anaesthesia with and without nitrous oxide: a feasibility study in adults and comparison with an intravenous bolus of propofol. *Anaesthesia* 1997; **52**: 410–15.

12. Peyton PJ, Stuart-Andrews C, Deo K, *et al.* Persisting concentrating and second gas effects on oxygenation during N_2O anaesthesia. *Anaesthesia* 2006; **61**: 322–9.

13. Barr G, Jakobsson JG, Owall A, Anderson RE. Nitrous oxide does not alter bispectral index: study with nitrous oxide as sole agent and as an adjunct to IV anaesthesia. *Br J Anaesth* 1999; **82**: 827–30.

14. Sanders RD, Franks NP, Maze M. Xenon: no stranger to anaesthesia. *Br J Anaesth* 2003; **91**: 709–17.

15. Joshi GP, Gertler R. Fast track general anesthesia and ambulatory discharge criteria. In: Steele SM, Nielsen KC, Klein SM, eds. *Ambulatory Anesthesia and Perioperative Analgesia.* New York: McGraw-Hill; 2005, pp. 233–8.

16. Ghoneim MM. Awareness during anesthesia. *Anesthesiology* 2001; **92**: 597–602.

17. Practice advisory for intraoperative awareness and brain function monitoring: a report by the American Society of Anesthesiologists Task Force on Intraoperative Awareness. *Anesthesiology* 2006; **104**: 847–64.

18. Sebel PS, Browdle TA, Ghoneim MM, Rampil IJ, Padilla RE, Gan TJ, Domino KB. The incidence of awareness during anesthesia: multicenter United States study. *Anesth Analg* 2004; **99**: 833–9.

19. Sandin RH, Enlund G, Samuelsson P, Lennmarkken C. Awareness during anesthesia: a prospective case study. *Lancet* 2000; **355**: 707–11.

20. Niedhart DJ, Kaiser HA, Jacobsohn E, Hantler CB, Evers AS, Avidan MS. Intrapatient reproducibility of the BISxp(R) monitor. *Anesthesiology* 2006; **104**: 242–8.

21. White PF. Use of cerebral monitoring during anaesthesia: effect on recovery profile. *Best Prac Res Clin Anaesthesiol* 2006; **20**: 181–9.

22. Cammu G, De Witte J, De Veylder J, Byttebier G, Vandeput D, Foubert L, Vandenbroucke G, Deloof T. Postoperative residual paralysis in outpatients vs. inpatients. *Anesth Analg* 2006; **102**: 426–9.

23. Sundman E, Witt H, Olsson R, Ekberg O, Kuylenstierna R, Eriksson LI. The incidence and mechanisms of pharyngeal and upper esophageal dysfunction in partially paralyzed humans. *Anesthesiology* 2000; **92**: 977–84.

24. Eriksson LI, Sato M, Severinghaus JW. Effect of a vecuronium-induced partial neuromuscular block on hypoxic ventilatory response. *Anesthesiology* 1993; **78**: 693–9.

25. Kopman AF, Yee PS, Neuman GG. Relationship of the train-of-four fade ratio to clinical signs and symptoms of residual paralysis in awake volunteers. *Anesthesiology* 1997; **86**: 765–71.

26. Naguib M, Kopman AF, Ensor JE. Neuromuscular monitoring and postoperative residual curarisation: a meta-analysis. *Br J Anaesth* 2007; **98**: 302–316.

27. Naguib M. Sugammadex: another milestone in clinical neuromuscular pharmacology. *Anesth Analg* 2007; **104**: 575–81.

28. Groudine SB, Soto R, Lien C, Drover D, Roberts K. Randomized, dose-finding, phase II study of the selective relaxant binding drug, sugammadex, capable of safely reversing profound rocuronium-induced neuromuscular block. *Anesth Analg* 2007; **104**: 555–62.

29. Suy K, Morias K, Cammu G, Hans P, van Duijnhoven WG, Heeringa M, Demeyer I. Effective reversal of moderate rocuronium- or vecuronium-induced neuromuscular block with sugammadex, a selective relaxant binding agent. *Anesthesiology* 2007; **106**: 283–8.

30. de Boer HD, van Egmond J, van de Pol F, Bom A, Booij LH. Sugammadex, a new reversal agent for neuromuscular block induced by rocuronium in the anaesthetized Rhesus monkey. *Br J Anaesth* 2006; **96**: 201–6.

31. Zaric D, Christiansen C, Pace N, Punjasawadwong Y. Transient neurolgic symptoms after spinal anesthesia with lidocaine versus other local anesthetics: a systematic review of randomized, controlled trials. *Anesth Analg* 2005; **100**: 1811–16.

32. Kouri ME, Kopacz DJ. Spinal 2-chloroprocaine: a comparison with lidocaine in volunteers. *Anesth Analg* 2004; **98**: 75–80.

33. Smith KN, Kopacz DJ, McDonald SB. Spinal 2-chloroprocaine: a dose-ranging study and the effect of added epinephrine. *Anesth Analg* 2004; **98**: 81–8.

34. Casati A, Danelli G, Berti M, Fioro A, Fanelli A, Benassi C, Petronella G, Fanelli G. Intrathecal 2-chloroprocaine for lower limb outpatient surgery: a prospective, randomized, double-blind, clinical evaluation. *Anesth Analg* 2006; **103**: 234–8.

35. Joshi GP: Multimodal analgesia techniques for ambulatory surgery. *Intern Anesthesiol Clin* 2005; **43**: 215–18.

36. Apfelbaum JL, Chen C, Shilpa S, Gan TJ. Postoperative pain experience: results from a national survey suggest postoperative pain continues to be undermanaged. *Anesth Analg* 2003; **97**: 534–40.

37. American Society of Anesthesiologists Task Force on Acute Pain Management: Practice guidelines for acute pain management in the perioperative setting: an updated report by American Society of Anesthesiologists Task Force on Acute Pain Management. *Anesthesiology* 2004; **100**: 1573–81.

38. Acute Pain Guidelines: Scientific Evidence; 2005. Available at: www.nhmrc.gov.au/publications/synopses/cp104syn.htm.

39. McQuay H, Moore RA. *An Evidence-based Resource for Pain Relief*. Oxford: Oxford University Press, 1998.

40. Gray A, Kehlet H, Bonnet F, Rawal N. Predicting postoperative analgesia outcomes: NNT league tables or procedure-specific evidence? *Br J Anaesth* 2005; **94**: 710–14.

41. Neugebauer E, Wilkinson R, Kehlet H, Schug SA. PROSPECT: a practical method for formulating evidence-based expert recommendations for the management of postoperative pain. *Surg Endosc* 2007; **21**:

42. Wu CL, Berenholtz SM, Pronovost PJ, Fleisher LA. Systematic review and analysis of postdischarge symptoms after outpatient surgery. *Anesthesiology* 2002; **96**: 994–1003.

43. Apfel CC, Kortilla K, Abdalla M, Kerger H, Turan A, Veddar I, *et al*. A factorial trial of six interventions for the prevention of postoperative nausea and vomiting. *N Engl J Med* 2004; **350**: 2441–51.

44. Henzi I, Walder B, Tramer MR. Dexamethasone for the prevention of postoperative nausea and vomiting: a quantitative systematic review. *Anesth Analg* 2000; **90**: 186–94.

45. Romundstad L, Breivik H, Roald H, Skolleborg K, Haugen T, Narum J, Stubhaug A. Methylprednisolone reduces pain, emesis, and fatigue after breast augmentation surgery: a single-dose, randomized, parallel-group study with methylprednisolone 125 mg, parecoxib 40 mg, and placebo. *Anesth Analg* 2006; **102**: 418–25.

46. Rubin GJ, Hotopf M. Systematic review and meta-analysis of interventions for postoperative fatigue. *Br J Surg* 2002; **89**: 971–84.

47. Bisgaard T, Klarskov B, Khelet H, Rosenberg J. Preoperative dexamethasone improves surgical outcome after laparoscopic cholecystectomy: a randomized double blind placebo-controlled trial. *Ann Surg* 2003; **238**: 651–60.

48. Cole JW, Murray DJ, McAllister JD, Hirshberg GE. Emergence behaviour in children: defining the incidence of excitement and agitation following anaesthesia. *Paediatr Anaesth* 2002; **12**: 442–7.

49. Coté CJ, Zaslavsky A, Downes JJ, Kurth CD, Welborn LG, Warner LO, Malviya SV. Postoperative apnea in former preterm infants after inguinal herniorrhaphy. A combined analysis. *Anesthesiology* 1995; **82**: 809–22.

50. Kouri ME, Kopacz DJ. Spinal 2-chloroprocaine: a comparison with lidocaine in volunteers. *Anesth Analg* 2004; **98**: 75–80.

51. Smith KN, Kopacz DJ, McDonald SB. Spinal 2-chloroprocaine: a dose-ranging study and the effect of added epinephrine. *Anesth Analg* 2004; **98**: 81–8.

52. Kallio H, Snäll EVT, Luode T, Rosenberg PH. Hyperbaric articaine for day-case spinal anaesthesia. *Br J Anaesth* 2006; **97**: 704–9.

53. Ilfeld BM, Mariano ER, Williams BA, Woodard JN, Macario A. Hospitalization costs of total knee arthroplasty with a continuous femoral nerve block provided only in the hospital versus on an ambulatory basis: a retrospective, case-control, cost-minimization analysis. *Reg Anesth Pain Med* 2007; **32**: 46–54.

54. Lonnqvist PA, Morton NS. Paediatric day-case anaesthesia and pain control. *Curr Opin Anaesthesiol* 2006; **19**: 617–21.

Part II

Clinical pharmacology

What's new in anaesthetic pharmacology?

MICHEL STRUYS

Currently, the 'anaesthetic state' is considered to be a combination of three important clinical endpoints: hypnosis, antinociception and immobility. The hypnotic component of anaesthesia can be managed by both intravenous and/or inhaled hypnotic–anaesthetic drugs and aims to achieve a predefined level of 'unconsciousness' (sedation) and 'amnesia' (loss of explicit memory formation) [1]. Hypnotic drugs have a distinct effect on both, although the intensity and dose–effect relationship can be variable between molecules [2]. Secondly, the analgesic component of anaesthesia is considered crucial, too, as it might be related to clinical outcome [3,4]. Nociception caused by an injury or trauma during anaesthesia results in autonomic, hormonal and metabolic changes in the body. As the patient is unconscious during anaesthesia, conscious pain reactions are absent; however, activation of the sympathetic neural and autonomic humoral pathways results in various physiological changes, such as the haemodynamic status of the patient. This 'nociceptive cascade' can be blunted by administering anti-nociceptive medication [5]. Immobility can be considered the third endpoint to obtain an adequate surgical level of anaesthesia. Involuntary reflex movements can occur as a response of pain, also voluntary movement might but occur during periods of insufficient hypnotic drug effect. Immobility can be achieved by accurate combinations of hypnotics and analgesics; however, to facilitate surgical procedures, neuromuscular blocking agents are frequently used.

'Anaesthetic pharmacology' is classically related to the development of the three classes of drugs typically associated with anaesthesia practice: hypnotics, analgesics and neuromuscular blocking agents. However, their reversal agents (if required) should be studied too. In order to create successful drugs, a knowledge of the underlying physiological and pharmacological mechanisms is crucial to fully understand the potential drug action of a candidate drug. Recently, we have witnessed the start of a revolution in our understanding of how anaesthesia is produced and how drugs used by anaesthetists work at a molecular level that might lead to further drug discovery and use optimization. Drugs exert their effects in various ways ranging from the simple actions that depend on their physicochemical properties of a drug to specific actions at enzymes and receptors. In the quest to fully understand the mechanisms of the components of anaesthesia, receptors are considered important. In Chapter 8, David Lambert describes the most important recent findings in this area.

Progress has been made in the understanding of all three classes of 'anaesthesia-related drugs', although no new drugs have reached the market yet. We reported extensively on the development of new and 'renewed' hypnotic drugs in the previous edition of *The Year in Anaesthesia and Critical Care* |6|. Since then, clinical and preclinical studies have progressed slowly but no large studies have yet been published.

The control of the nociception–antinociception balance has been perhaps the most exciting area of pharmaceutical creativity and development related to the practice of anaesthesia. Many international organizations, such as the World Health Organization, consider an adequate treatment of pain as a basic human right; however, for about 80% of the world's population, pain relief when needed is a right yet to be realized |7|. Novel therapies for pain cover widespread clinical needs and therefore constitute a continued opportunity for major pharmaceutical drug research. New treatments are likely to arise from better understanding of both the pathophysiology of clinical pain conditions and the pharmacology of existing therapies. Our knowledge of nociception pathways and mechanisms is growing every day, leading to the discovery of potential new therapeutic molecules. In the field of anaesthesia, acute and chronic pain medicine and critical care, new reports can be found on both centrally and peripherally acting analgesics based on their underlying mechanisms of action. Additionally, for the opioids, better administration techniques for fentanyl and morphine have been described. Transdermal fentanyl is now used for cancer pain, and it was followed by the subsequent introduction of oral transmucosal fentanyl for 'breakthrough pain'. Furthermore, Lennernäs and co-workers |8| have reported on the pharmacokinetics and tolerability of different doses of fentanyl following sublingual administration of a rapid-dissolving tablet for the relief of cancer pain. And a device the size of a matchstick that delivers systemic sufentanil subdermally via an injectable osmotic pump has been introduced for the relief of chronic pain |9|. Older drugs, such as morphine, have been reintroduced in long-acting formulation by using liposomal techniques |10| The analgesic activity of other centrally acting substances such as melatonin and the cannabinoids have led to these drugs being reported as being potentially important new classes of analgesics |11|. Among peripherally acting analgesics, peripheral kappa-opioid agonists |12| and peripheral opioids acting through 'transient receptor potential V1' ion channels have been investigated. More details are revealed by Peter Goldstein in Chapter 5 of this book. He also focuses on other important areas, including ionotropic purinergic (P_{2X}) receptors, voltage-gated sodium (Na_V) channels, hyperpolarization-activated cyclic nucleotide (HCN)-gated channels, and bradykinin and cytokine receptors.

Although immobility during anaesthesia can be achieved by an optimal combination of hypnotics and analgesia, facilitation of laryngoscopy, intubation and surgical access in dedicated areas requires the use of neuromuscular blocking agents. The ideal neuromuscular blocking agent would be non-depolarizing, with a rapid onset and offset and without side-effects such as histamine release. So far, no such drug has reached the market. Some early development on a new fast-onset (although somewhat slower than succinylcholine), short-acting, non-depolarizing neuromuscular blocking agent, called GW280430A, has been reported by various authors |13–20|. GW280430A is an asymmetric mixed-onium chlorofumarate, which is a novel structure for a muscle relaxant, although it has many similarities to mivacurium. Rocuronium remains the drug with the most rapid onset of action but, unfortunately, it is a medium- to long-acting agent. Improper titration of rocuronium, leading to a potential residual block at recovery of anaesthesia, is still subject to reversal with an anticholinesterase such as neostigmine. The side-effects of these reversal drugs are well known; unfortunately, we do not have better solutions commercially available today |21|. This might change with the introduction of a new reversal drug, called sugammadex (Org 25969, Organon, Oss, The Netherlands), which is a gamma-cyclodextrin designed to chelate or encapsulate the rocuronium. As recently stated by Hunter and Flockton |21| in an editorial in the *British Journal of Anaesthesia*, it looks like 'a doughnut and a hole' because it has a pocket that specifically binds the available rocuronium, thereby rapidly and completely reversing neuromuscular blockade, even in the presence of a deep block. If suggamadex does not have some yet non-discovered toxicity or side-effects, it will render conventional pharmacological reversal of neuromuscular blockade obsolete. Various recent investigations on suggamadex have been reported and are detailed in Chapter 7 of this book by Mitchell and Hunter.

Alongside the development of new drugs, optimization in drug delivery of existing drugs can result in a beneficial therapeutic outcome. This can be done by optimizing the physicochemical characteristics of the existing drugs, thereby enhancing the pharmacokinetic and dynamic properties (e.g. longer duration of action by using liposomal techniques), avoiding side-effects by introducing novel pharmaceutical formulations (e.g. avoiding pain on injection with propofol |22,23|) or by studying the possibilities of alternative routes of administration other than intravenous. Over the last few years, anaesthetists have asked for alternatives routes of administration to the classical (painful) intramuscular and intravenous administration, certainly in the paediatric populations. Intranasal administration of fentanyl, sufentanil, diamorphine and ketamine has been successfully applied under various conditions |24–27|. Orally administered fentanyl has been studied; however, success has been limited because of the large variability of the time to peak concentration, making it difficult to suggest a minimum interval between administration and the start of the painful stimulus |28|.

Thanks to the miniaturization of electronics in combination with new pharmaceutical techniques, various 'electronically' controlled drug delivery systems have been developed. In this area, transdermal drug delivery can be viewed as another alternative. The potential benefits of transdermal delivery have inspired several companies to overcome the challenges the skin presents as a barrier by developing active delivery technology. These systems use energy to enhance compounds crossing the 10- to 20-μm dead layer of the stratum corneum, which represents the major barrier. The technologies currently under development can be divided into two categories. The first uses iontophoresis, which allows particles to move across the skin by applying an electric current over two skin electrodes. A little reservoir holds the drug. The other type of active transdermal delivery systems, known as poration technologies, uses high-frequency pulses of energy temporarily to 'disrupt' the stratum corneum |29|. More details of new administration and delivery systems are given by Robert Sneyd in Chapter 6.

In conclusion, it can be stated that even though anaesthesia and intensive care represent relatively small markets for pharmaceutical companies, interesting pharmacological developments are in progress and might result in some new exciting therapeutical solutions. In this way, the growing knowledge of underlying physiological and pharmacological mechanisms is playing an important role in new drug development.

References

1. Veselis RA, Reinsel RA, Feshchenko VA. Drug-induced amnesia is a separate phenomenon from sedation: electrophysiologic evidence. *Anesthesiology* 2001; **95**: 896–907.

2. Veselis RA. Gone but not forgotten – or was it? *Br J Anaesth* 2004; **92**: 161–3.

3. Riles TS, Fisher FS, Schaefer S, Pasternack PF, Baumann FG. Plasma catecholamine concentrations during abdominal aortic aneurysm surgery: the link to perioperative myocardial ischemia. *Ann Vasc Surg* 1993; 7: 213–19.

4. Parker SD, Breslow MJ, Frank SM, *et al.* Catecholamine and cortisol responses to lower extremity revascularization: correlation with outcome variables. Perioperative Ischemia Randomized Anesthesia Trial Study Group. *Crit Care Med* 1995; **23**: 1954–61.

5. Huiku M, Uutela K, van Gils M, *et al.* Assessment of surgical stress during general anaesthesia. *Br J Anaesth* 2006; **98**: 447–55.

6. Ihmsen H. New hypnotics. In: Hunter J, Cook T, Pribe H, Struys M, eds. *The Year in Anaesthesia and Intensive Care.* Oxford: Clinical Publishing; 2005, 123–32.

7. Scholten W, Nygren-Krug H, Zucker HA. The World Health Organization paves the way for action to free people from the shackles of pain. *Anesth Analg* 2007; **105**: 1–4.

8. Lennernäs B, Hedner T, Holmberg M, Bredenberg S, Nystrom C, Lennernäs H. Pharmacokinetics and tolerability of different doses of fentanyl following sublingual administration of a rapidly dissolving tablet to cancer patients: a new approach to treatment of incident pain. *Br J Clin Pharmacol* 2005; **59**: 249–53.

9. Fisher DM, Kellett N, Lenhardt R. Pharmacokinetics of an implanted osmotic pump delivering sufentanil for the treatment of chronic pain. *Anesthesiology* 2003; **99**: 929–37.

10. Viscusi ER, Martin G, Hartrick CT, Singla N, Manvelian G. Forty-eight hours of postoperative pain relief after total hip arthroplasty with a novel, extended-release epidural morphine formulation. *Anesthesiology* 2005; **102**: 1014–22.

11. Shafer S. The future of anesthetic pharmacology. *Anesth Analg* 2007; 104 (Suppl.): S69–S74.

12. Eisenach JC, Carpenter R, Curry R. Analgesia from a peripherally active kappa-opioid receptor agonist in patients with chronic pancreatitis. *Pain* 2003; **101**: 89–95.

13. Gyermek L. Development of ultra short-acting muscle relaxant agents: history, research strategies, and challenges. *Medicinal research reviews* 2005; **25**: 610–54.

14. Geldner GF, Blobner M. GW280430A. *Anesthesiology* 2005; **102**: 861; author reply 2–5.

15. Lien CA, Belmont MR, Heerdt PM. GW280430A: pharmacodynamics and potential adverse effects. *Anesthesiology* 2005; **102**: 861–2; author reply 2–3.

16. Heerdt PM, Kang R, The A, Hashim M, Mook RJ Jr, Savarese JJ. Cardiopulmonary effects of the novel neuromuscular blocking drug GW280430A (AV430A) in dogs. *Anesthesiology* 2004; **100**: 846–51.

17. Savarese JJ, Belmont MR, Hashim MA, Bradley E, Stein B, Patel SS, Savarese JJ. Preclinical pharmacology of GW280430A (AV430A) in the rhesus monkey and in the cat: a comparison with mivacurium. *Anesthesiology* 2004; **100**: 835–45.

18. Belmont MR, Lien CA, Tjan J, Bradley E, Stein B, Patel SS, Savarese JJ. Clinical pharmacology of GW280430A in humans. *Anesthesiology* 2004; **100**: 768–73.

19. Zhu H, Meserve K, Floyd A. Preformulation studies for an ultrashort-acting neuromuscular blocking agent GW280430A. I. Buffer and cosolvent effects on the solution stability. *Drug Development and Industrial Pharmacy* 2002; **28**: 135–42.

20. Zhu HJ, Sacchetti M. Solid state characterization of an neuromuscular blocking agent – GW280430A. *International Journal of Pharmaceutics* 2002; **234**: 19–23.

21. Hunter JM, Flockton EA. The doughnut and the hole: a new pharmacological concept for anaesthetists. *Br J Anaesth* 2006; **97**: 123–6.

22. Gibiansky E, Struys MM, Gibiansky L, Vanluchene AL, Vornov J, Mortier EP, Burak E, Van Bortel L. AQUAVAN injection, a water-soluble prodrug of propofol, as a bolus injection: a phase I dose-escalation comparison with DIPRIVAN (part 1): pharmacokinetics. *Anesthesiology* 2005; **103**: 718–29.

23. Struys MM, Vanluchene AL, Gibiansky E, Gibiansky L, Vornav J, Mortier EP, Van Bortel L. AQUAVAN injection, a water-soluble prodrug of propofol, as a bolus injection: a phase I dose-escalation comparison with DIPRIVAN (part 2): pharmacodynamics and safety. *Anesthesiology* 2005; **103**: 730–43.

24. Hallett A, O'Higgins F, Francis V, Cook TM. Patient-controlled intranasal diamorphine for postoperative pain: an acceptability study. *Anaesthesia* 2000; **55**: 532–9.

25. Paech MJ, Lim CB, Banks SL, Rucklidge MW, Doherty DA. A new formulation of nasal fentanyl spray for postoperative analgesia: a pilot study. *Anaesthesia* 2003; **58**: 740–4.

26. Weber F, Wulf H, Gruber M, Biallas R. S-ketamine and S-norketamine plasma concentrations after nasal and i.v. administration in anesthetized children. *Paediatr Anaesth* 2004; **14**: 983–8.

27. Mathieu N, Cnudde N, Engelman E, Barvais L. Intranasal sufentanil is effective for postoperative analgesia in adults. *Can J Anaesth* 2006; **53**: 60–6.

28. Wheeler M, Birmingham PK, Dsida RM, Wang Z, Cote CJ, Avram MJ. Uptake pharmacokinetics of the Fentanyl Oralet in children scheduled for central venous access removal: implications for the timing of initiating painful procedures. *Paediatr Anaesth* 2002; **12**: 594–9.

29. Wang YT, Q, Fan Q, Michniak B. Transdermal ionotophoresis strategies to improve transdermal iontophoretic drug delivery. *Eur J Pharmacol and Biopharm* 2005; **60**: 179–91.

5

Mechanisms of pain pharmacology: what's new?

PETER A. GOLDSTEIN

Introduction

In general terms, pain is the subjective and emotional experience of a nociceptive stimulus; such a stimulus has the potential to produce injury at the cellular and/ or tissue level. But not all pain is created equally; hence, there is *nociceptive (*or *inflammatory)* pain, which results from the direct activation of nociceptors in the skin or soft tissue in response to injury and inflammation, and *neuropathic pain*, which results from pathology or injury within the nervous (peripheral or central) system |1–3|. There are qualitative differences between the two (Table 5.1), and these differences result in part from differences in the underlying cellular pathways leading to the development and maintenance of the two pain states. Thus, one cannot reasonably discuss mechanisms of pain pharmacology without considering the nature of the pain to be relieved. As the title of this chapter is 'Mechanisms of pain pharmacology', I have selected articles that examine various underlying molecular targets that contribute to inflammatory and neuropathic pain. I have chosen to emphasize one group of ligand-activated ion channels, called transient receptor

Table 5.1 Characteristic features of neuropathic and inflammatory pain

	Neuropathic pain	Inflammatory pain
Positive symptoms and signs		
Spontaneous pain in damaged area	Yes	Yes
Heat hyperalgesia	Rarely	Often
Cold allodynia	Often	Rarely
Hyperpathia	Often	Never
Aftersensations	Often	Rarely
Paroxysms	Often	Rarely
Burning pain	Often	Rarely
Throbbing pain	Rarely	Often
Negative symptoms and signs		
Sensory loss in damaged nerve territory	Yes	No
Motor deficit in damaged nerve territory	Often	No

Source: Kehlet *et al. Lancet* 2006; **367**: 1618–25.

potential (TRP) channels, as some of the most interesting and exciting work in the field of nociceptive signal transduction that has recently focused on these channels. Obviously, other mechanisms contribute to pain sensation and are reasonable therapeutic targets for novel analgesics. Other important areas include ionotropic purinergic (P_{2X}) receptors, voltage-gated sodium (Na_V) channels, hyperpolarization-activated cyclic nucleotide (HCN)-gated channels, and bradykinin and cytokine receptors, and articles discussing these pathways as potential molecular targets for the treatment of pain are also presented.

Cyclin-dependent kinase 5 modulates nociceptive signalling through direct phosphorylation of transient receptor potential vanilloid 1

Pareek TK, Keller J, Kesavapany S, *et al. Proc Natl Acad Sci USA* 2007; **104**: 660–5

BACKGROUND. The transient receptor potential vanilloid 1 (TRPV1) channel belongs to the transient receptor potential (TRP) ion channel family; like other TRPV channels, TRPV1 is expressed in dorsal root and trigeminal ganglion neurons, where it is activated by capsaicin, resiniferatoxin, heat (temperature $\geq 43°C$), hydrogen ions, endocannabinoid lipids (such as anandamide), eicosanoids and 2-aminoethyl diphenylborate. Phosphorylation of TRPV1 is essential for its proper functioning in response to nociceptive stimuli. Here, the authors examined the role of cyclin-dependent kinase 5 (Cdk5) phosphorylation of TRPV1 using *in vitro* assays (including Western blotting and Ca^{2+} imaging) for protein phosphorylation in stably transfected cells and sensory neurons expressing TRPV1, and nociceptive behavioural testing in mice with a restricted Cdk5 pattern of expression (conditional Cdk5 knockout).

INTERPRETATION. Using immunoprecipitation and Western blotting, Pareek and colleagues demonstrate that Cdk5 phosphorylates TRPV1 in fibroblast cells stably transfected with TRPV1 and cultured primary dorsal root ganglion (DRG) neurons at threonine-407; the extent of TRPV1 phosphorylation was markedly decreased in Cdk5 knockout mice. Assessment of the function of phosphorylated TRPV1 was determined using a $^{45}Ca^{2+}$ uptake assay, and inhibition of Cdk5 activity with roscovitine decreases capsaicin-induced $^{45}Ca^{2+}$ uptake in DRG neurons in a concentration-dependent manner. The authors also created a conditional Cdk5 knockout mouse in which the deletion was restricted to C-fibre-specific primary afferent neurons; TRPV1 phosphorylation in dorsal root and trigeminal ganglia neurons was markedly decreased, and conditional Cdk5 knockout mice showed marked increases in paw and tail withdrawal latency times in response to noxious heat stimuli. The authors conclude that TRPV1 phosphorylation by Cdk5 is important in the regulation of pain signalling.

Comment

Capsaicin, the pungent compound contained in spicy ('hot') peppers (spp. *capsicum*), was long known to modulate nociceptive transmission in the superficial dorsal horn of the spinal cord, but the underlying mechanism remained elusive. In a landmark study in 1997, Michael Caterina, working in the laboratory of David Julius at the University of California, San Francisco, identified and cloned the gene coding for the vanilloid capsaicin receptor, which they named VR1 |4|, and which was subsequently found to belong to the superfamily of TRP channels and was renamed TRPV1 |5,6|. Not only was the channel gated by capsaicin, it was also directly activated by heat |7|. In the logical follow-up study, Caterina and co-authors |8| created a mouse lacking the TRPV1 channel, and they very elegantly demonstrated that the channel was a critical component of the signal transduction pathway responsible for sensing noxious thermal, but not mechanical, stimuli.

To date, six subfamilies of TRP receptors have been identified, which in turn have a variable number of named channels: TRPC(1–7), TRPV(1–6), TRPM(1–7), TRPA(1), TRPP(2,3,5) and TRPM(1–3) |9|. TRPV, TRPM and TRPA channels have drawn extensive attention over the past decade as critical components in various signal transduction pathways in pain signalling, and a number of studies from the recent literature are discussed here. For readers seeking a more comprehensive understanding of TRP channels and their role in nociception, there are a number of excellent review articles worth reading |6,9,10|.

Phosphorylation is a critical step in the functional regulation of many proteins, and phosphorylation of TRPV1 is essential for its proper functioning in response to nociceptive stimuli |11–13|. The study by Pareek *et al.* not only reconfirms the role of TRPV1 in mediating nociceptive signalling, and again points to the TRPV1 channel itself as a putative analgesic target site but, more importantly, it demonstrates that regulatory mechanisms for TRPV1 channel function, specifically Cdk5-dependent phosphorylation, are potentially worthwhile targets as well. Cdk5 phosphorylates both neuronal and non-neuronal substrates |14,15|, so the challenge here will be finding an analgesic that selectively targets Cdk5 in sensory neurons.

Spider toxins activate the capsaicin receptor to produce inflammatory pain

Siemens J, Zhou S, Piskorowski R, *et al. Nature* 2006; **441**: 208–12

BACKGROUND. The authors examined whether peptide toxin from the West Indies tarantula (*Psalmopoeus cambridgei*) could activate, rather than inhibit, TRPV1 channels, using Ca^{2+} imaging, patch clamp electrophysiology and *in vivo* behavioural studies in wild-type and TRPV1 null (knockout) mice.

INTERPRETATION. Vertebrate and invertebrate toxins contain a plethora of peptide toxins that can inhibit channel function by blocking and/or inactivating mechanisms. Here, the authors asked whether an invertebrate toxin could activate the heat-sensitive channel, TRPV1. *P. cambridgei* toxin was commercially obtained, and the crude toxin was shown to increase intracellular Ca^{2+} concentration ([Ca^{2+}]$_i$) in HEK293 cells expressing TRPV1, but not TRPA1 or TRPM8, channels. Three purified vanillotoxins were isolated from the crude toxin: VaTx1, VaTx2 and VaTx3, of which VaTx3 is the most potent. Interestingly, increasing ambient temperature to 34 °C (from 24 °C) shifted the concentration-[Ca^{2+}]$_i$

response curve for VaTx3 to the left, and is consistent with the fact that TRPV1 is heat sensitive |4|. VaTx3 increased $[Ca^{2+}]_i$ in HEK293 cells expressing TRPV1, but not TRPV2, TRPV3 or TRPV4 channels. Finally, the authors demonstrate that VaTx3 could increase $[Ca^{2+}]_i$ in trigeminal ganglia sensory neurons from TRPV1 wild-type (+/+) mice, but not in neurons from TRPV1 knockout (–/–) mice; *in vivo*, plantar injection of VaTx3 produced significant increases in pain-associated responses (paw licking and paw thickness – a measure of neurogenic inflammation) in TRPV1+/+, but not TRPV1–/– mice. The authors concluded that peptide toxins target TRP channels, and that peptide toxic-activated channels on sensory nerve fibres elicit pain and inflammation.

Comment

Although TRPV1 channels have been shown to be involved in nociception, this study demonstrates for the first time that they are targets for animal peptide toxins that produce pain upon envenomation. Clearly, VaTx3 is unlikely to have value as an novel analgesic; rather, its value lies in its use as a probe to explore the structure–function relationship of the TRPV1 channel using traditional approaches (molecular biology, site-direct mutagenesis, patch clamp electrophysiology) as well as newer 3-D quantitative structure–activity relationship (QSAR) modelling techniques |16–19|. If we can elucidate the structural requirements that define VaTx3 as an agonist at TRPV1 channels then it may be possible to design either a selective inverse agonist or antagonist which, in theory, would have considerable analgesic value in treating the hypersensitivity associated with inflammatory pain as well as neuropathic pain |20|.

Noxious compounds activate TRPA1 ion channels through covalent modification of cysteines

Macpherson LJ, Dubin AE, Evans MJ, *et al. Nature* 2007; **445**: 541–5

BACKGROUND. TRPA1 belongs to the TRP ion channel family, is expressed in nociceptive sensory neurons, and is activated by a variety of noxious stimuli, including cold temperatures (temperature ≤18°C), pungent natural compounds (e.g. menthol, mustard oil, cinnamon oil) and environmental irritants |6,20|. Taking advantage of the fact that alkyne groups are rarely observed *in vivo*, Macpherson and colleagues used 'click chemistry' (which monitors a covalent modification of proteins via a copper(I)-catalysed cycloaddition reaction between alkyne and azide groups), mass spectrometry, electrophysiology and Ca^{2+} imaging to identify specific cysteine residues in the TRP1A required for channel activation.

INTERPRETATION. TRPA1 channels were expressed in HEK293 cells and covalent modification following treatment with iodoacetamide alkyne (IAA), super cinnamaldehyde alkyne (SCA) or mustard oil alkyne (MOA) demonstrated using rhodamine fluorescence and Western blotting. Fourteen cytosolic TRPA1 cysteines labelled by iodoacetamide (IA) were identified using mass spectroscopy; site-directed mutagenesis was performed (producing a cysteine → serine substitution), and three cysteines, C415, C422 and

C622, appeared to be necessary for normal channel function as measured by whole-cell voltage clamp recordings; of the three mutations, C622S appeared to produce the greatest loss of function. Using Ca^{2+} imaging and single-channel recordings, the authors also demonstrate that reactive compounds (mustard oil, super cinnamaldehyde) can produce sustained activation of TRPA1 channels and that compound-activated channels demonstrate open/closed transitions consistent with the existence of open and desensitized channel configurations. These results indicate that covalent modification of specific reactive cysteines within the TRPA1 channel can produce channel activation.

Comment

TRPA1 channels are expressed in nociceptive sensory neurons and are activated by a variety of noxious stimuli, including cold temperatures and pungent natural compounds such as those found in clove, ginger and spearmint, mustard and cinnamon oils and bradykinin [21]. In the present study, the authors, using a variety of techniques, demonstrate that three specific intracellular cysteine residues – C415, C422 and C622 – are required for normal functioning of the TRPA1 channel. These cysteines are located near (C622) or in (C415, C422) the intracellular N-terminal ankyrin domains that are a hallmark of the TRPA1 channel. As shown in the study by Macpherson and colleagues (and in a different study by Hinman *et al.* [22]), covalent modification of these residues by mustard oil or cinnamaldehyde derivatives leads to channel activation, and channel activation is associated with the perception of noxious stimuli [21,23,24]. As the authors note, 'by tuning TRPA1 to respond to covalent modification by reactive compounds, the nervous system can directly assess the noxious environment of sensory neurons'. It is tempting to speculate that selective block of covalent modification of specific residues in TRPA1 might have analgesic potential, in particular C622, but it is unclear whether or not all three residues must be modified for there to be a meaningful effect *in vivo*. On the other hand, it may be equally effective to find a less targeted, but still selective, blocker for TRPA1 channels and still provide meaningful pain relief (more of a howitzer than a fly-swatter approach), and this requires further investigation.

Protease-activated receptor 2 sensitizes the transient receptor potential vanilloid 4 ion channel to cause mechanical hyperalgesia in mice

Grant AD, Cottrell GS, Amadesi S, *et al. J Physiol* 2007; **578**: 715–33

BACKGROUND. Proteases that are generated during pathologic processes cleave protease-activated receptor 2 (PAR$_2$) on afferent nerves to cause mechanical hyperalgesia by unknown mechanisms. The authors hypothesized that PAR$_2$-mediated mechanical hyperalgesia requires sensitization of TRPV4. TRPV4 is another member of the TRP channel family, and is activated at cool temperatures (temperature $\geq 25°C$), as well as by noxious mechanical stimuli. Using immunohistochemistry, confocal microscopy, Ca^{2+} imaging, enzyme immunoassay,

electrophysiology and behavioural testing of TRPV4 gene knockout mice, the authors demonstrate that TRPV4 mediates PAR$_2$-induced mechanical allodynia and hyperalgesia, and that this process depends on the activation of phosholipase (PL) Cβ, protein kinase (PK) A and C, and possibly PKD.

INTERPRETATION. Using Ca^{2+} imaging, the authors demonstrated that activation of TRPV4 channels (using hypotonic stimuli or 4αPDD, a selective TRPV4 agonist) in either human bronchial epithelial or HEK293 cells increased intracellular Ca^{2+} concentration ([Ca^{2+}]$_i$); prior application of the protease-activated receptor 2 agonist PAR$_2$-AP augmented this response. PAR$_2$-AP-induced enhancement of the TRPV4-generated [Ca^{2+}]$_i$ signal could be blocked by inhibitors of PLCβ, PKA, PKC, and possibly PKD. In dorsal root ganglion (DRG) neurons grown in culture, PAR$_2$-AP similarly sensitized TRPV4 [Ca^{2+}]$_i$ signals and currents. TRPV4 immunoreactivity co-localized with that for substance P (SP) and calcitonin gene-related peptide (CGRP), both of which are mediators of nociceptive transmission, in DRG neurons and in the superficial dorsal horn of the spinal cord, and activation of TRPV4 with either hypotonic stimuli or 4αPDD increased SP and CGRP release in rat spinal cord slices; pretreatment with PAR$_2$-AP increased release of both peptides. Finally, intraplanar injection of 4αPDD (or hypotonic solution), PAR$_2$-AP or 4αPDD (or hypotonic solution) + PAR$_2$-AP increased the frequency of paw withdrawal in response to von Frey hair application in mice expressing TRPV4 (TRPV4+/+), but not in TRPV4–/– littermates. The authors conclude that sensitization of TRPV4-dependent release of nociceptive peptides and induction of mechanical hyperalgesia by PAR2-activated second messengers may underlie inflammatory hyperalgesia in pathologic states where proteases are activated and released.

Comment

As noted in a commentary |25| accompanying the article by Grant *et al.*, PAR$_2$ is expressed in nociceptive neurons, its activation leads to the release of pro-nociceptive peptides from afferent nerve terminals in the superficial spinal cord dorsal horn, which results in both thermal and mechanical hyperalgesia, and it is activated by tryptase released by mast cells onto neighbouring neurons under inflammatory conditions or following neuronal damage. Of equal importance, PAR$_2$ is not activated by thrombin and thus selective blockers of PAR$_2$ may lack prothrombotic properties and have an improved safety profile relative to other recently marketed non-steroidal anti-inflammatory drugs. Consequently, PAR$_2$ is perceived as a promising molecular target in the management of inflammatory and/or chronic pain by pharmaceutical companies. Because PAR$_2$ is upstream to a number of second-messenger pathways, PAR$_2$ antagonists may be more effective in treating neuropathic or inflammatory pain than selective TRPV channel antagonists.

TRPM8 is required for cold sensation in mice

Dhaka A, Murray AN, Mathur J, *et al*. *Neuron* 2007; **54**: 371–8

BACKGROUND. TRMP8 is activated at low to moderate temperatures (≤ 25–$27°C$) and by 'cooling-mimetic' compounds such as menthol and icilin, and is strongly expressed in a subset of small-diameter unmyelinated sensory neurons. Previous work suggested that TRMP8 might have a role in analgesia, but the function of TRMP8 with respect to thermosensation *in vivo* remained in doubt. Dhaka and colleagues generated a TRMP8 gene deletion mouse to explicitly address this question. TRPM8 knockout mice show reduced avoidance of cool temperatures compared with wild-type littermates, but have preserved nociceptive-like responses to temperatures $<0°C$. In addition, the authors found that TRPM8 mediates the analgesic effect of moderate cooling.

INTERPRETATION. Dhaka and colleagues disrupted the TRMP8 gene such that amino acid residues 2–29 were deleted and an enhanced green fluorescent protein and an SV40polyA tail in frame with the start codon of TRPM8 inserted; the approach led to the generation of mice lacking TRPM8 mRNA as measured by *in situ* hybridization. Ca^{2+} imaging demonstrated a marked decrease in the number of dorsal root ganglion neurons from TRPM8 knockout mice that were sensitive to either cold or menthol, while the number of capsaicin-sensitive neurons was unchanged when compared with neurons from wild-type littermates. At the behavioural level, sensitivity to cool temperature ($10°C<T<31°C$) was significantly reduced (as measured by two-temperature choice assay), as was sensitivity to formalin and cooling compounds (as measured by latency to paw lift/paw licking/'wet dog shakes'). The authors conclude that TRMP8 functions in a context-sensitive manner to detect unpleasant cold and to mediate the effect of cold-induced analgesia.

Comment

In the same issue, a second study reported a similar role for TRPM8 in mediating cold sensation |26|. Until the publication of these two studies, a clear role for TRMP8 in mediating cold nociception was in doubt |6|. The accompanying commentary by Man-Kyo Chung and Michael Caterina |27| summarizes the results of the two studies and draws the following conclusions: (i) TRPM8 contributes to avoidance of innocuous cold (~ 22–$30°C$); (ii) TRPM8 participates in nociceptive-related behaviours induced by extreme cold ($\sim 0°C$); and (iii) TRPM8 mediates cold-induced analgesia. Together, the results reported by Dhaka *et al.* and Colburn *et al.* |26| should dispel any questions as to whether or not TRPM8 is involved in cold perception. Blocking cold sensation *per se* may or may not have therapeutic value to individuals with heightened sensitivity to cold temperature; one could argue that knowing when to get out of the cold is protective against the development of frostbite, for example. However, TRPM8 does appear to contribute to cold hypersensitivity ('cold allodynia') following chronic constriction nerve injury |26| and may have potential, therefore, as a novel analgesic target in the treatment of some types of neuropathic pain.

Dynorphin A activates bradykinin receptors to maintain neuropathic pain

Lai J, Luo MC, Chen Q, *et al. Nat Neurosci* 2006; **9**: 1534–40

BACKGROUND. Dynorphin A, a major proteolytic fragment of prodynorphin, exhibits high affinity for μ, δ and κ opioid receptors, and in the spinal cord it produces opioid receptor-mediated neuronal inhibition. Dynorphin A also has excitatory effects, and has been shown to stimulate the release of excitatory amino acids in the lumbar spinal cord *in vivo* |28| and to increase $[Ca^{2+}]_i$ in cortical neurons *in vitro* |29|. Intrathecal administration is associated with pathological pain and motor dysfunction |30–33|; the mechanism(s) underlying these excitatory effects are unknown. Using Ca^{2+} imaging, Lai and co-authors first screened the known receptors present on dorsal root ganglion neurons to determine which receptor(s) mediated dynorphin A-induced increases in $[Ca^{2+}]_i$; they confirmed the sensitivity of the identified (bradykinin) receptor to dynorphin A modulation using a heterologous expression (F-11) system. Finally, they establish that bradykinin receptors contribute to the tactile hypersensitivity and thermal hyperalgesia induced by intrathecal dynorphin A administration or sciatic nerve ligation.

INTERPRETATION. The authors demonstrate that dynorphin A increases $[Ca^{2+}]_i$ due to Ca^{2+} influx through voltage-gated calcium channels in DRG neurons and F-11 cells expressing either B1 or B2 bradykinin receptors. Tactile hypersensitivity was measured using a series of von Frey hairs and thermal hyperalgesia was measured by latency to paw withdrawal in response to infrared heat application in rats and bradykinin B2 receptor knockout mice. *In vivo* testing indicated that spinal B2 receptor activation was required for maintaining, but not initiating, neuropathic pain. Following sciatic nerve ligation, quantitative polymerase chain reaction analysis demonstrated a significant increase in bradykinin B2 receptor mRNA levels in L5–6 DRGs ipsilateral to nerve ligation. The data indicate that selective antagonism of dynorphin A at bradykinin receptors blocks the pronociceptive effects of spinal dynorphin without altering the peripheral function of bradykinin or of dynorphin A at opioid receptors.

Comment

Upregulation of spinal dynorphin facilitates the maintenance of neuropathic pain states |34–36|. Under physiological conditions, spinal levels of dynorphin are low and bradykinin is absent |37|, so spinal bradykinin receptors are not activated. Here, Lai and colleagues demonstrate that dynorphin A increases, rather than decreases, pain due to bradykinin B2 receptor activation *in vivo*. Sciatic nerve ligation (SNL), one *in vivo* model for neuropathic pain |38|, results in a time-dependent upregulation of spinal dynorphin |35|, and the reversal of neuropathic pain by the bradykinin B2 receptor blocker DOE 140 reported here indicates that spinal B2 receptor activation is required for the maintenance, but not initiation, of neuropathic pain induced by SNL. As noted |37|, the ability of dynorphin A to bind to non-opioid receptors, such as bradykinin B1 and B2, opens new approaches for therapeutic intervention in the management of neuropathic pain. In this study, bradykinin receptor antagonists were administered intrathecally; it will be important to determine whether other routes of administration are equally effective. The results reported by Lai *et al.* raise additional issues, such as the nature of the molecular interaction between dynorphin A and bradykinin receptors and how this interaction leads to receptor activation as well as whether other opioids, both endogenous and exogenous, can replicate the effects of dynorphin A. Although further work remains to be done, it appears that dynorphin A-mediated activation of bradykinin receptors is a novel mechanism underlying the maintenance of neuropathic pain and thus represents a fresh target with respect to the development of new therapies for the treatment of neuropathic pain.

Repeated intrathecal injections of plasmid DNA encoding interleukin 10 produce prolonged reversal of neuropathic pain

Milligan ED, Sloane EM, Langer SJ, *et al. Pain* 2006; **126**: 294–308

BACKGROUND. Glial proinflammatory cytokines, including tumour necrosis factor (TNF), interleukin 1 (IL-1) and interleukin 6 (IL-6) appear to contribute to neuropathic pain |39|. Glial inhibitors and selective TNF, IL-1 and IL-6 inhibitors have been shown to acutely reverse neuropathic pain in relevant animal models. Selectively blocking a single pathway is unlikely to treat the underlying condition successfully in the long run due to the contribution of alternative pathways; on the other hand, non-selective inhibition of proinflammatory cytokines might prove successful. Interleukin 10 (IL-10) suppresses the production and function of all proinflammatory cytokines |40|; here, the authors intrathecally delivered naked plasmid DNA vectors encoding IL-10 (pDNA-IL-10) to test its ability to relieve neuropathic pain in a chronic nerve constriction injury (CCI) rat model.

INTERPRETATION. The authors created naked plasmid vectors for human and rat IL-10 (pDNA-hIL-10 and pDNA-rIL-10, respectively). Mechanical sensitivity was determined using von Frey hairs, and CCI surgery performed after baseline mechanical threshold values obtained. Intrathecal administration of pDNA-rIL-10 transiently reversed CCI-induced mechanical allodynia with increasingly longer therapeutic intervals with each subsequent pDNA injection when subsequent doses were administered after the initial effect had resolved; notably, if the second injection occurred while mechanical allodynia was fully resolved (within 3 days of the first injection), then a long-acting (~ 40 days) effect was observed. Intrathecal administration of pDNA-rIL-10 reliably reversed CCI-induced mechanical allodynia 2 months after initial nerve injury without producing additional analgesia. The data suggest that intrathecal IL-10 gene therapy may be a novel approach to successfully treating neuropathic pain.

Comment

In some respects, this article should generate the most excitement of all the articles presented for review; it provides valuable information indicating that intrathecal administration of pDNA-rIL-10 can not only alleviate neuropathic pain shortly after its induction (within 7 days of surgery), but, of potentially greater importance, can *reverse* well-established neuropathic pain (at least in a chronic nerve constriction animal model). Risk factors have been identified to predict the likelihood of developing severe, early postoperative pain |41–43| and, while it can be difficult to extrapolate from this information and identify those individuals who will eventually develop chronic, or neuropathic pain |3,44|, the severity of acute postoperative pain appears to correlate with the risk for developing chronic pain |44–47|. The ability to disrupt/alleviate established neuropathic pain is an important goal and, although this paper is limited to rats, it has significant implications for the treatment of neuropathic pain in humans. Another important advance is the use of a naked DNA plasmid to deliver the IL-10 gene; traditional delivery vehicles have used retroviral vectors, and their use has been shown to have mutagenic and oncogenic effects |48,49|. Since the technique employed uses a non-viral transfer vector, the risk of developing a viral vector-mediated cancer is markedly reduced and, in theory, may be non-existent.

Inhibitory role of supraspinal $P2X_3$/$P2X_{2/3}$ subtypes on nociception in rats

Fukui M, Nakagawa T, Minami M, *et al. Mol Pain* 2006; **2**: 19

BACKGROUND. Extracellular adenosine triphosphate (ATP) acts as a neurotransmitter at ionotropic (i.e. ligand-gated ion channels) P_{2X} and metabotropic (i.e. ligand-activated second messenger-coupled) P_{2Y} receptors. Of the seven identified P_{2X} receptors, the P_{2X3} subtype contributes to ATP-mediated excitatory nociceptive transmission at peripheral and spinal sites; conversely, supraspinal P_{2X} receptors appear to play an inhibitory role in nociceptive transmission, but the subtype identity of these supraspinal P_{2X} receptors is unknown. The authors administered (via intracerebroventricular [i.c.v.] injection), $\alpha,\beta,$-methylene-ATP (an agonist at P_{2X3} and $P_{2X2/3}$, but not P_{2X2} receptors), A-317491 (a novel, selective antagonist for P_{2X3} homomeric and $P_{2X2/3}$ heteromeric receptors) and P_{2X3} receptor antisense oligodeoxynucleotide to rats and measured the change in nocifensive behaviours elicited by application of accelerating pressure (32 g/s) to the hind paw, or by formalin (intraplantar) or acetic acid (i.p.) injection.

INTERPRETATION. In the paw pressure test, the nociceptive threshold before the i.c.v. injection served as control; injection of $\alpha,\beta,$-methylene-ATP significantly increased the nociceptive threshold, and A-317491 significantly reduced the antinociceptive effect of $\alpha,\beta,$-methylene-ATP in a dose-dependent fashion, and this effect was replicated by injection of P_{2X3} antisense oligodeoxynucleotide. Inflammatory pain induced by formalin or acetic acid injection elicited typical nociceptive behaviours (formalin: paw elevation/licking/biting/shaking; acetic acid: writhing), and i.c.v. injection of A-317491 significantly increased those behaviours. The results indicate that activation of supraspinal $P_{2X3}/P_{2X2/3}$ receptors produces antinociception.

Comment

The relatively recent cloning of the genes coding for P_{2X} receptor subunits has enabled researchers to better define the role of specific receptor subtypes in nociceptive signal transduction |**50**|. The P_{2X3} receptor appears to be a key player amongst P_{2X} receptors in contributing to inflammatory and neuropathic pain. At the level of the spinal cord, activation of P_{2X3} and $P_{2X2/3}$ receptors has a pronociceptive effect such that pharmacological block or gene knockdown/knockout of the receptor has analgesic properties |**51**|. Interestingly, at supraspinal levels, activation of P_{2X3} and $P_{2X2/3}$ receptors appears to have an analgesic effect as the P_{2X3} receptor antagonist A-317491 inhibits α,β-methylene-ATP-induced analgesia while increasing inflammatory agent-induced nociceptive behaviours |**52**|. Published data suggest that P_{2X3} receptor expression is restricted to primary afferent neurons, which, if true, would suggest that the compounds tested here are less selective than thought, although the results obtained with P_{2X3} antisense oligodeoxynucleotide make a fairly compelling argument that the effects observed are indeed due to P_{2X3} receptor blockade. That caveat notwithstanding, this study adds to a growing body of literature implicating P_{2X} receptors in general, and P_{2X3} receptors in specific, in pain pathways. The trick now, of course, is to develop compounds that can selectively target supraspinal rather than spinal receptors.

Role of peripheral hyperpolarization-activated cyclic nucleotide-modulated channel pacemaker channels in acute and chronic pain models in the rat

Luo L, Chang L, Brown SM, *et al. Neuroscience* 2007; **144**: 1477–85

BACKGROUND. Hyperpolarization-activated cyclic nucleotide (HCN) gated channels, also known as pacemaker channels, contribute to spontaneous oscillatory electrical activity in the brain and heart and have been implicated in the development and maintenance of acute and chronic hyperalgesia, as well as allodynia. Four HCN channel isoforms (HCN1–4) have been identified, and these channels may contribute to spontaneous pain, which can occur following peripheral nerve injury, although direct evidence for this has been lacking. Here, the authors investigated whether HCN channels were involved in the development of spontaneous pain induced by mild thermal injury and tactile allodynia induced by sciatic nerve ligation and mild thermal injury in rats. The data indicate that expression and modulation of HCN channels in the peripheral nervous system may play a role in sensory processing and contribute to spontaneous pain and tactile allodynia.

INTERPRETATION. Pain models (in adult male rats) used were: (i) mild thermal injury (MTI) – uniform first-degree burn was produced across the paw plantar surface in anaesthetized rats by placing the paw on a 56°C hotplate for 20s, under constant pressure, and (ii) sciatic nerve ligation (SNL) – unilateral ligation of lumbar fifth and sixth spinal nerves. Systemic (i.p.) administration of the HCN-channel blocker ZD7288 significantly reduced tactile allodynia following MTI and both local and systemic administration of ZD7288 reduced spontaneous nocifensive behaviours (elevating, licking/ mouthing, shaking affected paw). Both locally and systemically administered ZD7288 significantly decreased SNL-induced tactile allodynia, although systemic administration did so for a longer time. Fluorescent immunostaining demonstrated labelling for HCN1, HCN2, HCN3 and HCN4 in Meissner's corpuscles and Merkel cells in plantar skin.

Comment

Abnormal electrical activity in dorsal root ganglion neurons following peripheral nerve injury is thought to contribute to the development of spontaneous pain, allodynia and hyperalgesia |53|. While much work related to ectopic activity in DRG neurons has focused on fast sodium (Na$_V$) channels |54–58|, it is clear that other ion channels are also involved in generating ectopic signals, including HCN channels |59,60|. In the present work, Luo *et al.* demonstrate that HCN channels contribute to the development of allodynia and spontaneous pain behaviours in rats following sciatic nerve ligation. The authors found that systemic and local administration of the HCN channel blocker ZD7288 suppressed tactile allodynia following mild thermal injury and sciatic nerve ligation; the efficacy of intraplantar injection of ZD7288 in suppressing tactile allodynia indicates that the site of action was not just at the level of the DRG soma, but was also in peripheral mechanosensory structures (e.g. Meissner's corpuscles, Merkel cells). This group has previously shown that, at the systemic dose used here (10 mg/kg), the resulting peak plasma concentration for ZD7288 is 3.6 ± 0.3 μmol/l |59|, which is unlikely to have non-specific channel effects; for i.p. injection, however, 50 μl of 30 mmol/l ZD7288 was injected, so it is possible that the peripheral effects were mediated by other additional ion channels due to non-specific block as a consequence of high local tissue concentrations. That caveat notwithstanding, HCN channels are likely to be important targets in the pursuit of new analgesics for the treatment of both inflammatory and neuropathic pain.

An SCN9A channelopathy causes congenital inability to experience pain

Cox JJ, Reimann F, Nicholas AK, *et al. Nature* 2006; **444**: 894–8

BACKGROUND. Cox and colleagues examined three consanguineous families from northern Pakistan, members of which displayed a congenital absence of any form of pain sensation. They identified three novel and distinct nonsense mutations (S459X, I767X and W897X) in SCN9A, which is the gene coding for the α-subunit of the voltage-gated sodium channel, Na$_v$1.7. Individuals with any one of the mutations had a complete inability to perceive, or feel, pain. Heterologous expression of mutant Na$_v$1.7 channels in HEK293 cells led to the formation of non-functional sodium channels. The data indicate that SCN9A is an essential and non-redundant requirement for nociception in humans.

INTERPRETATION. The authors used a positional cloning strategy to identify the mutated gene; an initial genome-wide scan using 400 polymorphic microsatellite markers identified an 11.7-megabase region of chromosome 2q24 as a region of interest. There are ~50 genes in this linkage region, and a subsequent bioinformatics scan identified SCN9A as the most promising gene underlying the phenotype. SCN9A codes for the α-subunit of the voltage-gated sodium channel, Na$_v$1.7, and this protein is strongly expressed in nociceptive neurons.

Comment

Nine voltage-gated sodium channels have been identified (Na$_v$1.1–1.9), and Na$_v$ channels contain both a pore-forming α-subunit and an auxiliary β-subunit; the α-subunit will form functional homomeric channels in heterologous expression systems, but it is the β-subunit that determines the kinetics and voltage dependence of channel gating |**61**|. These channels are responsible for action potential generation and propagation in excitable cells, and indiscriminate block (as produced by amide and ester local anaesthetics) can produce profound sensory and motor deficits. The Na$_v$1.7 channel is found in peripheral sensory neurons, where it generates a tetrodotoxin-sensitive current, I_{Na}. Previous work has shown that several point mutations in SCN9A are associated with the development of erythermalgia |**62,63**|, an inherited neuropathy that is characterized by recurrent episodes of severe pain associated with redness and warmth in the feet or hands, and at least one of those mutations (I484T) results in a gain-of-function in expressed channels containing that mutation |**64**|. Additional mutations in SCN9A are associated with paroxysmal extreme pain disorder |**65**|, an inherited condition characterized by paroxysms of rectal, ocular or submandibular pain with flushing; these mutations lead to marked deficits in sodium channel fast inactivation. In marked contrast to those studies, the present report by Cox and co-authors provides clear evidence that a different set of mutations in SCN9A (compared with those associated with neuropathic pain states) can produce a loss-of-function in expressed sodium channels, and that those mutations are associated with the complete absence of pain *in vivo*. Furthermore, and of equal importance, although transmission of nociceptive (painful) information was abolished, motor function was fully preserved as was normal (i.e. not painful) tactile sensation. Thus, as noted by Stephen Waxman |**66**| in the commentary on the article by Cox *et al.*, 'these findings should stimulate the search for novel analgesics that selectively target this sodium channel subunit'.

Conclusion

In writing this chapter, I am reminded of the story of the passer-by who encounters a thoroughly inebriated fellow one night who was searching for his keys under a street lamp – not because he lost them there, but because that was where the light was brightest. The biological pathways, and there are many, that contribute to the development of inflammatory and neuropathic pain are still being uncovered. We need to 'shine the light' on the molecular and cellular events that enable us to perceive pain in order to find the 'keys' that will permit the development of new therapies for its prevention and treatment. The past year has seen exciting developments that provide new insights into the channels and second messenger pathways that contribute to inflammatory and neuropathic pain. The articles describing the contribution of various ion channels (TRP, P_{2X}, HCN and Na_V channels) as well as second messenger-coupled receptors (bradykinin and cytokine receptors) to inflammatory and neuropathic pain enhance our understanding of how these specific molecules contribute to pain perception. It is likely that additional targets will be uncovered in the future. Clearly, the promising results obtained in laboratory animal studies need to be replicated in human subject trials. A search of the clinical trials database maintained by the US National Institutes of Health (http://clinicaltrials.gov/ct; keywords – neuropathic, pain; database searched 25 June 2007) uncovered 68 registered human trials, and many of those trials were testing drugs already in the marketplace (including lamotrigine [Lamictal™], pregabalin [Lyrica™] and gabapentin [Neurontin™]). The absence of active clinical trials investigating the safety and efficacy of novel analgesics aimed at the molecules reviewed here indicates that there is much work yet to be done.

References

1. Basbaum AI, Jessell TM. The perception of pain. In: Kandel ER, Schwartz JH, Jessell TM, eds. *Principles of Neural Science*, 4th edn. New York: McGraw-Hill; 2000, 472–91.

2. Campbell JN, Meyer RA. Mechanisms of neuropathic pain. *Neuron* 2006; **52**: 77–92.

3. Kehlet H, Jensen TS, Woolf CJ. Persistent postsurgical pain: risk factors and prevention. *Lancet* 2006; **367**: 1618–25.

4. Caterina MJ, Schumacher MA, Tominaga M, Rosen TA, Levine JD, Julius D. The capsaicin receptor: a heat-activated ion channel in the pain pathway. *Nature* 1997; **389**: 816–24.

5. Montell C, Birnbaumer L, Flockerzi V, Bindels RJ, Bruford EA, Caterina MJ, *et al.* A unified nomenclature for the superfamily of TRP cation channels. *Mol Cell* 2002; **9**: 229–31.

6. Dhaka A, Viswanath V, Patapoutian A. TRP ion channels and temperature sensation. *Annu Rev Neurosci* 2006; **29**: 135–61.

7. Tominaga M, Caterina MJ, Malmberg AB, Rosen TA, Gilbert H, Skinner K, Raumann BE, Basbaum AI, Julius D. The cloned capsaicin receptor integrates multiple pain-producing stimuli. *Neuron* 1998; **21**: 531–43.

8. Caterina MJ, Leffler A, Malmberg AB, Martin WJ, Trafton J, Petersen-Zeitz KR, *et al*. Impaired nociception and pain sensation in mice lacking the capsaicin receptor. *Science* 2000; **288**: 306–13.

9. Ramsey IS, Delling M, Clapham DE. An introduction to TRP channels. *Annu Rev Physiol* 2006; **68**: 619–47.

10. Wang H, Woolf CJ. Pain TRPs. *Neuron* 2005; **46**: 9–12.

11. Bhave G, Zhu W, Wang H, Brasier DJ, Oxford GS, Gereau RW IV. cAMP-dependent protein kinase regulates desensitization of the capsaicin receptor (VR1) by direct phosphorylation. *Neuron* 2002; **35**: 721–31.

12. Jung J, Shin JS, Lee SY, Hwang SW, Koo J, Cho H, Oh U. Phosphorylation of vanilloid receptor 1 by Ca^{2+}/calmodulin-dependent kinase II regulates its vanilloid binding. *J Biol Chem* 2004; **279**: 7048–54.

13. Premkumar LS, Ahern GP. Induction of vanilloid receptor channel activity by protein kinase C. *Nature* 2000; **408**: 985–90.

14. Dhavan R, Tsai LH. A decade of CDK5. *Nat Rev Mol Cell Biol* 2001; **2**: 749–59.

15. Kim Y, Sung JY, Ceglia I, Lee KW, Ahn JH, Halford JM, *et al*. Phosphorylation of WAVE1 regulates actin polymerization and dendritic spine morphology. *Nature* 2006; **442**: 814–17.

16. Mekenyan O. Dynamic QSAR techniques: applications in drug design and toxicology. *Curr Pharm Des* 2002; **8**: 1605–21.

17. Swaan PW, Ekins S. Reengineering the pharmaceutical industry by crash-testing molecules. *Drug Discov Today* 2005; **10**: 1191–200.

18. Norinder U. *In silico* modelling of ADMET – a minireview of work from 2000 to 2004. *SAR QSAR Environ Res* 2005; **16**: 1–11.

19. Ognyanov VI, Balan C, Bannon AW, Bo Y, Dominguez C, Fotsch C, *et al*. Design of potent, orally available antagonists of the transient receptor potential vanilloid 1. Structure-activity relationships of 2-piperazin-1-yl-1H-benzimidazoles. *J Med Chem* 2006; **49**: 3719–42.

20. Levine JD, Alessandri-Haber N. TRP channels: Targets for the relief of pain. *Biochim Biophys Acta* 2007; doi: 10.1016/j.bbadis.2007.01.008.

21. Bandell M, Story GM, Hwang SW, Viswanath V, Eid SR, Petrus MJ, Earley TJ, Patapoutian A. Noxious cold ion channel TRPA1 is activated by pungent compounds and bradykinin. *Neuron* 2004; **41**: 849–57.

22. Hinman A, Chuang HH, Bautista DM, Julius D. TRP channel activation by reversible covalent modification. *Proc Natl Acad Sci USA* 2006; **103**: 19564–8.

23. Bautista DM, Jordt SE, Nikai T, Tsuruda PR, Read AJ, Poblete J, Yamoah EN, Basbaum AI, Julius D. TRPA1 mediates the inflammatory actions of environmental irritants and proalgesic agents. *Cell* 2006; **124**: 1269–82.

24. Kwan KY, Allchorne AJ, Vollrath MA, Christensen AP, Zhang DS, Woolf CJ, Corey DP. TRPA1 contributes to cold, mechanical, and chemical nociception but is not essential for hair-cell transduction. *Neuron* 2006; **50**: 277–89.

25. Surprenant A. Pain TRP-ed up by PARs. *J Physiol* 2007; **578**: 631.

26. Colburn RW, Lubin ML, Stone DJ Jr, Wang Y, Lawrence D, D'Andrea MR, Brandt MR, Liu Y, Flores CM, Qin N. Attenuated cold sensitivity in TRPM8 null mice. *Neuron* 2007; **54**: 379–86.

27. Chung MK, Caterina MJ. TRP channel knockout mice lose their cool. *Neuron* 2007; **54**: 345–7.

28. Skilling SR, Sun X, Kurtz HJ, Larson AA. Selective potentiation of NMDA-induced activity and release of excitatory amino acids by dynorphin: possible roles in paralysis and neurotoxicity. *Brain Res* 1992; **575**: 272–8.

29. Tang Q, Lynch RM, Porreca F, Lai J. Dynorphin A elicits an increase in intracellular calcium in cultured neurons via a non-opioid, non-NMDA mechanism. *J Neurophysiol* 2000; **83**: 2610–5.

30. Walker JM, Moises HC, Coy DH, Baldrighi G, Akil H. Nonopiate effects of dynorphin and des-Tyr-dynorphin. *Science* 1982; **218**: 1136–8.

31. Faden AI, Jacobs TP. Dynorphin-related peptides cause motor dysfunction in the rat through a non-opiate action. *Br J Pharmacol* 1984; **81**: 271–6.

32. Stevens CW, Weinger MB, Yaksh TL. Intrathecal dynorphins suppress hindlimb electromyographic activity in rats. *Eur J Pharmacol* 1987; **138**: 299–302.

33. Vanderah TW, Laughlin T, Lashbrook JM, Nichols ML, Wilcox GL, Ossipov MH, Lai J, Porreca F, Malan TP Jr. Single intrathecal injections of dynorphin A or des-Tyr-dynorphins produce long-lasting allodynia in rats: blockade by MK-801 but not naloxone. *Pain* 1996; **68**: 275–81.

34. Wang Z, Gardell LR, Ossipov MH, Vanderah TW, Brennan MB, Hochgeschwender U, Hruby VJ, Malan TP Jr, Lai J, Porreca F. Pronociceptive actions of dynorphin maintain chronic neuropathic pain. *J Neurosci* 2001; **21**: 1779–86.

35. Malan TP, Ossipov MH, Gardell LR, Ibrahim M, Bian D, Lai J, *et al.* Extraterritorial neuropathic pain correlates with multisegmental elevation of spinal dynorphin in nerve-injured rats. *Pain* 2000; **86**: 185–94.

36. Burgess SE, Gardell LR, Ossipov MH, Malan TP Jr, Vanderah TW, Lai J, Porreca F. Time-dependent descending facilitation from the rostral ventromedial medulla maintains, but does not initiate, neuropathic pain. *J Neurosci* 2002; **22**: 5129–36.

37. Altier C, Zamponi GW. Opioid, cheating on its receptors, exacerbates pain. *Nat Neurosci* 2006; **9**: 1465–7.

38. Wang LX, Wang ZJ. Animal and cellular models of chronic pain. *Adv Drug Deliv Rev* 2003; **55**: 949–65.

39. Watkins LR, Milligan ED, Maier SF. Glial activation: a driving force for pathological pain. *Trends Neurosci* 2001; **24**: 450–5.

40. Moore KW, de Waal Malefyt R, Coffman RL, O'Garra A. Interleukin-10 and the interleukin-10 receptor. *Annu Rev Immunol* 2001; **19**: 683–765.

41. Kalkman CJ, Visser K, Moen J, Bonsel GJ, Grobbee DE, Moons KG. Preoperative prediction of severe postoperative pain. *Pain* 2003; **105**: 415–23.

42. Pavlin DJ, Sullivan MJ, Freund PR, Roesen K. Catastrophizing: a risk factor for postsurgical pain. *Clin J Pain* 2005; **21**: 83–90.

43. Katz J, Poleshuck EL, Andrus CH, Hogan LA, Jung BF, Kulick DI, Dworkin RH. Risk factors for acute pain and its persistence following breast cancer surgery. *Pain* 2005; **119**: 16–25.

44. Perkins FM, Kehlet H. Chronic pain as an outcome of surgery. A review of predictive factors. *Anesthesiology* 2000; **93**: 1123–33.

45. Macrae WA. Chronic pain after surgery. *Br J Anaesth* 2001; **87**: 88–98.

46. Bisgaard T, Rosenberg J, Kehlet H. From acute to chronic pain after laparoscopic cholecystectomy: a prospective follow-up analysis. *Scand J Gastroenterol* 2005; **40**: 1358–64.

47. Katz J, Jackson M, Kavanagh BP, Sandler AN. Acute pain after thoracic surgery predicts long-term post-thoracotomy pain. *Clin J Pain* 1996; **12**: 50–5.

48. Baum C, von Kalle C, Staal FJ, Li Z, Fehse B, Schmidt M, Weerkamp F, Karlsson S, Wagemaker G, Williams DA. Chance or necessity? Insertional mutagenesis in gene therapy and its consequences. *Mol Ther* 2004; **9**: 5–13.

49. Baum C, Kustikova O, Modlich U, Li Z, Fehse B. Mutagenesis and oncogenesis by chromosomal insertion of gene transfer vectors. *Hum Gene Ther* 2006; **17**: 253–63.

50. North RA. Molecular physiology of P2X receptors. *Physiol Rev* 2002; **82**: 1013–67.

51. North RA. The P2X$_3$ subunit: a molecular target in pain therapeutics. *Curr Opin Investig Drugs* 2003; **4**: 833–40.

52. Fukui M, Nakagawa T, Minami M, Satoh M, Kaneko S. Inhibitory role of supraspinal P2X$_3$/P2X$_{2/3}$ subtypes on nociception in rats. *Mol Pain* 2006; **2**: 19.

53. Liu CN, Michaelis M, Amir R, Devor M. Spinal nerve injury enhances subthreshold membrane potential oscillations in DRG neurons: relation to neuropathic pain. *J Neurophysiol* 2000; **84**: 205–15.

54. Waxman SG, Dib-Hajj S, Cummins TR, Black JA. Sodium channels and pain. *Proc Natl Acad Sci USA* 1999; **96**: 7635–9.

55. Waxman SG. The molecular pathophysiology of pain: abnormal expression of sodium channel genes and its contributions to hyperexcitability of primary sensory neurons. *Pain* 1999; **6** (Suppl.): S133–40.

56. Waxman SG, Cummins TR, Dib-Hajj SD, Black JA. Voltage-gated sodium channels and the molecular pathogenesis of pain: a review. *J Rehabil Res Dev* 2000; **37**: 517–28.

57. Waxman SG. Channel, neuronal and clinical function in sodium channelopathies: from genotype to phenotype. *Nat Neurosci* 2007; **10**: 405–9.

58. Wood JN, Akopian AN, Baker M, Ding Y, Geoghegan F, Nassar M, *et al.* Sodium channels in primary sensory neurons: relationship to pain states. *Novartis Found Symp* 2002; **241**: 159–68; discussion 168–72.

59. Chaplan SR, Guo HQ, Lee DH, Luo L, Liu C, Kuei C, Velumian AA, Butler MP, Brown SM, Dubin AE. Neuronal hyperpolarization-activated pacemaker channels drive neuropathic pain. *J Neurosci* 2003; **23**: 1169–78.

60. Yao H, Donnelly DF, Ma C, LaMotte RH. Upregulation of the hyperpolarization-activated cation current after chronic compression of the dorsal root ganglion. *J Neurosci* 2003; **23**: 2069–74.

61. Catterall WA, Goldin AL, Waxman SG. International Union of Pharmacology. XLVII. Nomenclature and structure-function relationships of voltage-gated sodium channels. *Pharmacol Rev* 2005; **57**: 397–409.

62. Yang Y, Wang Y, Li S, Xu Z, Li H, Ma L, *et al.* Mutations in SCN9A, encoding a sodium channel α subunit, in patients with primary erythermalgia. *J Med Genet* 2004; **41**: 171–4.

63. Drenth JP, te Morsche RH, Guillet G, Taieb A, Kirby RL, Jansen JB. SCN9A mutations define primary erythermalgia as a neuropathic disorder of voltage gated sodium channels. *J Invest Dermatol* 2005; **124**: 1333–8.

64. Cummins TR, Dib-Hajj SD, Waxman SG. Electrophysiological properties of mutant Nav1.7 sodium channels in a painful inherited neuropathy. *J Neurosci* 2004; **24**: 8232–6.

65. Fertleman CR, Baker MD, Parker KA, Moffatt S, Elmslie FV, Abrahamsen B, Ostman J, Klugbauer N, Wood JN, Gardiner RM, Rees M. SCN9A mutations in paroxysmal extreme pain disorder: allelic variants underlie distinct channel defects and phenotypes. *Neuron* 2006; **52**: 767–74.

66. Waxman SG. Neurobiology: a channel sets the gain on pain. *Nature* 2006; **444**: 831–2.

6

Drug administration techniques

ROBERT SNEYD

Introduction

In order for a patient to benefit from a pharmaceutical the compound needs to be present in the right tissue compartment at the necessary concentration for the appropriate time period. Currently, most drugs are administered intermittently and the vagaries of absorption, distribution and elimination mean that actual achieved concentrations are suboptimal or even subtherapeutic for significant proportions of the treatment period.

In the case of analgesics, the lack of an adequate tissue concentration translates into an unsatisfactory patient experience (pain), with the possibility of adverse clinical consequences as well. Stable or pseudo-stable drug concentrations may be achieved by repeated administration at appropriate intervals or by continuous administration. These techniques require repeated intervention and may be expensive when staffing and other related costs are considered.

Recently, the development of novel pharmaceutical formulations offers the possibility of a single administration, with drugs subsequently released into tissues from a depot. In theory, a sustained period of appropriate tissue concentrations can follow, with improved patient experience and outcomes and reduced staffing costs. Such novel presentations typically require advanced pharmaceutical technology for the vehicle/administration system but this may also permit the development of new intellectual property around 'old' drugs, such as morphine, fentanyl and oxycodone, and possibly permit marketing at a premium price with the high procurement cost potentially offset by reduced staffing, improved patient experience and possibly decreased duration of hospital stay.

Single administration is not without its risks. Once a depot presentation is embedded within the patient it usually cannot be removed, although some early projects did attempt this. Thus, the Norplant contraceptive could be cut out from the subcutaneous tissue into which it was injected [1] and a prototype slow-release morphine suppository had an attached string with which it could be extracted [2] per rectum.

Both drug distribution/elimination (i.e. pharmacokinetics) and the dose–response relationship (i.e. pharmacodynamics) are variable between patients and may even vary within a single patient across time. Thus, a frail elderly woman will probably achieve different concentrations and possibly respond differently to a young man, even though both receive a similar dose (expressed as mg/kg). Further, improving cardiac output during recovery from surgery or decreasing renal clearance during the progressive development of acute renal failure may cause drug concentrations for decrease or increase respectively.

Finally, if the release profile is unsuitable when set against even the 'typical' pharmacokinetics of a drug then progressively increasing concentrations may produce toxic effects, possibly well after administration. Thus, were a slow-release morphine preparation to cause gradually increasing blood concentrations then a patient who appeared comfortable and stable at 20:00 h might develop respiratory depression in the middle of the night.

It is against this background that candidate technologies must be assessed and clinicians should ask critically whether, in their own practice, the novel formulation will be safe and efficacious and to what extent it can actually improve outcomes or decrease costs. Typically, the realization of efficiency savings in the care of surgical patients requires the re-engineering of care pathways, and without this the introduction of expensively reformulated versions of old compounds may simply increase cost without discernible improvement.

Closed-loop and patient-controlled drug administration take a different approach. In each case the administration of the drug is in response to an effect measure. In closed-loop systems something has to be measured – for example, twitch height, bispectral index or arterial blood pressure. In patient-controlled systems the patient's own experience is the effect measure and patients determine for themselves whether or not supplementary drug is required and administer it, subject to system-based controls.

Novel depots of buprenorphine prodrugs have a long-acting antinociceptive effect

Liu KS, Tzeng JI, Chen YW, *et al. Anesth Analg* 2006; **102**: 1445–51

BACKGROUND. The partial agonist buprenorphine attracts some use in perioperative medicine and is more widely used in primary care and chronic pain presentations. Synthesis of a pro-drug adds a second stage to the slow-release process, with the molecule first requiring release from the delivery system and subsequently metabolism to the active form. Buprenorphine and three buprenorphine pro-drugs – buprenorphine propionate, enanthate and decanoate (Fig. 6.1) – were formulated in a lipid vehicle (sesame oil) and injected i.m. into rats. A control group received the sesame oil but no buprenorphine and further animals received buprenorphine dissolved in saline, that is the standard method of administration without the depot. Antinociceptive effect was measured using a paw withdrawal test, in which the animal was placed on a glass floor and infrared light shone onto a hindpaw. The endpoint was the time to paw withdrawal and the total exposure was limited to avoid tissue damage if the paw was not withdrawn by 20 s.

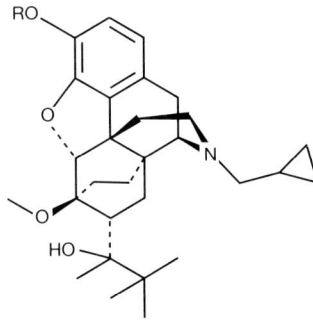

Buprenorphine base	R = H
Buprenorphine propionate	R = CH₃CH₂CO
Buprenorphine enanthate	R = CH₃(CH₂)₅CO
Buprenorphine decanoate	R = CH₃(CH₂)₈CO

Fig. 6.1 Chemical structures of buprenorphine base and its ester derivatives. Reproduced with permission from |3|.

INTERPRETATION. Buprenorphine in saline produced analgesia from 30 min to 5 h. The use of the oil depot delayed the onset of analgesia to 2 h and extended analgesia to 26 h. Substitution of the propionate, enanthate and decanoate pro-drugs extended analgesia to 28, 52 and 70 h respectively.

Comment

Both the lipid vehicle and the pro-drug presentations were effective in extending the period of analgesia in this animal model. However, sesame oil is not a recognized vehicle for drug administration to humans. Further, the presentation of a compound as a pro-drug introduces a further source of variability, i.e. the process of conversion to the active form. Because buprenorphine is a partial agonist, it may attenuate the subsequent effects of an administered pure agonist. This could, theoretically, cause problems were a patient receiving slow-release buprenorphine to require reoperation with use of morphine or fentanyl. Nevertheless, if the pro-drugs are stable and non-toxic, they might be useful in the pain clinic.

Evaluation of a single-dose, extended-release epidural morphine formulation for pain after knee arthroplasty

Hartrick C, Martin G, Kantor G, et al. J Bone Joint Surg 2006; **88**: 273–281

BACKGROUND. Lamellar liposome technology has been used for several decades to produce sustained-release drug formulations for parenteral administration. Multivesicular liposomes are foam-like structures with large numbers of liposomal compartments. **A commercial preparation, DepoDur®, presents morphine in a liposomal formulation, which is now widely approved for single-dose lumbar epidural administration as a perioperative analgesic. Recently, case reports of intrathecal administration followed by prolonged respiratory depression have precipitated an FDA warning |4| 'cases of intrathecal administration of DepoDur® have been reported ... In all cases, signs of prolonged respiratory depression were observed requiring narcotic antagonist (naloxone) administration or ventilatory support.'**

INTERPRETATION. A total of 168 patients received either DepoDur® or a placebo (sham) epidural injection 30 min before knee arthroplasty. Intraoperative opioid was restricted to a maximum of fentanyl 250μg and after surgery, breakthrough pain was treated with i.v. bolus hydromorphone with placebo (saline) patient-controlled analgesia (PCA) in the DepoDur® group and i.v. morphine then morphine using patient-controlled analgesia (PCA) in the control group. Patients receiving DepoDur® had significantly reduced mean pain intensity recall scores at 4–8, 4–12, 4–24 and 4–30h and used less opioid in the perioperative period. Opioid-related adverse events were frequent in all groups: nausea (78%), vomiting (43%) and pruritus (43%). Five of 61 patients receiving DepoDur® 30mg and 4 of 51 receiving 20mg developed respiratory depression. All were aged over 65 years. The respiratory depression was described as serious in four patients. Sixteen of the 112 DepoDur® patients required an opioid antagonist, always within the first 24h.

Comment

Achieving blinding in a study comparing two very different treatments – in this case, an epidural foam and an intravenous solution – is extremely difficult. These authors used sham epidurals and placebo PCA – a technique known as 'double-blind, double-dummy' – with additional staffing to accomplish it. An additional limitation is the restriction of clinical practice around the interventions being studied. In this case, intraoperative fentanyl was limited to 250 μg, regardless of the duration of surgery. A high level of patient observation was applied, with 'brief neurologic checks and sedation assessments performed throughout 48 h'; thus, the environment was closer to a high-dependency unit than a typical surgical ward.

Conclusion

DepoDur® is certainly efficacious as an analgesic; that is, it reduces pain. However, it did not produce comprehensive analgesia – supplementary PCA was still necessary for most patients. In this study, as is commonly the case in the drug development process, the investigators were restricted to a rather artificial treatment package. Thus, in the study period the use of paracetamol, non-steroidal anti-inflammatory drugs (NSAIDs) and other agents, such as clonidine, was prohibited. Typically, contemporary analgesic practice is multimodal and it is possible that, had adjunctive agents been allowed in this study, the supplementary PCA would have been unnecessary. The occurrence of serious respiratory depression is alarming. A high proportion of surgical patients are over 65 years and any episode of respiratory depression is a potential catastrophe. Against this background, many clinicians would not be prepared to use the formulation outside a high-dependency environment, thereby adding substantially to the cost of care. Further studies are needed to determine the role of DepoDur® in more realistic clinical scenarios and to determine if it can be safely used on general wards.

The rationale for DepoDur® is that a single sustained-release epidural injection avoids the use of indwelling epidural catheters (which may reduce complications) and possibly avoid the need for PCA. Thus, a single relatively expensive medication given once might decrease the complexity of care, improve quality and possibly save money. This study does not use necessary detailed methodology to address the issue of whether DepoDur® is value for money. Any attempt to study this would need to include the costs of additional nursing, if that were considered necessary.

Analgesic efficacy of DepoDur® alone, or in combination with bupivacaine, for low abdominal surgery: a randomized, placebo-controlled trial

Gamblinga D, Hughesa T, Campbella J, et al. The Journal of Pain 2007; **8** (Suppl. 1): S45

BACKGROUND. Fentanyl and preservative-free morphine are commonly mixed with bupivacaine for epidural administration.

INTERPRETATION. A prospective study was conducted to evaluate the effect of bupivacaine admixture on DepoDur®. Patients undergoing elective surgery received epidural DepoDur® 15 mg or placebo as a separate injection 15, 30 or 60 min after 0.25% epidural bupivacaine 20 ml. Postoperative analgesia was provided by fentanyl PCA. For all analgesia efficacy endpoints, DepoDur® with bupivacaine was superior to bupivacaine alone. Combined treatment was not different from DepoDur® alone. Nausea and vomiting were more frequent after DepoDur® with bupivacaine (75% and 37%) compared with DepoDur® (59% and 19%) or bupivacaine alone (52% and 13%). Respiratory depression related to DepoDur® occurred in one patient receiving DepoDur® alone vs. six patients receiving DepoDur® with bupivacaine. The improved analgesia and increased incidence of typical opioid side-effects suggest that bupivacaine may accelerate the release of morphine from the DepoDur® foam, possibly by destabilizing the micelles, and raises concerns about the safety of such practice in general clinical use.

Liposomal formulations of prilocaine, lidocaine and mepivacaine prolong analgesic duration

Cereda C, Brunetto G, de Araujo D, et al. Canad J Anesth 2006; **53**: 1092

BACKGROUND. Local anaesthesia is widely used for surgical procedures as the sole anaesthetic and is also a key supplement to general anaesthesia techniques, especially in day surgery. Extending the duration of action of local anaesthetics might increase patient comfort and satisfaction after surgery or even make practicable as a day-case procedures type of surgery, which would previously have required a hospital stay. Liposomes are tiny spherical vesicles comprising a phospholipid bilayer membrane and contain a liquid core within which drugs may be delivered. Liposomes are potential vehicles for slow release delivery of local anaesthetics.

INTERPRETATION. Two per cent liposomal formulations of prilocaine, lidocaine and mepivacaine were prepared and compared with standard 2% aqueous solutions by measuring the duration of infraorbital nerve blockade when the formulations were injected into rats. A control preparation of liposomes without local anaesthetic was without anaesthetic effect. The liposomal formulation increased the intensity of the block by 26–57% and its duration by 23–55%.

Comment

These results indicate that liposomes provide effective drug delivery systems for intermediate-duration local anaesthetics. Mepivacaine was affected to the greatest extent, while lidocaine benefited least from liposome encapsulation. Recently, a similar study has demonstrated prolonged local anaesthetic effect of a liposomal bupivacaine preparation in mice |5|. We can anticipate further, probably rapid, development of liposomal local anaesthetic formulations for use in man. Given that the drugs themselves are well understood and widely used, there will be pressure to accelerate the processes of clinical study and regulatory approval. Nevertheless, a cautious approach may be appropriate as the consequences of prolonged local anaesthetic block at tissue level (as opposed to neuraxial block) are unclear. Further, the practical implications of patients with prolonged local anaesthesia in a home environment need comprehensive consideration and safe working practices must be established.

Iontophoretic transdermal system using fentanyl compared with patient-controlled intravenous analgesia using morphine for postoperative pain management

Grond S, Hall J, Spacek A, *et al. Br J Anaesth* 2007; **98**: 806–15

BACKGROUND. Iontophoresis drug application uses an electrical current to facilitate the movement of a pharmaceutical through the skin. This avoids first-pass hepatic metabolism and permits the development of a needle-free application system. Although iontophoresis has been researched for years, the emergence of a viable commercial application has lagged theoretical developments. Recently, a single-use self-contained iontophoresis system for administration of fentanyl has been developed and its principles and potential described elsewhere |6|.

INTERPRETATION. This large-scale multicentre European phase III study compared the fentanyl iontophoretic transdermal system (fentanyl ITS) with morphine-based PCA in patients undergoing elective major orthopaedic or abdominal surgery. The study design was pragmatic with no restrictions on intraoperative management and no restrictions on the use of non-opioid analgesics, including paracetamol and NSAIDs, either during or after surgery. After patients had regained consciousness, initial analgesia was provided, with intermittent bolus injections of morphine. When patients were awake and comfortable (pain score less than 4 on a 10-point scale) they were randomly allocated to the fentanyl ITS ($n = 325$) or to morphine PCA ($n = 335$). The fentanyl ITS provided fentanyl $40\,\mu g$ over 10 min up to six times per hour, the morphine PCA dosage schemes varied between institutions. If necessary, supplementary intravenous morphine was administered during the first 3 h after initiation of fentanyl ITS or morphine PCA. The study was designed to test for non-inferiority of fentanyl ITS to morphine PCA with the patient global assessment (PGA) at 24 h as the primary endpoint. PGA describes the pain control as poor, fair, good or excellent with responses of good or excellent defined as success. The patients studied were mainly white and in the PCA group the morphine bolus dose varied between 1 and 3 mg, with lockout intervals of 5 to 20 min. The proportion of PGA at 24 h that were either good or excellent were 86.2% and 87.5% for fentanyl ITS and morphine PCA, respectively. Supplemental morphine analgesia was required by 11% of patients in each group. Withdrawals for inadequate analgesia and adverse events were similar between the two treatments. Application-site reactions, primarily erythema, were seen in 44% of the fentanyl ITS group.

Comment

This was a large study with a practical design allowing the new technology, fentanyl ITS, to be evaluated in a real-world application. The widespread distribution of trial centres ensured a broad exposure, although the average number of patients per site was low (13 per centre), and in many ways this could be regarded as a pre-marketing seeding study as much as a formal clinical trial. Nevertheless, the incorporation of supplementary analgesics is a crucial enhancement and allows us to interpret the outcomes in a real-world way – in contrast to the constrained protocols of many analgesia studies in which supplementary analgesics are prohibited and prophylactic anti-emetics withheld in favour of symptomatic treatment. The latter, more rigorous, approach yields more homogeneous patient treatments and eases interpretation of efficacy, but the corollary is outcome data that is divorced from clinical reality.

An earlier comparison of fentanyl ITS with morphine PCA |7| permitted enrolment of patients with high pain scores and subsequently described higher rates of patient withdrawal and lower PGAs for fentanyl ITS. In the present trial, the use of supplementary analgesics with titration of patients to satisfactory analgesia before enrolment probably allowed sufficient time for the ITS to become effective before severe pain developed.

This study was not blinded. In practice, the development of a double-blind, double-dummy methodology for comparing fentanyl ITS and morphine PCA would have been difficult, and it is conceivable that the subsequent complexity might have compromised patient safety. Accordingly, an element of the patient's satisfaction might be attributable to the perceived newness of the fentanyl ITS, investigator enthusiasm and other placebo effects. Overall, this was a robust and reasonably convincing study of the iontophoretic technology and suggests that fentanyl ITS may be a useful alternative to morphine PCA. Further studies might sensibly investigate whether the system can save cost, enhance patients' outcomes, permit early discharge or, possibly, be suitable for domiciliary use with subsequent early discharge from hospital.

Pharmacokinetics and pharmacodynamics of a new intranasal midazolam formulation in healthy volunteers

Wermeling DP, Record KA, Kelly TH, et al. Anesth Analg 2006; **103**: 344–9

BACKGROUND. Intranasal application midazolam is not new and the water-soluble intravenous formulation has been used in this way since at least 1988 |8| to sedate children and adult patients who have special needs. However, the standard injectable formulation is not optimized for nasal administration.

INTERPRETATION. A specially formulated intranasal formulation of midazolam was compared with intramuscular (i.m.) and intravenous (i.v.) administration in 12 adult volunteers using a crossover design in which all subjects received the drug by all three routes at 1-week intervals. Intranasal doses were delivered as 0.1-ml unit-dose sprays of a novel formulation. The mean midazolam bioavailabilities and percentage coefficient of variation were 72.5 (12) and 93.4 (12) after the intranasal and i.m. doses, respectively. Following intranasal administration, the maximum blood concentration was at 10 min. Nasopharyngeal irritation, eye watering and a bad taste were reported after intranasal doses.

Comment

The adverse events reported after the intranasal presentation were typical of those described when the standard i.v. presentation is given nasally. The reported pharmacokinetics suggest that the novel formulation works but give us no idea whether it represents an improvement. What is missing from the present study is a direct comparison between the novel nasal formulation and the 'standard' technique, that is, using the i.v. formulation inappropriately. Further, such a comparison should be in the intended patient population, i.e.. children, not adults, as were studied here.

Control of muscle relaxation during anesthesia: a novel approach for clinical routine

Stadler KS, Schumacher PM, Hirter S, et al. IEEE Trans Biomed Eng 2006; **53**: 387–98

BACKGROUND. Closed-loop administration of a drug to produce a stable desired clinical effect exploits biomedical engineering, pharmacokinetics and

pharmacodynamics. Neuromuscular block is an especially attractive target for such a development because the effect – paralysis – is readily measured.

INTERPRETATION. The authors describe enhancements of the engineering approach to closed-loop control of neuromuscular block using two separate measures within the train-of-four, i.e. the twitch count and the t1/t4 ratio. By integrating these responses within a physiologically based pharmacokinetic and pharmacodynamic model, in this case for 28 patients receiving vecuronium, effective closed-loop control was achieved without an initial period of stabilization – which was typical of earlier systems. Only three patients required pharmacological reversal of neuromuscular blockade.

Comment

Claims for closed-loop control of neuromuscular block include stable block, minimization of drug consumption, reduction of clinician workload and the possibility of avoiding the need to reverse paralysis at the end of the case. In practice, such systems, which have been described for many years |9|, may represent the technical solution to something of a non-problem.

Most clinicians already feel comfortable using neuromuscular blockers and do so when necessary. However, clinical practice is changing and the overall requirements for intraoperative paralysis appear to be decreasing. At the same time, the problems associated with prolonged paralysis in the critically ill are now well documented.

Closed-loop control of rocuronium infusion was considered as an enhancement to the product profile of an in-patent pharmaceutical much as target-controlled infusion was offered to users of propofol i.v. anaesthesia. In the latter case the development addressed a real clinical need – the reluctance of clinicians to use i.v. anaesthesia because of its perceived complexity. In the case of paralysis the clinical need is not clearly defined and closed-loop systems such as this one are unlikely to become a commercial reality.

References

1. Shihata AA, Salzetti RG, Schnepper FW, Deutsch G. Innovative technique for Norplant implants removal. *Contraception* 1995; **51**: 83–5.

2. Hanning CD, Vickers AP, Smith G, Graham NB, McNeil ME. The morphine hydrogel suppository. A new sustained release rectal preparation. *Br J Anaesth* 1988; **61**: 221–7.

3. Liu KS, Tzeng JI, Chen YW, Huang KL, Kuei CH, Wang JJ. Novel depots of buprenorphine prodrugs have a long-acting antinociceptive effect. *Anesth Analg* 2006; **102**: 1445–51.

4. Anonymous. Detailed view: safety labeling changes approved by FDA Center for Drug Evaluation and Research (CDER) – February 2007.

5. Shikanov A, Domb AJ, Weiniger CF. Long acting local anesthetic-polymer formulation to prolong the effect of analgesia. *J Control Release* 2007; **117**: 97–103.

6. Power I. Fentanyl HCl iontophoretic transdermal system (ITS): clinical application of iontophoretic technology in the management of acute postoperative pain. *Br J Anaesth* 2007; **98**: 4–11.

7. Viscusi ER, Reynolds L, Chung F, Atkinson LE, Khanna S. Patient-controlled transdermal fentanyl hydrochloride vs. intravenous morphine pump for postoperative pain: a randomized controlled trial. *JAMA* 2004; **291**: 1333–41.

8. Wilton NC, Leigh J, Rosen DR, Pandit UA. Preanesthetic sedation of preschool children using intranasal midazolam. *Anesthesiology* 1988; **69**: 972–5.

9. de Vries JW, Ros HH, Booij LH. Infusion of vecuronium controlled by a closed-loop system. *Br J Anaesth* 1986; **58**: 1100–3.

7

New reversal agents in anaesthesia: what's on the horizon?

SARAH MITCHELL, JENNIFER HUNTER

Introduction

Why do we need a new reversal agent to antagonize neuromuscular block? We have all been using neostigmine (an anticholinesterase) as a competitive antagonist of non-depolarizing neuromuscular blocking agents for many years. Although effective, it produces unwanted muscarinic effects such as bronchospasm, bradyarrhythmias and increased gut motility (which may be harmful in the presence of a potentially weak gut anastomosis). It is generally given with antimuscarinics, such as glycopyrrolate or atropine, which also have side-effects (tachyarrhythmias, dry mouth and blurred vision). Neostigmine in high doses (>2.5 mg) may increase the risk of postoperative nausea and vomiting [1,2]. More importantly, recovery from neuromuscular blockade should have commenced before neostigmine is given – reappearance of the second twitch (T2) of the train-of-four (TOF) is recommended and it takes at least 7 min to achieve a TOF ratio of 0.7 [3,4]. Although Ali *et al.* [5] stated that a TOF ratio of at least 0.7 was necessary prior to extubation, it is now thought that satisfactory recovery from block requires the return of the TOF ratio to be >0.9 [6,7]. There is evidence of significant residual effects with TOF ratios below 0.9 [6,8]. For example, Eriksson *et al.* [8] showed pulmonary aspiration in volunteers with a TOF ratio less than 0.9. Importantly, residual block is often poorly recognized [9]. In a study of patients given intermediate-duration neuromuscular blocking drugs, in those patients receiving rocuronium the incidence of residual block (TOF ratio <0.8) on arrival in the postoperative care unit was 39% [9]. Even with reversal, the incidence of residual block in the rocuronium group was 37% [9]. One reason may be that the duration of neuromuscular block with rocuronium varies widely compared with that with the benzylisoquinolones [10,11]. However, inadequate recovery from block has also been reported in the recovery room after atracurium [9].

For rapid-sequence induction, suxamethonium is the drug of choice: 1.0 mg/kg provides good intubating conditions within 60 s and spontaneous recovery from block to T1 of 90% occurs within 11 min (mean 9.3 min, with a small SD of 1.2 min) in the presence of normal plasma cholinesterase |12|. This is too long, however, to protect the brain from irreversible damage if tracheal intubation fails and the patient becomes hypoxic. There are also relative contraindications to using suxamethonium (such as hyperkalaemia and malignant hyperpyrexia), and the side-effects are numerous (including anaphylaxis, hyperkalaemia and myalgia). Rocuronium, in large doses, is also used for rapid-sequence induction: studies have shown equivalent intubating conditions with rocuronium 1.0 mg/kg to suxamethonium, although the standard deviation (SD) is greater with the non-depolarizer |13|. In addition, in these doses, rocuronium exerts its clinical effects for a long time – one study showed spontaneous recovery to a TOF ratio of 0.7 after rocuronium 0.9 mg/kg during halothane anaesthesia took 93 (SD 11.7) min |14|. The main reason for the continued use of suxamethonium in these circumstances is its short duration of action |15|. Ideally, a fast-acting non-depolarizing neuromuscular blocking agent would be available: one with a short duration of action, that could be easily reversed at any time, even in the presence of profound block. Such a muscle relaxant would be suitable to reverse in the 'cannot intubate, cannot ventilate' scenario.

Sugammadex (Org 25969)

Sugammadex is a new *selective relaxant binding agent* for rocuronium that acts by *chelation* or *encapsulation*. Early studies suggest that it is able to reverse profound neuromuscular block from this aminosteroid within 2 min (see Gijsenbergh, 2005). This may enable large doses of rocuronium to be used for rapid-sequence induction, avoiding the side-effects of suxamethonium, and allowing rescue reversal within a few minutes if necessary.

Sugammadex is designed for antagonizing neuromuscular block produced only by the aminosteroids. Does it have the same efficacy in reversing other aminosteroidal neuromuscular blocking agents such as vecuronium and pancuronium? Although primarily designed to reverse rocuronium, work has also shown its use in reversing vecuronium-induced neuromuscular block (see Suy, 2007). Animal studies suggest it is not as effective at antagonizing pancuronium |16|. Benzylisoquinolones, such as atracurium and mivacurium, have a completely different chemical structure, which will *not* be encapsulated by sugammadex |16|. One of the major benefits of this selective relaxant binding agent is that antimuscarinics do not need to be co-administered.

Pharmacology

Sugammadex is one of the γ-cyclodextrin group of oligosaccharides. It consists of eight glucose units in a ring-like structure with a molecular weight of 1297 |17| (Fig. 7.1). Cyclodextrin molecules have a hollow core, which is lipophilic. They are soluble in water.

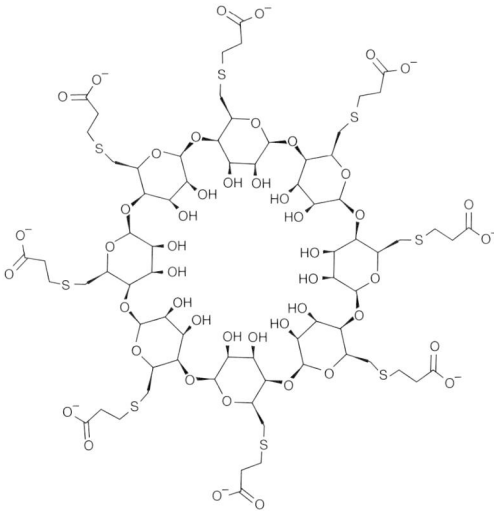

Fig. 7.1 The structure of sugammadex (per-6-(2-carboxyethylthio)-per-6-deoxy-γ-cyclodextrin sodium salt). The negative hydrophilic charges on the tails of the molecule attract and bind the positive charge on the quaternary ammonium group of rocuronium. Source: Epemolu *et al.* (2003) (published with permission).

Sugammadex (first known as Org 25969) acts by encapsulating rocuronium within its ring-like structure. The hydrophilic charged exterior draws rocuronium into sugammadex's core to form a tight, irreversible inclusion complex. The negatively charged extensions electrostatically bind to the positively charged quaternary ammonium groups of an aminosteroid neuromuscular blocking drug. Encapsulation decreases the levels of free rocuronium, promoting passive diffusion of the drug from the post-synaptic nicotinic receptors back into the plasma.

The complex is so tightly bound that even in the presence of very low levels of free rocuronium in the plasma it does not dissociate. The complex is excreted unchanged in the urine, with a mean clearance of 93 ml/min |18|, 38% less than average creatinine clearance (136 ml/min). Sparr *et al.* |18| suggest that this may be due to plasma protein binding of the complex or that sugammadex is partly reabsorbed through the renal tubule lumen. Alternatively, under general anaesthesia, this may equate with the patient's creatinine clearance. Termination of the action of rocuronium is achieved by redistribution of the complex, not by metabolism or excretion. The effect of sugammadex in patients with renal failure is still uncertain: early studies suggest that it is unaltered, but as yet only a small number of such patients (just 15) have been given the drug |19|.

Side-effects

Few adverse events have been reported with sugammadex, but they include prolongation of the QT interval of the electrocardiogram (ECG). This finding is of uncertain significance as it is common with many anaesthetic agents, including sevoflurane |**20,21**|. Episodes of hypotension have been reported with sugammadex in the Sorgenfrei study (2006). Increased urinary levels of N-acetyl-glucosaminidase (a lysosomal enzyme that may be an indicator of proximal tubule damage |**22**|) have been recorded in at least two studies in seven patients (see Sorgenfrei *et al.* 2006) |**18**|. Even though the drug has undergone significant development, it will probably take many more patient exposures before the true side-effects are realized. They would not be expected to be common if a drug has successfully reached the marketing stage. There are some questions about the potential of sugammadex to encapsulate endogenous steroids such as glucocorticoids, sex hormones and aldosterone, as well as other exogenous steroidal drugs, such as hydrocortisone |**23**|. More work needs to be carried out in humans in this respect.

First human exposure of Org 25969, a novel agent to reverse the action of rocuronium bromide

Gijsenbergh F, Ramael S, Houwing N, *et al. Anesthesiology* 2005; **103**: 695–703

BACKGROUND. This study describes the first administration of Org 25969 to 29 human volunteers. The primary objective was to explore the safety and tolerability of Org 25969 in man. The pharmacokinetics and efficacy were also assessed. In part 1 of the study, 19 healthy volunteers were given varying doses of Org 25969 (0.1–8.0 mg/kg) or placebo in this double-blind trial. Plasma and urinary levels were measured over 480 min. In part 2, 10 volunteers were each anaesthetized twice and received placebo or Org 25969 in a crossover manner. Neuromuscular monitoring was established using the TOF-Watch® SX. Total intravenous anaesthesia was induced and maintained with propofol and remifentanil. Rocuronium 0.6 mg/kg was followed 3 min later by either placebo or Org 25969 (0.1–8.0 mg/kg).

INTERPRETATION. *Part 1*: Org 25969 plasma concentrations showed dose-linear pharmacokinetics over the range 0.1–8.0 mg/kg (i.e. the half life of the drug is independent of plasma concentration and its clearance is independent of dose and dosing interval). Volume of distribution was 18 l (which is less than rocuronium: V_{ss} = 233 ml/kg |**24**|) and plasma clearance 120 ml/min (similar to glomerular filtration rate in healthy humans). *Part 2*: No reversal of neuromuscular blockade was seen with doses of Org 25969 below 1.0 mg/kg, and a plateau in its effect was seen between 4.0 and 8.0 mg/kg, suggesting that doses greater than 4.0 mg/kg are not advantageous (except perhaps for immediate reversal within a few minutes of giving the relaxant). In the two subjects who received Org 25969 8.0 mg/kg, times from administration to recovery of the TOF ratio to 0.9 were 1.0 and 1.2 min. No signs of recurarization were observed in the 90 min of TOF monitoring following Org 25969. Fig. 7.2 shows a train-of-four TOF-Watch® SX trace from a volunteer during Part 2 of the study, demonstrating a rapid and sustained return of twitch height with Org 25969 8.0 mg/kg following rocuronium 0.6 mg/kg given 3 min earlier.

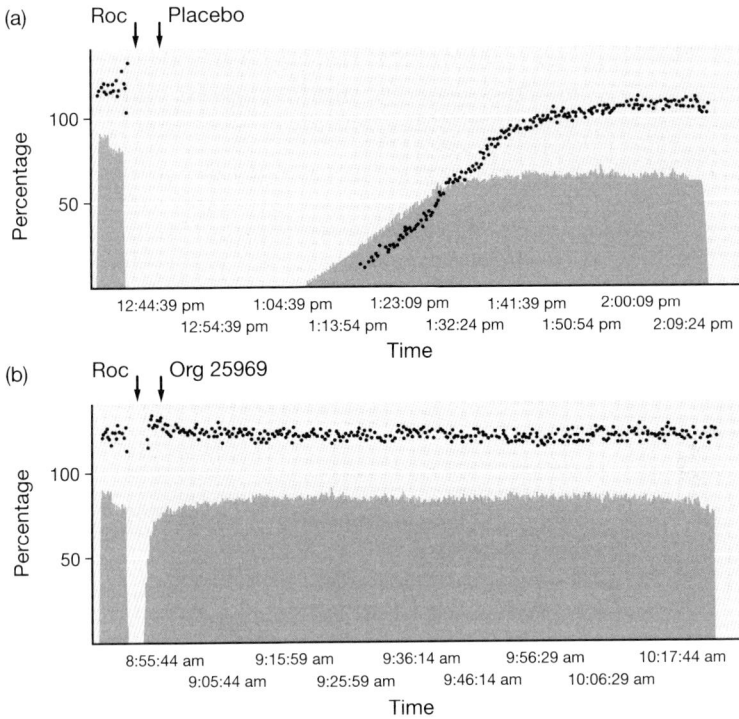

Fig. 7.2 Train-of-four TOF-Watch® SX tracing from a volunteer who participated in Part 2 of the Gijsenbergh study. The vertical lines represent the height of the twitch response and the dots are the value of the TOF ratio. The volunteer received rocuronium 0.6 mg/kg (Roc) followed by placebo at 3 min in one treatment period (a), or Org 25969 8.0 mg/kg in another treatment period (b). The very rapid effect of Org 25969 is clearly demonstrated in (b) compared with the slow spontaneous recovery from rocuronium in (a) (which is little appreciated). Source: Gijsenbergh *et al.* (2005).

Comment

This study highlighted the possibility of immediate reversal of profound rocuronium-induced neuromuscular blockade with large doses of Org 25969 in humans, mimicking the 'cannot intubate, cannot ventilate' scenario, and providing a possible escape route. The sugammadex was well tolerated in 29 healthy volunteers. Adverse events were mild, including anosmia (which may not be of import in surgical patients), taste perversion and a dry mouth. This was a small phase I study but it was the first to clarify the pharmacokinetics of Org 25969, albeit complexed with rocuronium. An assay for sugammadex itself is not yet available. This study noted eight episodes of QT interval prolongation in six subjects, but five of these were in the placebo group, so it is questionable that these findings could be attributed to sugammadex.

Reversal of rocuronium-induced neuromuscular block by the selective relaxant binding agent sugammadex. A dose-finding and safety study

Sorgenfrei IF, Norrild K, Larsen PB, et al. Anesthesiology 2006; **104**: 667–74

BACKGROUND. This study aimed to investigate the dose–response, pharmacogenetics and safety profile of reversing rocuronium-induced block with sugammadex. Twenty-seven male surgical patients received either placebo or sugammadex (at doses varying between 0.5 mg/kg and 4.0 mg/kg) for reversal of rocuronium-induced neuromuscular block at reappearance of T2 of the TOF. Intravenous anaesthesia was induced and maintained with fentanyl and propofol. The time taken for recovery of the TOF ratio to 0.9 was the primary variable recorded.

INTERPRETATION. Sugammadex produced a dose-dependent reduction in the time taken for the TOF ratio to recover to 0.9. Median recovery time in the placebo group was 21 min, compared with 1.1 min in those receiving sugammadex 4.0 mg/kg. Plasma levels of rocuronium were increased in all patients treated with sugammadex compared with placebo, suggesting that sugammadex promoted the displacement of rocuronium from the postsynaptic nicotinic receptor. Renal excretion of rocuronium was increased by the use of sugammadex. In the placebo group, the amount of rocuronium excreted in the urine at 16 h was a median of 19% of the initial dose (similar to previous reports of the urinary excretion of rocuronium |24|), but in the sugammadex 4.0 mg/kg group the median value at 16 h was 53%. Adverse events occurred in 22 out of 27 patients. Two patients developed significant hypotension. In one patient the blood pressure dropped from 100/50 mmHg to 60/27 mmHg 17 min following sugammadex 2.0 mg/kg, which may not be of significance. In another patient given sugammadex 3.0 mg/kg the blood pressure fell within 10 min from 120/80 mmHg to 61/30 mmHg, being attributed possibly to sugammadex or to the administration of fentanyl and propofol in the preceding 5 min. Neither patient developed any sequelae. Minor effects included coughing and movement during surgery and parosmia, nausea, vomiting and vertigo postoperatively. What is the mechanism for the repeatedly reported parosmia? We cannot explain it. Haematological and biochemical markers remained unchanged except for an increase in urinary N-acetyl-glucosaminidase in five patients. This was also found to be increased in some of the placebo patients and the authors did not consider it clinically relevant. No recurarization was seen in any patient.

Comment

This phase II trial demonstrated the effectiveness of sugammadex when given at the same time as an anticholinesterase is administered in current practice. It demonstrates that sugammadex in doses of 2.0 mg/kg or greater antagonizes moderate rocuronium-induced neuromuscular block, from which recovery had begun, to a TOF ratio of 0.9 within 3 min. This is impressive: time to reversal of rocuronium with neostigmine given at the same recovery point varies widely; it was reported as over 20 min in one study |25|.

As in the previous study, plasma levels of rocuronium were seen to increase in patients given sugammadex. As yet, the sugammadex–rocuronium complexes cannot be differentiated from free rocuronium molecules by the assay method, increasing the apparent levels of rocuronium in the plasma.

The study confirmed that sugammadex increased excretion of rocuronium in the urine within the first 16 h. A variety of minor adverse events were identified: it remains unclear as to how many of these were related to sugammadex. The significance of an increased N-acetyl-glucosaminidase is, as yet, uncertain.

Org 25969 (sugammadex), a selective relaxant binding agent for antagonism of prolonged rocuronium-induced neuromuscular block

Shields M, Giovannelli M, Mirakhur RK, *et al. Br J Anaesth* 2006; **96**: 36–43

BACKGROUND. The previous study by Sorgenfrei (2006) examined dose ranges and recovery times from sugammadex, following a single bolus dose of rocuronium. This study aimed to calculate the dose requirements and time to maximum recovery using sugammadex for antagonism of profound neuromuscular blockade produced by repeated doses of rocuronium. Thirty patients were anaesthetized with propofol, nitrous oxide and supplementary opiates. Rocuronium 0.6 mg/kg was administered and supplementary doses given to maintain profound block at a post-tetanic count (PTC) of <10. At recovery of T2, following at least 2 h of neuromuscular block, patients were randomized to receive sugammadex (0.5, 1.0, 2.0, 3.0, 4.0 or 6.0 mg/kg). Thus, antagonism was initiated at a moderate degree of block. The time to achieve a TOF ratio of 0.9 using the TOF-Watch® SX was recorded.

INTERPRETATION. Recovery was faster with larger doses of sugammadex (as in the Sorgenfrei study). Time to attain a TOF of 0.9 with sugammadex 0.5 mg/kg was 6.49 min (which is no benefit over neostigmine) but 1.22 min with sugammadex 4.0 mg/kg. Even after prolonged block, the effective reversal dose appears to be 2–4 mg/kg, as after a single bolus dose of rocuronium. In this study, surprisingly, sugammadex 6.0 mg/kg produced a longer recovery time than sugammadex 4.0 mg/kg (1 min 22 s in the 4.0 mg/kg compared with 2 min 32 s in the 6.0 mg/kg group). This may be due to the small number of patients (six) studied in each subgroup. No serious adverse events were recorded.

Comment

Shields *et al.* have confirmed, in this phase II study, that the effective dose of sugammadex to reverse profound block is 2.0–4.0 mg/kg. This dose is independent of whether a single bolus dose of rocuronium or repeated doses have been used. Again, there was no evidence of recurarization. Adverse events, which were judged to be related to sugammadex, were documented in 5 out of 24 patients. These were generally mild, self-limiting and not dose related. Table 7.1 documents the adverse

Table 7.1 Adverse events occurring in each human study

	Study (with dose of sugammadex used in mg/kg in parenthesis)							
	Gijsenbergh	Shields	Sorgenfrei	Suy	Sacan	Groudine	Vanacker	Total
Dry mouth	3 (8, 8, 4)	1 (0.5)			1 (4)			5
Taste perversion	2 (0.5, 4)							2
Parosmia	1 (4)		1 (3)					2
Nausea		2 (0.5, 6)	1 (3)		4 (4)		1 (2)	8
Vomiting		1 (0.5)	2 (3)				1 (2)	4
Atrial fibrillation		1 (0.5)						1
Tachycardia				1 (4)				1
Bradycardia						1 (8)	1 (2)	2
Hypotension			2 (2, 3)				2 (2)	4
Paraesthesiae	1 (8)							1
Pyrexia		1 (0.5)						1
Rigors		1 (6)						1
Agitation		1 (4)						1
Polyuria		1 (4)						1
Retention		1 (4)						1
Dyspnoea		1 (0.5)						1
Respiratory failure		1 (0.5)						1

Adverse event								
Coughing	1 (4)	NA	NA			1 (8)		5
Movement			3 (2, 3, 4)					3
Malaise			1 (2)					1
Rhinitis			1 (3)					1
Vertigo/dizziness			1 (3)			1 (2)		2
Change in temperature	1 (4)							1
Prolonged awakening				1 (2)				1
Erythema				1 (8)				1
Abdominal pain				1 (0.5)				1
Recurarization				1 (0.5)				1
Elevated creatine kinase						1 (8)		1
Hiccoughs							1 (2)	1
Elevated N-acetyl-glucosaminidase	NA	NA	NA	NA	NA	NA	NA	5
Total number of patients in study	29	30	27	79	20	43	42	61/270

Note that the events were not dose related and all resolved without sequelae. Many may be unrelated to sugammadex.
NA, not assessed.
Sources: Gijsenbergh (2005), Sorgenfrei (2006), Shields (2006), Suy (2007), Sacan (2007), Groudine (2007), Vanacker (2007).

events reported in human studies. Gijsenbergh documented QT prolongation in three patients given sugammadex. No major changes in heart rate were recorded in Shield's study but it is unclear whether the QT interval was looked at specifically.

Time course of action of sugammadex (Org 25969) on rocuronium-induced block in the rhesus monkey, using a simple model of equilibrium of complex formation

de Boer HD, van Egmond J, van de Pol F, et al. Br J Anaesth 2006; **97**: 681–6

BACKGROUND. Sugammadex is still undergoing phase III trials, and collection of data regarding its duration of action is ongoing. The aims of this study were to estimate the half life of sugammadex and determine whether a further dose of rocuronium can be given once neuromuscular block has already been reversed with sugammadex. Anaesthetized rhesus monkeys were given rocuronium 0.1 mg/kg and the degree of neuromuscular block determined. Recovery was allowed to occur spontaneously and 60 min later a dose of sugammadex 1.0 mg/kg was given. At intervals of 15, 30 or 60 min after sugammadex a further dose of rocuronium 0.1 μg/kg was administered and the neuromuscular effects documented. The first dose of rocuronium gave a mean neuromuscular block (depression of T1) of 93%. After sugammadex, rocuronium given 15, 30 and 60 min later produced neuromuscular blocks of 17%, 49% and 79% respectively.

INTERPRETATION. The authors estimate the half life of sugammadex in the rhesus monkey to be 30 min. They imply that it may be possible to produce neuromuscular block with rocuronium shortly after using sugammadex if necessary but this work also needs to be carried out in humans. Resistance to block may well be encountered in such circumstances.

Comment

This study is limited because the number of monkeys used was small (four monkeys used three times each). The authors have pointed out that rhesus monkeys are more sensitive to rocuronium than are humans (ED_{90} in humans is 0.3 mg/kg but in rhesus monkeys it is 0.1 mg/kg). The monkeys were, therefore, given a smaller dose of rocuronium than would be used in humans. However, the monkeys recovered spontaneously much faster than humans from an equipotent dose of rocuronium. Certainly, these findings suggest that rocuronium, given up to an hour after sugammadex administration, will be less efficacious than normal. It remains to be seen whether data from human studies reinforce these results.

Until more information has been collected on re-establishing neuromuscular block after reversal with sugammadex, one of the benzylisoquinolones (such as atracurium) that is unaffected by sugammadex should be used.

Reversal of neuromuscular blockade and simultaneous increase in plasma rocuronium concentration after the intravenous infusion of the novel reversal agent Org 25969

Epemolu O, Bom A, Hope F, et al. Anesthesiology 2003; **99**: 632–7

BACKGROUND. This guinea pig study looked at plasma rocuronium concentrations and reversal of neuromuscular block after intravenous infusions of sugammadex. Rocuronium 12–19 nmol/kg/min was infused for 1h to produce steady state 90% neuromuscular block in 12 anaesthetized guinea pigs. After the first 30 min, the guinea pigs received a concomitant infusion of either sugammadex 50 nmol/kg/min or saline. Twitch height was recorded and plasma levels of rocuronium measured at 10-min intervals. At the end of the study, rocuronium levels in the urine remaining in the bladder were measured.

INTERPRETATION. After 30 min, a steady-state plasma rocuronium concentration and 90% twitch depression were reached in each group. In the six guinea pigs then infused with saline there was no difference in twitch height or plasma rocuronium concentration over the next 30 min (Fig. 7.3). In contrast, with an infusion of sugammadex there was

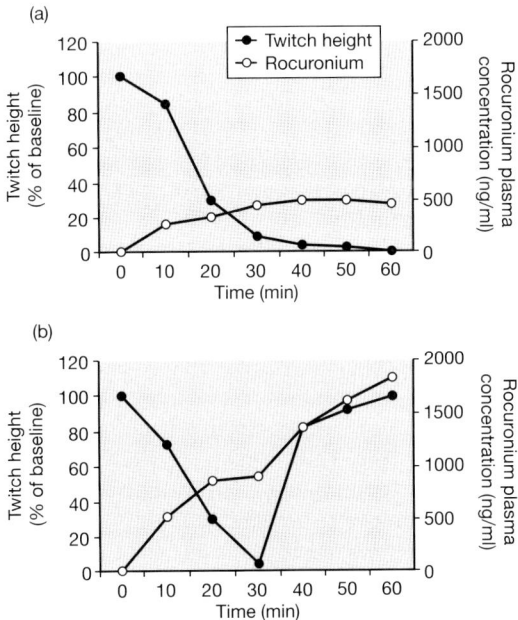

Fig. 7.3 Relationship between plasma rocuronium concentration and twitch height in the saline-treated (a) and sugammadex (b) groups. The plasma rocuronium concentration and twitch height dramatically increase with the start of the sugammadex infusion (b), compared with the saline group (a), suggesting rapid termination of neuromuscular block. Source: Epemolu et al. (2003).

rapid reversal of neuromuscular block, despite the ongoing rocuronium infusion, and an increase in the concentration of rocuronium in the plasma (see Fig. 7.3). The authors reported no significant changes in the heart rate or blood pressure in either group.

Comment

This is a small study of sugammadex in guinea pigs. Whether these results can be reproduced in humans is unknown. However, it confirms that sugammadex causes the reversal of profound rocuronium-induced neuromuscular block (recovery to 80% of control twitch height within 10 min). It is unlikely that an infusion of a reversal agent would be used in clinical practice, and this may have contributed to the absence of cardiovascular changes. We acknowledge, however, that infusions of relaxants are used to maintain steady state neuromuscular block. The doubling of plasma concentrations of rocuronium within 30 min of the start of the sugammadex infusion (see Fig. 7.3) suggests that redistribution is the main mechanism of recovery from block.

Effective reversal of moderate rocuronium- or vecuronium-induced neuromuscular block with sugammadex, a selective relaxant binding agent

Suy K, Morias K, Cammu G, et al. Anesthesiology 2007; **106**: 283–8

BACKGROUND. Previous studies showed that sugammadex is an effective selective relaxant binding agent for rocuronium. This phase II study also looked at the effects of sugammadex on vecuronium-induced neuromuscular blockade. Under total intravenous anaesthesia (with propofol and remifentanil), 80 surgical patients were randomly allocated to receive either rocuronium 0.6 mg/kg or vecuronium 0.1 mg/kg. Varying doses of sugammadex or placebo were given at reappearance of T2 (TOF-Watch® SX), and the time taken for recovery of the TOF ratio to 0.9 was recorded.

INTERPRETATION. Sugammadex reduced recovery times in both the rocuronium and vecuronium groups compared with placebo. Mean time in the rocuronium group to a TOF ratio of 0.9 was 3.7 min with sugammadex 0.5 mg/kg and 1.1 min with sugammadex 4.0 mg/kg. This is very fast indeed. In the vecuronium group, mean time to a TOF ratio of 0.9 was 2.5 min after sugammadex 1.0 mg/kg compared with 1.5 min in the 4.0 mg/kg group. Again, these are much faster recovery times than with neostigmine, albeit slightly longer than after rocuronium – unfortunately, no statistical comparison was given. Adverse events were recorded in 50% of the vecuronium group and 64% of the rocuronium group. One patient in the rocuronium/sugammadex 4.0 mg/kg group developed a tachycardia within 1 min of being given sugammadex, but this resolved within 1 min. Other adverse events possibly related to the drug were prolonged awakening (one patient: sugammadex 2.0 mg/kg) and postoperative erythema (one patient: sugammadex 8.0 mg/kg – the authors did not specify which part of the body). One case of abdominal discomfort was considered definitely related to sugammadex (0.5 mg/kg). Unfortunately, the authors make no further comment about this event. However, 57% of the placebo patients also experienced an adverse event. There was no apparent relationship between the dose of sugammadex and the adverse events reported. There was, however, one case of residual neuromuscular block in the vecuronium group. The patient received the lowest dose of sugammadex (0.5 mg/kg) and the TOF ratio initially rose to 0.9 but decreased to 0.8 (no mention of the time period over which this happened is made in the article). There were no clinical signs of residual block in this patient, but the low dose of sugammadex used was probably inadequate in these circumstances.

Comment

This is the first report of sugammadex effectively reversing vecuronium-induced neuromuscular block when recovery has commenced (not profound block). With sugammadex 4.0 mg/kg, the mean time to recovery of the TOF ratio to 0.9 was similar in both the vecuronium and rocuronium groups (1.1 min in the rocuronium group and 1.5 min in the vecuronium group).

No mention of analysis of the ST segments was made during this study, although one patient developed a tachycardia. The adverse events thought to be related to sugammadex were mild or moderate in nature and resolved spontaneously. However, serious adverse events were reported in six patients (haematoma, small bowel perforation in two patients, haemorrhage at incision site, constipation and muscle haemorrhage). These were thought by the safety assessor to be unrelated to sugammadex.

For the first time in a prospective study, the efficacy of sugammadex in reversing vecuronium- as well as rocuronium-induced neuromuscular block when recovery has commenced was demonstrated.

Sugammadex reversal of rocuronium-induced neuromuscular blockade: a comparison with neostigmine–glycopyrrolate and edrophonium–atropine

Sacan O, White PF, Tufanogullari B, *et al. Anesth Analg* 2007; **104**: 569–74

BACKGROUND. This open, parallel study recruited 60 patients undergoing elective surgical procedures and divided them into three groups. Induction was with fentanyl and propofol and anaesthesia was maintained with an infusion of remifentanil and desflurane. Muscle relaxation was obtained with rocuronium 0.6 mg/kg and further doses as necessary. At the end of the operation, reversal drugs were given at least 15 min after the last dose of rocuronium. This was considered to be in the presence of moderate block. The initial twitch height on reversal was 12 ± 8% in the edrophonium group, 12 ± 14% in the neostigmine group and 6 ± 7% in the sugammadex group. The first group received edrophonium 1 mg/kg and atropine 10 μg/kg, the second group were given neostigmine 70 μg/kg

and glycopyrrolate 14 µg/kg, and the third group sugammadex 4 mg/kg. Train-of-four responses and haemodynamic variables were recorded throughout. A blinded observer recorded any adverse events during and after surgery.

INTERPRETATION. The results were impressive: 20/20 in the sugammadex group achieved a TOF ratio of 0.9 in less than 5 min, compared with 0/20 in the edrophonium and 1/20 in the neostigmine group. The TOF was monitored for 30 min after giving the reversal drug. The mean time to reach a TOF ratio of 0.9 in the sugammadex group was 1 min 47 s (SD 61 s) compared with 5 min 31 s (SD 27 s) and 17 min 24 s (SD 590 s) in the edrophonium and neostigmine groups respectively (based on only two patients in the edrophonium group and five in the neostigmine group who reached a TOF = 0.9 in the 30-min period).

Comment

These results again demonstrate the effectiveness of sugammadex in reaching a TOF ratio of 0.9 in less than 5 min after moderate blockade from rocuronium. It is the first study to directly compare its speed of action with the currently available reversal agents, neostigmine and edrophonium. It highlights some of the inadequacies of the drugs used presently: namely, the length of time taken to reach a TOF value of 0.9, the variability in the speed of response, and the unpleasant side-effects (such as dry mouth and tachycardia). The adverse events recorded were few – there were no significant changes in pulse rate, QT interval or blood pressure, and minimal side-effects were noticed postoperatively. Perhaps not surprisingly, the incidence of a dry mouth in the recovery unit was 1/20 in the sugammadex group and 19/20 and 17/20 in the edrophonium and neostigmine groups respectively ($P < 0.05$).

The study can be criticized – the authors admit it would have been better to perform a randomized controlled trial but they state the drug company protocol requirements prevented this. The doses of neostigmine (70 µg/kg) and glycopyrrolate (14 µg/kg) used seem larger than those used in the UK – which may have contributed to the tachycardias seen in this group. The dose of sugammadex used was based on the Sorgenfrei study: it would have been useful to also compare the effect of a lower dose, for example sugammadex 2 mg/kg. Usefully, this study included a volatile agent for maintenance of anaesthesia – all the previous studies have used intravenous anaesthesia. Another study published in the same issue of *Anesthesia and Analgesia* investigates the efficacy of sugammadex during sevoflurane or propofol anaesthesia (see Vanacker *et al.* 2007).

A randomized, dose-finding, phase II study of the selective relaxant binding drug, sugammadex, capable of safely reversing profound rocuronium-induced neuromuscular block

Groudine SB, Soto R, Lien C, et al. Anesth Analg 2007; **104**: 555–62

BACKGROUND. Reversal of profound neuromuscular block is potentially one of the more exciting uses of sugammadex. This small study compared varying doses of sugammadex in reversing rocuronium-induced neuromuscular block at a post-tetanic count (PTC) of 1 or 2 in elective surgery patients. Propofol was used for induction and maintenance, with nitrous oxide and fentanyl or remifentanil for analgesia. Thirty-seven patients were randomized to receive either rocuronium 0.6 mg/kg or 1.2 mg/kg, with maintenance doses to keep a PTC of 1 or 2. For reversal, a dose of sugammadex (0.5, 1.0, 2.0, 4.0 or 8.0 mg/kg) was given. The times taken to reach a TOF ratio of 0.9 after giving the sugammadex were compared.

INTERPRETATION. At doses of sugammadex 0.5 or 1.0 mg/kg, the time taken to reach a TOF ratio of 0.9 varied widely (4.5–84.1 min). In some cases, a TOF of 0.9 had not been reached after 30 min and a dose of neostigmine was given. As the dose of sugammadex was increased, the speed of recovery increased, with a reduction in variability. At a dose of 2.0 mg/kg given when the PTC was 1 or 2, the time taken to reach a TOF ratio of 0.9 was between 1.8 and 15.2 min, and in the 4.0 mg/kg and 8.0 mg/kg group a TOF of 0.9 was reached between 1.5 and 4.7 min or between 0.8 and 2.1 min, respectively. The adverse events thought possibly to be related to sugammadex included coughing on the tracheal tube (8.0 mg/kg – likely to be secondary to rapid reversal), dizziness (2.0 mg/kg) and bradycardia (8.0 mg/kg). The most serious reported adverse event was a significantly elevated creatine kinase (CK) level (5400 iu/l) in one of the nine patients in the 8.0 mg/kg group. This patient had a total abdominal hysterectomy. Such a finding is not uncommon in postoperative patients but more modest increases of 250–300 iu are normally found |26|. Otherwise, the patient had an uncomplicated recovery. All the other patients appeared to have had CK levels measured in this study, but in no other patient was any change in this variable reported as an adverse event.

Comment

This small, open-label study showed that doses of sugammadex 4.0 mg/kg and above are capable of rapidly reversing profound rocuronium-induced block. Doses less than 1.0 mg/kg are not sufficient to reverse block from a PTC of 1 or 2. Only 43 patients received sugammadex in this study out of 50 who were enrolled, and only 37 patients were included in the efficacy analysis because of protocol violations. All 43 patients were included in the safety analysis. There were no significant changes in blood pressure or QT interval in these patients, which is reassuring compared with the earlier trials. Interestingly, a TOF ratio of 0.9 from profound block was achieved in 2 min in the patient with a raised plasma CK but, unfortunately, no comparison is provided with the CK levels in the other patients. Again, this phase II study was not a randomized controlled trial and involvement of the sponsors was acknowledged by the authors as a limitation.

Reversal of rocuronium-induced neuromuscular block with the novel drug sugammadex is equally effective under maintenance anesthesia with propofol or sevoflurane

Vanacker BF, Vermeyen KM, Struys MMRF, et al. Anesth Analg 2007; **104**: 563–8

BACKGROUND. Sevoflurane has been shown to prolong the duration of action of rocuronium compared with propofol |27|, and so far the majority of studies of sugammadex have used total intravenous anaesthesia. This study compared the efficacy of sugammadex in reversing rocuronium-induced block to a TOF ratio of 0.9 during sevoflurane or propofol anaesthesia. After induction with an opioid and propofol, 42 patients were randomized to receive sevoflurane or propofol for maintenance of anaesthesia. Neuromuscular block was measured using acceleromyography (TOF-Watch® SX) and rocuronium 0.6 mg/kg given for intubation. No further doses of rocuronium were used. The time taken for reappearance of T2 was recorded and sugammadex 2.0 mg/kg was then given. Anaesthesia and neuromuscular monitoring were continued until a TOF ratio of 0.9 had been reached.

INTERPRETATION. This study demonstrated the increased duration of action of rocuronium during sevoflurane anaesthesia very clearly. Mean recovery time from administration of rocuronium to reappearance of T2 was 33 min in the propofol group and 51.8 min in the sevoflurane group ($P = 0.002$). After sugammadex, the mean time to reach a TOF ratio of 0.9 was the same in both groups (1.8 min) and less than 3 min in all but two patients (one in each group). The adverse events thought to be related to sugammadex were minimal. The QT interval was prolonged to varying extents in all patients in both treatment groups but to a more significant degree in patients in the sevoflurane compared with the propofol group. This is not unexpected as it has been shown that sevoflurane prolongs the QT interval |20,21|. There was no residual paralysis or recurarization in either group. Adverse events possibly related to sugammadex included two cases of hypotension (values not given), one case of hiccoughs, and one patient with bradycardia, nausea and vomiting.

Comment

This trial demonstrates that sugammadex is equally effective in reversing moderate rocuronium-induced neuromuscular block with maintenance anaesthesia from propofol or sevoflurane. Sugammadex 2 mg/kg, given at reappearance of the second twitch of the TOF, produced a TOF ratio of 0.9 in under 5 min in all 41 patients (one patient in the sevoflurane group was excluded for a protocol violation). This is significantly quicker than currently available reversal agents, such as neostigmine and edrophonium [25]. The prolongation of the QT interval was thought to be related to the anaesthetic agents, and other adverse events were mild and self-limiting.

Conclusion

These studies show the impressive effects of sugammadex in reversing rocuronium-induced neuromuscular block. For a summary of the effects of varying doses of sugammadex see Table 7.2. The recommended dose is 2–4 mg/kg for reversal of both rocuronium and vecuronium-induced moderate block (reappearance of T2). For rocuronium, this appears to be independent of whether a bolus dose or repeated doses initially producing profound block (to a PTC < 10) have been given. No studies looking at profound block with vecuronium have yet been reported. Gijsenbergh et al. (2005) also suggest from studies in volunteers that sugammadex 8.0 mg/kg can be used for immediate rescue reversal of block, which would make use of large doses of rocuronium more appealing for rapid-sequence induction. A plateau in the speed of recovery is reached at doses higher than sugammadex 8.0 mg/kg.

Table 7.2 Mean predicted doses of sugammadex required to reverse rocuronium- or vecuronium-induced neuromuscular block

Dose of sugammadex (mg/kg)	Mean time to reach TOF = 0.9 (min)	Reference
Immediate reversal (within 3–5 min of rocuronium)		Gijsenbergh (2005)
4	2.6–3.0	
8	1.0–1.2	
Profound block (PTC 1 or 2)		Groudine (2007)
2	4.85	
4	2.6	
8	2.25	
Profound block (twitch height 6%)		Sacan (2007)
4	1.8 min	
Moderate block (reappearance T2)		Mean results from Sorgenfrei (2006), Suy (2007) and Vanacker
2	1.6	(2007
4	1.1	
Moderate block (reappearance T2) with vecuronium		Suy (2007)
2	2.3	
4	1.5	

Sources: Gijsenbergh (2005), Sorgenfrei (2006), Suy (2007), Groudine (2007), Sacan (2007) and Vanacker (2007).

It is interesting to note that inhalational anaesthesia does not appear to affect the duration of recovery from neuromuscular block after sugammadex. The effects of sugammadex in the presence of renal impairment have also yet to be reported in detail |19|. One case report describes an accidental overdose of sugammadex 40 mg/kg given 5 min after rocuronium 0.6 mg/kg which produced a TOF ratio of 0.9 in 1 min 19 s |28|. Fortunately, the patient suffered no adverse signs or symptoms and all investigations were reported as normal after this incredible incident (how could one draw up such a large volume of drug unquestioningly?).

Adverse events were common in all these studies and although they had no lasting sequelae, there did seem to be a particularly high incidence of them in the earlier studies (see Table 7.2). Two studies noticed a significant number of episodes of coughing and movement after giving sugammadex (Sorgenfrei *et al.* |18|). These signs may well be associated with an insufficient depth of anaesthesia at a time of continuing surgical stimulus and incomplete block. As with any new drug, we need to be vigilant in observing for adverse signs and symptoms after the use of sugammadex. Throughout these studies, the significance of the recording of adverse events could be criticized: they do not seem to be good discriminators.

The cost of sugammadex is likely to be a major factor in its success: it is as yet unknown. The benefits of sugammadex over neostigmine (especially for immediate reversal and reversal of profound block) may well make clinicians choose to use rocuronium for all routine cases, with further cost implications.

References

1. King MJ, Milazkiewicz R, Carli F, Deacock AR. Influence of neostigmine on postoperative vomiting. *Br J Anaesth* 1988; **61**: 403–6.

2. Tramer MR, Fuchs-Buder T. Omitting antagonism of neuromuscular block: effect on postoperative nausea and vomiting and risk of residual paralysis. A systematic review. *Br J Anaesth* 1999; **82**: 379–86.

3. Hunter JM, Jones RS, Utting JE. Use of atracurium during general surgery monitored by the train-of-four stimuli. *Br J Anaesth* 1982; **54**: 1243–50.

4. McCourt KC, Mirakhur RK, Kerr CM. Dosage of neostigmine for reversal of rocuronium block from two levels of spontaneous recovery. *Anaesthesia* 1999; **54**: 651–5.

5. Ali HH, Utting JE, Gray TC. Quantitative assessment of residual antidepolarizing block. II. *Br J Anaesth* 1971; **43**: 478–85.

6. Kopman AF, Yee PS, Neuman GG. Relationship of the train-of-four fade ratio to clinical signs and symptoms of residual paralysis in awake volunteers. *Anesthesiology* 1997; **86**: 765–71.

7. Viby-Mogensen J. Postoperative residual curarization and evidence-based anaesthesia. *Br J Anaesth* 2000; **84**: 301–3.

8. Eriksson LI, Sundman E, Olsson R, Nilsson L, Witt H, Ekberg O, *et al.* Functional assessment of the pharynx at rest and during swallowing in partially paralyzed humans: simultaneous videomanometry and mechanomyography of awake human volunteers. *Anesthesiology* 1997; **87**: 1035–43.

9. Hayes AH, Mirakhur RK, Breslin DS, Reid JE, McCourt KC. Postoperative residual block after intermediate-acting neuromuscular blocking drugs. *Anaesthesia* 2001; **56**: 312–18.

10. Maybauer DM, Geldner G, Blobner M, Pühringer F, Hofmockel R, Rex C, Wulf HF, Eberhart L, Arndt C, Eikermann M. Incidence and duration of residual paralysis at the end of surgery after multiple administrations of cisatracurium and rocuronium. *Anaesthesia* 2007; **62**: 12–17.

11. Arain SR, Kern S, Ficke DJ, Ebert TJ. Variability of duration of action of neuromuscular-blocking drugs in elderly patients. *Acta Anaesthesiol Scand* 2005; **49**: 312–15.

12. Kopman AF, Zhaku B, Lai KS. The 'intubating dose' of succinylcholine: the effect of decreasing doses on recovery time. *Anesthesiology* 2003; **99**: 1050–4.

13. Andrews JI, Kumar N, van den Brom RH, Olkkola KT, Roest GJ, Wright PM. A large simple randomized trial of rocuronium vs. succinylcholine in rapid-sequence induction of anaesthesia along with propofol. *Acta Anaesthesiol Scand* 1999; **43**: 4–8.

14. Cooper RA, Mirakhur RK, Maddineni VR. Neuromuscular effects of rocuronium bromide (Org 9426) during fentanyl and halothane anaesthesia. *Anaesthesia* 1993; **48**: 103–5.

15. Tornero-Campello G. Rapid-sequence induction: rocuronium or suxamethonium? *Anesth Analg* 2006; **103**: 1579.

16. Miller S, Bom A. Org 25969 causes selective reversal of neuromuscular blockade induced by steroidal NMBs in the mouse hemi-diaphragm preparation. *Eur J Anaesthesiol* 2001; **18** (Suppl. 23): 100.

17. Hunter JM, Flockton EA. The doughnut and the hole: a new pharmacological concept for anaesthetists. *Br J Anaesth* 2006; **97**: 123–6.

18. Sparr HJ, Vermeyen KM, Beaufort AM, Rietbergen H, Proost JH, Saldien V, *et al.* Early reversal of profound rocuronium-induced neuromuscular blockade by sugammadex in a randomized multicenter study: efficacy, safety, and pharmacokinetics. *Anesthesiology* 2007; **106**: 935–43.

19. Staals L, Snoeck MMJ, Flockton EA, Heeringa M, Driessen JJ. The efficacy of sugammadex in subjects with impaired renal function. *Eur J Anaesthesiol* 2007; **2**: 122–3.

20. Paventi S, Santevecchi A, Ranieri R. Effects of sevoflurane vs. propofol on QT interval. *Minerva Anestesiol* 2001; **67**: 637–40.

21. Kleinsasser A, Loeckinger A, Lindner KH, Keller C, Boehler M, Puehringer F. Reversing sevoflurane-associated Q-Tc prolongation by changing to propofol. *Anaesthesia* 2001; **56**: 248–50.

22. Westhuyzen J, Endre ZH, Reece G, Reith DM, Saltissi D, Morgan TJ. Measurement of tubular enzymuria facilitates early detection of acute renal impairment in the intensive care unit. *Nephrol Dial Transplant* 2003; **18**: 543–51.

23. Bom A, Bradley M, Cameron K, Clark JK, van EJ, Feilden H, MacLean EJ, Muir AW, Palin R, Rees DC, Zhang MQ. A novel concept of reversing neuromuscular block: chemical encapsulation of rocuronium bromide by a cyclodextrin-based synthetic host. *Angew Chem Int Ed Engl* 2002; **41**: 266–70.

24. Proost JH, Eriksson LI, Mirakhur RK, Roest G, Wierda JM. Urinary, biliary and faecal excretion of rocuronium in humans. *Br J Anaesth* 2000; **85**: 717–23.

25. Bevan JC, Collins L, Fowler C, Kahwaji R, Rosen HD, Smith MF, de Scheepers LD, Stephenson CA, Bevan DR. Early and late reversal of rocuronium and vecuronium with neostigmine in adults and children. *Anesth Analg* 1999; **89**: 333–9.

26. Charlson ME, MacKenzie CR, Ales KL, Gold JP, Fairclough GF Jr, Shires GT. The post-operative electrocardiogram and creatine kinase: implications for diagnosis of myocardial infarction after non-cardiac surgery. *J Clin Epidemiol* 1989; **42**: 25–34.

27. Lowry DW, Mirakhur RK, McCarthy GJ, Carroll MT, McCourt KC. Neuromuscular effects of rocuronium during sevoflurane, isoflurane, and intravenous anesthesia. *Anesth Analg* 1998; **87**: 936–40.

28. Molina AL, de Boer HD, Klimek M, Heeringa M, Klein J. Reversal of rocuronium-induced (1.2 mg kg⁻¹) profound neuromuscular block by accidental high dose of sugammadex (40 mg kg⁻¹). *Br J Anaesth* 2007; **98**: 624–7.

Declaration of interest

Jennifer Hunter received funding from Organon Teknika plc towards clinical (phase IIIa) research trials on Org 25969 (sugammadex) in 2006.

8

Receptors in anaesthesia: what's new?

DAVID LAMBERT

Introduction

From the outset this was a difficult chapter to prepare as a recent search on PubMed in the last 18 months of the proposed title 'Receptors in anaesthesia' yields ~247 hits! A separate search of 'Opioids and anaesthesia' gives a further 671 possible hits, probably making the original 247 a gross underestimate. My selection of only 10 papers (4% of 247) largely reflects my own personal interests and I apologize to those authors whose work I did not select. I have chosen work covering the 'practical stages of anaesthesia' and included: anaesthetic action (papers on xenon and Orexins); nicotinic receptors and neuromuscular blockade (mode of action of suxamethonium); pain (receptors in the transmission process and opioids); and intensive care (melanocortins and Toll-like receptors). I hope that you will find my personalized view of these papers interesting.

Basic receptor pharmacology is one of the main areas of interest in modern anaesthetic research. Indeed, the advancement of the $GABA_A$ receptor as a unifying target (with a couple of exceptions) of anaesthetic action laid the purely lipid hypothesis of Meyer-Overton to rest and $GABA_A$ receptors remain an active area of interest [1].

The identification of many orphan receptors and the application of reverse pharmacology (receptor first, ligand second) has added a fourth opioid receptor, the nociceptin receptor (NOP), to our probably most well-known anaesthetic family, the opioids. From identification of NOP in c. 1994 and its endogenous peptide ligand nociceptin/orphanin FQ (N/OFQ) in 1995 to the present date, there has been rapid advancement in knowledge of this interesting system, including some clinical trials. I have included a study from the anaesthetic literature of this receptor–peptide system in which analgesia and hypnosis are described – an attractive feature of an agent used in anaesthesia. On the opioid theme the application of genetic approaches to the study of MOP (μ) opioid receptor single nucleotide polymorphisms (in particular the A118G polymorphism) as an explanation for varying opioid requirements and the interaction of MOP and capsaicin (TRPV1) receptors is also included.

Protection of neurons and organ systems has been the subject of many anaesthetic-related studies and there is currently a large volume of literature on preconditioning, particularly with respect to the heart |2,3|. Indeed, over the review period for this article there were 21 papers on 'Anaesthesia and preconditioning'. I have, therefore, selected three papers that describe protection from different standpoints: Xenon for neuroprotection, with emphasis on possible use in neonates; and the role of melanocortin and Toll-like receptors in organ protection. These latter two receptor types may be important during sepsis and systemic inflammatory response system (SIRS). Suxamethonium has been in successful clinical use for many years, yet its precise mode of action with regard to non-muscle effects is addressed in the paper of Jonsson *et al.*, who show that this agent does not interact with neuronal nicotinic receptors.

Xenon mitigates isoflurane-induced neuronal apoptosis in the developing rodent brain

Ma D, Williamson P, Januszewski A, *et al*. Anesthesiology 2007; **106**: 746–53

BACKGROUND. There can be few less obvious anaesthetic agents than xenon, yet this agent has been used in the clinical setting for half a century. Xenon displays low blood–gas partition coefficient, low cardiovascular side-effect profile, analgesic properties and neuroprotective actions |4,5|, making it a particularly interesting/useful anaesthetic agent. However, the low abundance and costs involved in production require rational decisions as to indications for use. In this study the authors show that isoflurane-induced apoptosis in the developing rat brain can be prevented by co-administration of 75% xenon. Are the authors justified to suggest that this agent might be of use in anaesthesia for neonates?

INTERPRETATION. Exposure of 7-day-old rat pups to 0.75% isoflurane (but not 75% nitrous oxide or xenon) produced an increase in cortical caspase-3 staining (indicating apoptosis). When nitrous oxide and isoflurane were combined, apoptosis was enhanced. However, when xenon was co-administered with isoflurane, apoptosis returned to that produced by air alone. Similar data were observed in the hippocampus. The authors also examined a range of apoptotic markers in organotypic hippocampal slices from 8- to 9-day-old mice pups exposed to the various gases for 6 h. These *in vitro* studies confirm and extend the *in vivo* findings to show that isoflurane increases the expression of markers of both intrinsic and common apoptotic pathways that were enhanced by nitrous oxide but reduced by xenon.

Comment

Xenon (and nitrous oxide) are NMDA receptor antagonists and xenon is known to produce neuroprotection |4,5|. This study clearly shows that isoflurane and nitrous oxide alone or in combination are neurotoxic and xenon can protect against this effect. What does this mean for the clinical anaesthetist? As isoflurane and nitrous oxide are commonly administered in combination, then increased neurodegeneration might be anticipated, although this is not universally accepted |6|. Whilst there are a number of problems with this study that complicate extrapolation to humans, including long exposure and the use of non-human tissue, this study give a tantalizing insight into a potential novel therapeutic strategy. So are the authors justified to suggest that xenon might be of use in neonates? Based on the data presented, further studies (and licensing issues in neonates) are certainly warranted.

Orexins increase cortical acetylcholine release and electroencephalographic activation through orexin-1 receptor in the rat basal forebrain during isoflurane anesthesia

Dong H-L, Fukuda S, Murat E, *et al. Anesthesiology* 2006; **104**: 1023–32

BACKGROUND. Orexins are involved in the control of sleep and arousal. There are two orexins (A and B) and two receptors (OX-1 and OX-2), with OX-1 showing some selectivity for orexin A. In this study the authors show that injection of orexin A and B into the basal forebrain (BF) of the rat increases acetylcholine efflux in the somatosensory cortex and increases arousal. When the pedinculopontine tegmentum (PPTg) was stimulated, acetylcholine was released and the electroencephalogram (EEG) activated, and this was blocked by the OX-1 receptor antagonist SB334867. The authors conclude that OX-1 receptors in the BF are involved in arousal.

INTERPRETATION. The authors have used a microdialysis technique coupled with discrete brain stimulation. Injection and microdialysis cannulae were placed into the BF, electrical-stimulating electrodes were placed into the PPTg and EEG recording screws were placed over the skull. All experiments were performed under 1MAC isoflurane (1.2% in rat). Injection of orexin A and higher doses of orexin B into BF stimulated acetylcholine release. EEG changes (burst suppression ratio, BSR) followed a similar pattern with a decrease in BSR from 10 pmol orexin-A and at 100 pmol all animals showed EEG arousal. For orexin B the effects were less potent and weaker. When the OX-1 receptor antagonist SB334867 was injected into BF and the PPTg electrically stimulated, acetylcholine release was inhibited, indicating endogenous orexinergic control. Similar data were observed in the EEG.

Comment

Using a number of complementary experimental strategies, the authors show that orexins (also called hypocretins) cause arousal in isoflurane-anaesthetized rats. It is already well known that orexins cause arousal and stabilize wakefulness |7|, so what is interesting about this paper? This paper suggests that, in addition to the control of 'physiological wakefulness', orexins may be involved in arousal from anaesthesia and that this involves cholinergic ventral ascending pathways originating in the

PPTg. Whilst the pathway in itself is interesting, from a receptor point of view the authors have made good use of the potency difference in OX-1 and OX-2 for orexins A and B (OX-1 show some selectivity for orexin A over orexin B but are equipotent at OX-2) and the selective OX-1 antagonist SB334867. It is also interesting that the clinical sleep disturbance, narcolepsy, is due to reduced OX-2 receptor activation (reduced spinal orexin A levels are a diagnostic criterion for narcolepsy) and that pharmacologically induced sleep (anaesthesia in this paper) might be due to reduced OX-1 receptor activation. The role of OX-2 receptors in narcolepsy comes from studies using OX-2 and orexin knockout animals |8|. It would have been nice to repeat the studies of Dong *et al.* on isoflurane-anaesthetized OX-1 and orexin knockout animals.

Activation and inhibition of human muscular and neuronal nicotinic acetylcholine receptors by succinylcholine

Jonsson M, Dabrowski M, Gurley DA, *et al. Anesthesiology* 2006; **104**: 724–33

BACKGROUND. Succinylcholine is a depolarizing neuromuscular blocking drug (NMBD), widely used in anaesthesia and emergency medicine whenever rapid relaxation and intubation are required. Despite this widespread use, its mechanism of action (particularly with respect to side-effects) is poorly understood. In this paper the authors examine the action of succinylcholine at recombinant human muscle and neuronal nicotinic receptors transiently expressed in *Xenopus* oocytes. This NMBD activates then desensitizes the muscle nicotinic receptor. In contrast the neuronal subtypes are not activated at concentrations as high as 1 mM. There was some inhibition at $> 10^{-5}$ mol/l.

INTERPRETATION. *Xenopus* oocytes were injected with mRNA encoding human muscle ($\alpha 1\beta 1\delta\epsilon$) nicotinic receptor, the presynaptic nicotinic autoreceptor ($\alpha 3\beta 2$), the ganglionic nicotinic receptors ($\alpha 3\beta 4$ and $\alpha 7$) and the central nicotinic receptor ($\alpha 4\beta 2$). There is some overlap in the locations of these receptors. The muscle type nicotinic receptor was potently activated by succinylcholine (EC_{50} 10.8 μM, Fig. 8.1) and succinylcholine inhibited the response to acetylcholine (IC_{50} 126 μM). Over the 1–10 mmol/l range there was a small activation of neuronal nicotinic receptors. There was a weak and complex inhibition of acetylcholine activation of neuronal nicotinic receptors.

Comment

There is much controversy as to the precise mode of action of the depolarizing neuromuscular blocker succinylcholine. An interaction with a muscle-type nicotinic receptor of the form $\alpha 1\beta 1\delta\epsilon$ is to be expected and this study confirms that over the clinical range of plasma concentrations such an interaction occurs. What is particularly interesting about this paper is that, by examining the interaction of succinylcholine with a range of neuronal nicotinic receptors, it is possible to draw

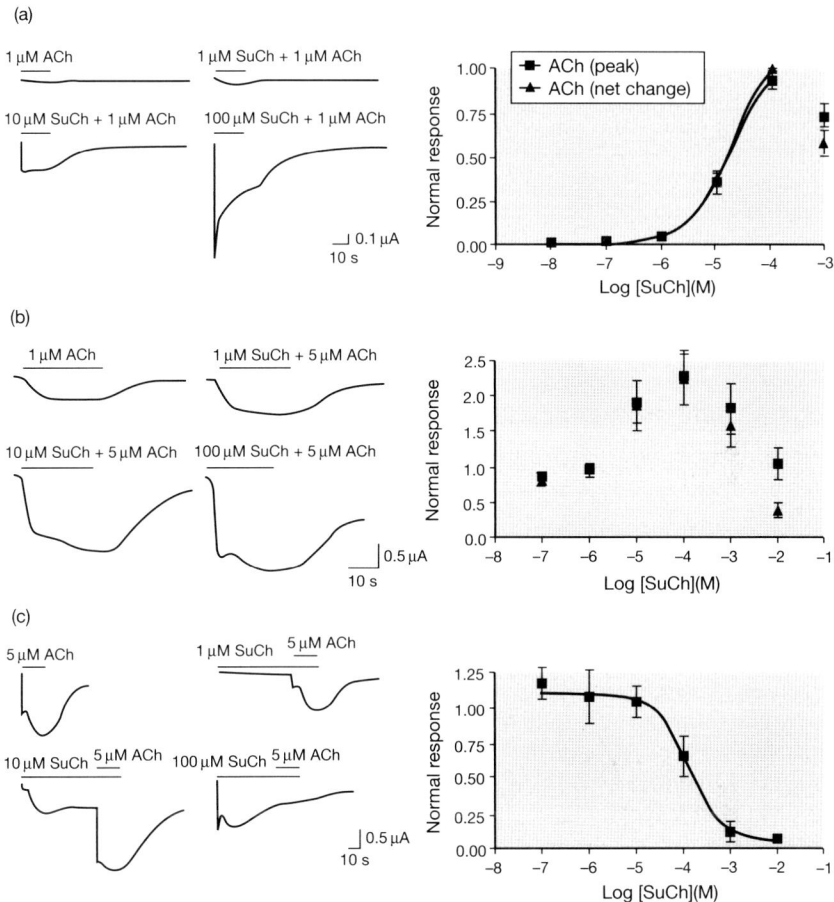

Fig. 8.1 The effect of succinylcholine (SuCh) on acetylcholine (ACh)-mediated responses in human $\alpha 1 \beta 1 \gamma 1$ nicotinic ACh receptor expressed in *Xenopus* oocytes voltage clamped at -60 mV. (a) ACh, 1 μmol/l, was coapplied with various concentrations of SuCh. Current responses in each oocyte were normalized to the peak current and maximal net charge response to ACh in each oocyte yielding the concentration–response relations shown on the right. ACh 5 μmol/l was coapplied (b) or preapplied (c) for 55 s with SuCh. The ACh responses in each oocyte were normalized to the ACh precontrols. The preapplication SuCh current was subtracted from the ACh current in preapplication experiments. Representative current traces from a single oocyte are shown on the left with ACh and SuCh added as indicated by the horizontal bars. For concentration–response curves, data are presented as mean $\pm$ SEM. When no error bars are seen, they are smaller than the symbol. Source: Jonsson *et al.* (2006).

some conclusions regarding tetanic fade and the potential to produce arrhythmias. Tetanic fade is produced by block of the presynaptic autoreceptor $\alpha 3 \beta 2$, thereby reducing acetylcholine autofacilitation |**9,10**|. This study is the first to show that succinylcholine neither activates nor blocks $\alpha 3 \beta 2$ receptors at clinically relevant concentrations and provides some molecular clues as to why tetanic fade is not observed in the clinical setting. Effects of succinylcholine on heart rhythm (ventricular tachyarrhythmias) may be caused by stimulation of ganglionic ($\alpha 3\beta 4$ and $\alpha 7$) nicotinic receptors. Again, the authors clearly show that succinylcholine neither activates nor blocks these subtypes at clinically relevant concentrations. As this agent produces a weak interaction with muscarinic receptors, the cardiotoxic actions remain unclear. Whilst this is a detailed and very logical way to address these problems, a note of caution needs to be added. In an attempt to examine a receptor in isolation, all of us who work with recombinant receptors/proteins have effectively removed the target of interest from its native environment and prevented any signalling interactions. Some of these concerns have been covered in an accompanying editorial |11|.

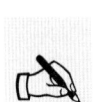

Human opioid receptor A118G polymorphism affects intravenous patient-controlled analgesia morphine consumption after total abdominal hysterectomy

Chou W-Y, Wang C-H, Liu P-H, *et al*. Anesthesiology 2006; **105**: 334–7

BACKGROUND. The efficacy of morphine in the clinic may have an underlying genetic component. Mu (*μ* or MOP) opioid receptors are the main clinical targets for opioids, including morphine and several single nucleotide polymorphisms (SNPs) have been identified for this receptor. The authors have examined PCA morphine requirements in women undergoing total abdominal hysterectomy and carrying the common SNP A118G. There was in increase in morphine requirements in A118G homozygotes.

INTERPRETATION. The authors recruited 80 Taiwanese women (46 ± 6 years), all of whom were genotyped by PCR using a 10-ml blood sample. Forty-three (53.7%) patients were homozygous for A118 (AA, this is what would be found in 'normal' MOP), 19 (23.8%) were heterozygous (AG) and 18 (22.5%) were homozygous G118 (GG). There were no demographic differences between the three genotypes. At the end of surgery, each patient received 0.08 mg/kg loading dose of morphine and then PCA for 48 h. Morphine consumption in the first 24 h was 27 mg, 29 mg and 33 mg in groups AA, AG and GG respectively; that is, there was a significant (22%) increase in morphine consumption (and morphine *demand*) in patients homozygous for the A118G SNP. There was no difference in morphine consumption over the second 24-h period. There were no significant differences in nausea or sedation scores or the numbers of patients who vomited.

Comment

The A118G mutation is an exon 1 A to G substitution changing asparagine to aspartate in position 40 of the receptor and there is some evidence of *in vitro* functional differences (although this has been disputed) |12,13| and an association of A118G with alcohol and opiate addiction has also been reported |12|. This is a relatively small study of 80 patients, of whom only 18 were homozygous A118G and the increased morphine requirements were limited to the first 24 h. So why was this paper selected? MOP receptors have been the study of intense basic research over the last two decades with (i) the suggestion that two subtypes underlie analgesia and respiratory depression, which was refuted by (ii) the molecular cloning of MOP and (iii) the identification of a highly selective MOP endogenous peptide endomorphin |14|. Variability in morphine requirements is well known and is often attributed to varying pharmacokinetics in different patient groups, but genetic variability is also a possible contributory factor. With the introduction of simple cost-effective genotyping platforms and a wealth of information available on MOP polymorphisms |12| the time for anaesthesia to exploit these technologies is here. This small study is, therefore, the beginning of these efforts and in the accompanying editorial, Landau |15| states that this is 'one of the first bench to bedside reports to examine the association of MOP polymorphism and post-op analgesia'.

Synthesis and characterization of potent and selective μ-opioid receptor antagonists, [Dmt^1, D-2-Nal^4] endomorphin-1 (Antanal-1) and [Dmt^1, D-2-Nal^4] endomorphin-2 (Antanal-2)

Fichna J, do-Rego J-C, Chung NN, *et al. J Med Chem* 2007; **50**: 512–20

BACKGROUND. The clinical 'holy grail' in opioid pharmacology and use is the design of an ultra-potent morphine-like molecule without respiratory side-effects or tolerance |11|. Endomorphin is the endogenous peptide agonist for the MOP receptor and there are two isoforms |11|. Here, the authors produce several modifications of endomorphin 1 and 2. Three of these, [Dmt^1, D-2-Nal^4] endomorphin-1 (Antanal-1), [Dmt^1, D-2-Nal^4]endomorphin-2 (Antanal-2) and [Dmt^1, D-1-Nal^4]endomorphin-1, display interesting pharmacological profiles. Antanal-1 and 2 are highly potent MOP antagonists and [Dmt^1, D-1-Nal^4]endomorphin-1 is a mixed MOP agonist and DOP antagonist.

INTERPRETATION. The structures of endomorphin 1 and 2 are Tyr-Pro-Trp-Phe-NH$_2$ and Tyr-Pro-Phe-Phe-NH$_2$. The authors have added two modifications known to produce antagonist activity: (1) addition of 2′,6′-dimethyltyrosine (Dmt) into position 1 (to replace 'normal' tyrosine) and either 3-(1-naphthyl)-D-alanine (D-1-Nal) or 3-(2-naphthyl)-D-alanine (D-2-Nal) into position 4. In total, eight peptoids were produced but Antanal-1 and 2 and [Dmt^1,D-1-Nal^4]endomorphin-1 were the most interesting. In a series of functional experiments Antanal-1 was a MOP antagonist with and antagonist potency or pA_2 of 7.61 and Antanal-2 with a pA_{22} of 8.89 *in vitro*. Both were antagonists *in vivo* in the hotplate test in mice. Interestingly, [Dmt^1,D-1-Nal^4]endomorphin-1 was a MOP agonist (*in vitro* EC$_{50}$ 1.15 nmol/l) and a DOP antagonist (*in vitro* pA_2 8.59).

Comment

The authors of this work probably feel that Antanal-1 and 2 are the more interesting, but I take a different view and find [Dmt^1,D-1-Nal^4]endomorphin-1 the more interesting molecule. DOP antagonists reduce the development of tolerance to MOP agonists without affecting analgesic efficacy (to put it in a clinical context, give a DOP antagonist and your patient may not develop tolerance to morphine). As such, a compound that can deliver both 'pharmacological profiles' goes some way to providing an opioid with a reduced side-effect profile |16|. In agreement with this strategy, animals in which the DOP has been genetically deleted (DOP knockout animals) did not become morphine tolerant |17|. The design of mixed MOP/DOP ligands is not new but use of this strategy with endomorphins is innovative and, as endomorphins are relatively small, the end peptidomimmetic product is also small and relatively easy to synthesize. It has also been demonstrated that the selective DOP antagonist naltrindole reversed MOP-mediated respiratory depression and also increased gastrointestinal transit |18,19|. Whilst it is premature to make any conclusive statements, a move away from the design and evaluation of opioids with single targets (i.e. better MOP agonists) to mixed MOP agonist/ DOP antagonists may pave the way to producing morphine-like analgesia without tolerance, respiratory depression and reduced GI motility. Indeed, such molecules might represent prototypes for a new class of analgesics.

Characterization of SB-705498, a potent and selective vanilloid receptor-1 (VR1/TRPV1) antagonist that inhibits the capsaicin-, acid-, and heat-mediated activation of the receptor

Gunthorpe MJ, Hannan SL, Smart D, *et al. J Pharmacol Exp Ther* 2007; **321**: 1183–92

BACKGROUND. TRPV1 receptors are non-selective cation channels which are sensitive to protons, noxious heat and capsaicin and are found on nociceptive afferents |20|. Development of high-potency selective TRPV1 antagonists capable of inhibiting the response to these stimuli represent a novel analgesic strategy, i.e. switching off nociceptive afferent traffic. In a series of experiments using recombinant TRPV1 and native TRPV1 of human and rat origin, the authors report a potent inhibitory action against capsaicin, pH reduced to 5.3 and increased temperature to 50°C. The authors suggest that this molecule would be suitable for clinical development.

INTERPRETATION. In HEK293 cells expressing human, rat or guinea pig TRPV1 receptors SB-705498 inhibited capsaicin mediated increase in Ca^{2+} with pK_i of 7.6, 7.5 and 7.3, respectively. In native rat dorsal root ganglion neurons a pK_i of 7.1 was measured. In response to changing pH from 7.3 to 5.3 (increased protons) pIC_{50} values for SB-705498 of 7.1 and 6.9 were obtained at human and rat receptors. The effects of elevating buffer temperature to 50°C at the human TRPV1 were inhibited by SB-705498 with a pIC_{50} of 8.2 (Fig. 8.2). There was little or no activity of SB-705498 against 39 other targets, including G-protein coupled receptors and other ion channels.

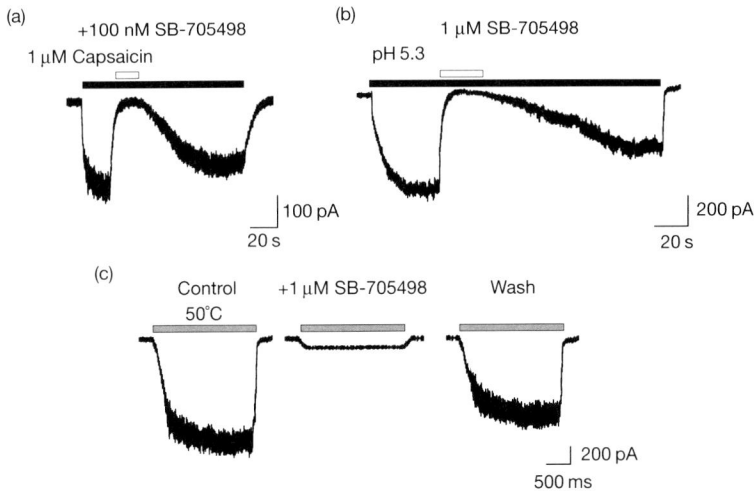

Fig. 8.2 Capsaicin ($1\,\mu M$) (a), reduced pH (5.3) (b) and increased temperature (50°C) (c) produce an inward current in HEK293 cells expressing the human TRPV1, consistent with activation. The response to these three activators was inhibited by SB-705498. Source: Gunthorpe *et al.* (2007).

Comment

TRPV1 receptors are often described as molecular integrators of inflammatory pain in as much as they respond to heat, acidosis and can be sensitized by several inflammatory mediators |20,21|. There is much debate as to whether the endocannabinoid, anandamide is an endogenous activator of this receptor and exogenous addition increases ion flux through the channel |22|. These receptors are a logical target in the pain pathway. Traditionally, capsaicin cream has been used for a range of indications including (but not limited to) diabetic neuropathy, osteoarthritis, psoriasis and overactive bladder where its use is often limited by its extreme pungency, leading to problems in patient compliance |20|. This paper explores a different approach by using an antagonist. The reasoning is that in several pain conditions abnormal TRPV1 firing might be present (via raised H^+, increased temperature or via sensitization) and that using an antagonist might switch off this signalling. SB-705498 represents a new TRPV1 antagonist with high potency and selectivity that could be used for this purpose. Moreover, this antagonist has good *in vivo* profile in terms of pharmacokinetics (in rat, guinea pig and dog) and ability to reverse capsaicin-induced secondary hyperalgesia in the rat. In the guinea pig the authors hint at reversal of inflammatory pain |23|. As a result, SB-705498 is now in clinical trials for (i) rectal hyperalgesia and irritable bowel syndrome (phase II), (ii) migraine pain (phase II) and (iii) dental pain (phase I). SB-705498 is not the only antagonist and GSK are not the only company involved in the development of TRPV1 antagonists for pain |20| and as such the future for this class as novel analgesics is bright.

μ-Opioid receptor activation modulates transient receptor potential vanilloid 1 (TRPV1) currents in sensory neurons in a model of inflammatory pain

Endres-Becker J, Heppenstall PA, Mousa SA, *et al. Mol Pharmacol* 2007; **71**: 12–18

BACKGROUND. TRPV1 receptors are involved in the development of inflammatory pain (hyperalgesia) and this can be treated with peripheral opioids |24|. TRPV1 and opioid receptors are both found in cells of the dorsal root ganglion |20,24|. This elegant study in rats examines whether opioid and TRPV1 receptors are upregulated in the DRG in inflammatory pain and whether opioid receptor activation can modulate TRPV1 function. Intraplantar injection of morphine reduced thermal hyperalgesia following intraplantar capsaicin. The authors report that both receptor types are upregulated and that morphine acting at MOP receptors reduces current flow through TRPV1 receptors.

INTERPRETATION. TRPV1 receptor mRNA levels did not change in DRG as a result of 96-h intraplantar complete Freund's adjuvant (CFA) inflammation. However, there was an approximate three-fold increase in TRPV1 protein expression measured using the radioligand [^{3}H]resiniferatoxin (although this ligand also interacts with protein kinase C), perhaps indicating that CFA increases translation rather than transcription. In an immunohistochemical paradigm 96-h CFA increased the expression of MOP and TRPV1 in DRG cells with co-expression in 14% of all neurons. In cultured DRG neurons both morphine and the experimental MOP opioid DAMGO reduced TRPV1 Ca^{2+} current. The inhibitory action of morphine was reversed by the non-selective opioid antagonist naloxone, by inhibiting G$_{i/o}$ signalling with pertussis toxin and by increasing cAMP with forskolin or 8-Br-cAMP. In whole animals i.p. capsaicin produced thermal hyperalgesia (decreased paw withdrawal latency, PWL: Fig. 8.3) and this was reduced by IP morphine.

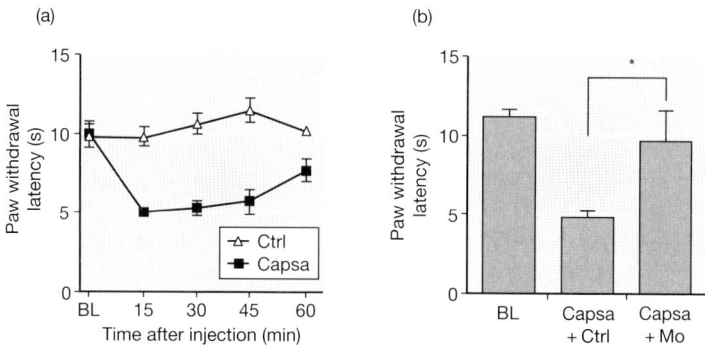

Fig. 8.3 Hyperalgesia to heat after plantar capsaicin injection in animals pretreated with morphine. The mean baseline PWL (BL, 10.4 ± 0.3 s) showed a time-dependent decrease after local capsaicin injection (Capsa) compared with control (Ctrl) animals (a). This hyperalgesia (Capsa + Crtl) was significantly reduced by local application of morphine (Capsa + Mo) (*t*-test,*P<0.05) (b). Source: Endres-Becker *et al.* (2007).

Comment

In essence this paper shows that both MOP and TRPV1 receptors are expressed on DRG neurons and that inflammation produces an up-regulation. Moreover, MOP activation modulates TRPV1 activity, indicating interplay between two disparate receptor types: G-protein-coupled opioid MOP and the ligand-gated ion channel TRPV1. This is the first study to report such a molecular interaction. Importantly, as demonstrated in the thermal hyperalgesia test, this action occurs *in vivo*. Opioid receptors couple to $G_{i/o}$ G-proteins to reduce cAMP formation and hence PKA activation, reduce Ca^{2+} channel activity and open K^+ channels to hyperpolarize. That G-protein signalling is involved in TRPV1 inhibition could be predicted but the authors show this conclusively via pertussis toxin pretreatment (which ADP-ribosylates $G_{i/o}$ to essentially uncouple opioid receptor signalling) experiments. Whilst it is possible that K^+ channel activation might hyperpolarize the DRG to reduce the TRPV1 signal, the authors have probed a role for adenylyl cyclase and cAMP by elevating intracellular cAMP with forskolin or by adding the membrane-permeable cAMP analogue 8-Br-cAMP. This treatment would activate protein kinase A and protein kinase A phosphorylates TRPV1 to increase its activity. Conversely, reduced pKA activity would reduce TRPV1 phosphorylation and reduce activity. Therefore, increased cAMP should reverse the effects of opioids and this is exactly what was reported. The authors conclude that their observations 'demonstrate an important mechanism underlying the, analgesic efficacy of peripherally acting MOP ligands in inflammatory pain'. The periphery represents an important analgesic target and, in common with research into other novel analgesic targets, offers a number of advantages with respect to side-effect profile.

The hypnotic, electroencephalographic, and antinociceptive properties of nonpeptide ORL1 receptor agonists after intravenous injection in rodents

Byford AJ, Anderson A, Jones PS, *et al*. Anesth Analg 2007; **104**: 174–9

BACKGROUND. The nociceptin/orphanin FQ peptide receptor NOP (previously termed ORL1) is currently classified as the fourth (but non-classical) opioid receptor |25|. From an anaesthetic point of view, there has been much interest in this peptide–receptor system as it affects pain processing but it also modulates a wide range of other responses including feeding, locomotion, mood and the cardiovascular system |25|. Here, the authors show two non-peptide NOP agonists, Ro 65–6570 and Org 26383, act as hypnotics and analgesics at similar doses in rodents.

INTERPRETATION. The authors measured hypnosis as loss of righting reflex (LRR) in mice and EEG burst suppression in rats and nociception via the formalin paw test in mice. The NOP agonists Ro 65–6570 and Org 26383 (given systemically) caused a dose-dependent LRR with HD_{50} values of 0.59 and 3.67 μmol/kg that was reversed by a NOP antagonist but not naloxone (Table 8.1). Both NOP agonists produced EEG burst

Table 8.1 Effects of Naloxone (3 mg/kg) or a proprietary ORL1 receptor antagonist (10 μmol/kg) on sleep times produced by Ro 65-6570 (1.2 μmol/kg) or Org 26383 (7.8 μmol/kg).

ORL1 receptor agonist	LRR (%)	Onset time (min)	Second injection	Sleep time (min)
Ro 65-6570	100	1.2 ± 0.04	Saline	38.9 ± 2.2
		1.4 ± 0.1	Naloxone	42.8 ± 1.6
Org 26383	100	1.4 ± 0.1	Saline	44.4 ± 4.8
		1.5 ± 0.4	Naloxone	45.3 ± 2.6
Ro 65-6570	100	1.3 ± 0.1	Saline	38.3 ± 3.9
		1.4 ± 0.1	ORL1 antagonist	11.8 ± 3.8
Org 26383	100	1.4 ± 0.1	Saline	31.0 ± 2.3
		1.3 ± 0.1	ORL1 antagonist	4.3 ± 2.3

LRR, percentage of mice losing their righting reflex. Data are mean $\pm$ SD ($n = 10$).
Source: Byford et al. (2007)

suppression and this corresponded with LRR. In the formalin paw test both NOP agonists inhibited formalin dependent nociceptive behaviour (licking, flinching, paw-lifting) in a dose-dependent manner. Calculated ED_{50} values (mean of phase I and II) were around 0.39 and 1.90 μmol/kg, respectively – these were close to LRR HD_{50} values. There were some technical problems with the PWL test in that high doses of NOP agonists produced LRR but this was reversed by formalin injection.

Comment

There is considerable interest in the development of NOP ligands for clinical use. That NOP ligands are hypnotic and modulate pain processing is not new |25| but this study adds a number of pieces of new and important information. Classical hypnotics interact with GABA receptors. In the present study, the effects of Ro 65–6570 and Org 26383 were reversed by NOP receptor selective antagonists, clearly indicating that the hypnotic action of these molecules was independent of a *direct* action on GABA receptors. The effect of NOP ligands, in particular the endogenous peptide N/OFQ on nociception, are complex, with pro-nociceptive and/or anti-opioid actions supraspinally and anti-nociceptive actions spinally |26|. As the authors point out, there are few published studies examining the effects of systemic administration on nociception. Non-peptide agonists offer clear advantages in this respect with regards to metabolism. In the present work systemic administration in mice produced an anti-nociceptive response with no evidence of pro-nociceptive actions. Finally, the doses required to produce hypnosis and anti-nociception for both compounds were similar.

Selective melanocortin MC$_4$ receptor agonists reverse haemorrhagic shock and prevent multiple organ damage

Giuliani D, Mioni C, Bazzani C, et al. Br J Pharmacol 2007; **150**: 595–603

BACKGROUND. Melanocortins (e.g. melanocyte-stimulating hormone [MSH] and adrenocorticotrophic hormone [ACTH]) activate the melanocortin receptor. The melanocortin receptor is a G-protein coupled receptor and a family of five isoforms (MC$_{1-5}$) with differing central and peripheral locations. In a rat model of haemorrhagic shock (withdrawal of 50% of circulating blood volume) activation of melanocortin receptors with the non-selective [Nle^4,D-Phe^7]α-melanocyte-stimulating hormone (NDP-α-MSH) or the selective MC$_4$ agonists RO27–3225 and PG-931 reversed the effects of shock. The MC4 agonist RO27–3225 protected the heart, lung, liver and kidney from damage. Pretreatment with a selective MC$_4$ antagonist HS024 prevented this protective action. The authors suggest that MC$_4$ agonists might be important in preventing organ failure following circulatory shock.

INTERPRETATION. Acute haemorrhage in rats was induced by reducing circulating blood volume over a 20- to 25-min period. This resulted in a fall of MAP to 20–25 mmHg and the death of all saline-treated animals. Treatment with NDP-α-MSH, RO27-3225 and PG-931 i.v., 5 min after the end of bleeding produced a dose-dependent increase in MAP and at the highest dose of each drug 100% survival. The effects of the highest dose (100% survival) were fully prevented by intraplantar injection of the MC$_4$ antagonist HS024 given 2 min prior to the start of bleeding. Haemorrhage increased free radical production, which was also reduced by RO27-3225 and PG-931 in a HS024-sensitive manner. Following haemorrhage there were 'substantial' changes in several organ systems, including swelling of the left ventricle, subendocardial and contraction band necrosis, low-level emphysematous changes to the lungs, scattered hepatic necrosis and enhanced bcl2 expression in the kidney. Treatment with the highest dose of RO27-3225, with measurements made at 25 min, prevented these changes. In addition, the authors studied a separate group of animals at 24 h with essentially identical results.

Comment

Melanocortins are an interesting group of peptides that include the well-known ACTH (the current MC$_2$ receptor located in the adrenal gland was previously known as the ACTH receptor) and MSH (with α, β and γ isoforms) the archetypal ligand for the MC$_1$ receptor. MC$_3$ and MC$_5$ are located both centrally and peripherally but the MC$_4$ receptor is located predominantly in the central nervous system. The authors have previously demonstrated an activation of the 'brain cholinergic anti-inflammatory pathway' |27| by MC$_4$ receptor activation and this system may be involved in the inflammatory response produced by haemorrhage. The role of these peptides in the control of feeding (obesity/cachexia) is well known but this peptide–receptor system is also involved in several other diseases, including erectile dysfunction and inflammation. The role of MC₄ receptors in haemorrhagic shock has not been explored clinically, although there is some evidence in humans that ACTH(1–14) protects against the cardiovascular effects of aortic-dissection-induced haemorrhagic shock and increased survival rates |28|. With the current interest in MC receptors and the availability of a number of selective MC agonists currently in clinical trials, it seems sensible that these drugs are tested in patients with, or at risk of, shock, where multiple organ failure might be anticipated.

Toll-like receptor 4 plays a crucial role in the immune-adrenal response to systemic inflammatory response syndrome

Zacharowski K, Zacharowski PA, Koch A, et al. Proc Natl Acad Sci USA 2006; **103**: 6392–7

BACKGROUND. Toll-like receptors (TLRs) are involved in the initial response to bacterial infection, in which they recognize components of different micro-organisms; they exhibit pattern recognition. The involvement of these receptors in sepsis and SIRS has been the subject of much work. In this study the authors have used a mixture of TLR4 knockout (KO) mice and lipopolysaccharide (LPS) to examine the role of TLR4 (and 2) in sepsis. In TLR4-KO animals there was an increase in adrenal size and an increase in several plasma cytokines. In LPS-treated wild-type animals there was an increase in these cytokines (although some of this may have been mediated by TLR2) and activation of NF-κB. This was not observed in TLR4-KO. The authors suggest that TLR4 is important in the cross talk between innate immunity and the endocrine stress response.

INTERPRETATION. In TLR-KO animals the adrenal was significantly enlarged compared with wild type, with the cortex making up this enlargement. There was a marked reduction in adrenal lipid droplets in TLR4-KO. There was a 4.5-fold increase in plasma corticosterone but adrenocorticotrophic hormone (ACTH) did not change. In TLR-KO, IL-12, TNFα and IL-1β increased, although the latter failed to reach statistical significance. Studies with LPS are confounded by the fact that some batches are contaminated with TLR2 ligands. In this study the authors used commercial (cLPS, non-pure) and pure LPS (pLPS) whose activity was confirmed in a reporter gene assay. In wild-type animals both LPS preparations increased adrenal corticosterone (measured at 6 h) and cLPS increased ACTH. No increase was observed in TLR4-KO. cLPS increased IL-1β, IL-6, IL-12, TNFα and IL10. This effect was not seen with pLPS and no response was seen with either LPS source in TLR4-KO. Both cLPS and pLPS activated the transcription factor NF-κB in wild-type but not TLR4-KO animals. From these data the authors conclude that in TLR4-KO the degree of immune–adrenal communication is impaired and that this may have important consequences in survival from sepsis and SIRS.

Comment

The ability to recognize an invading pathogen and mount a coordinated and appropriate response are critical to survival, especially in the extreme case of sepsis and SIRS. Toll-like receptors are important in this process |29|. This study examines a role for TLR4 in the response to its ligand LPS. The approach used by Zacharowski and colleagues is interesting and utilizes to good effect TLR4-KO and the LPS 'contamination' problem. In this latter approach cLPS will activate TLR4 (and TLR2 due to contamination) and pLPS will activate TLR4 only. They clearly show that TLR4 (and TLR2 from previous studies) is 'an essential mediator of the adrenal stress response'. TLR4 agonists and antagonists are at various stages of development and require evaluation in a critical care setting.

Conclusion

Receptor pharmacology, covering all of the areas of anaesthetic practice, has a great deal to offer our specialty. The '-omics' (genomics, proteomics, metabolomics) revolution, commonplace in pharmacology, is beginning to make its way into anaesthesia |30|, with studies like that of Chou et al., on the A118G SNP, exemplifying these beginnings.

It is also pleasing to note that some of the studies reviewed here involve the introduction of several new molecules to the clinic. If I had to pick one it would be the GSK capsaicin receptor (TRPV1) antagonist SB-705498, which is currently in phase II trials for pain. Most analgesics are agonists that activate receptors, for example morphine activating the MOP (μ) receptor. From a clinical perspective, receptor activation has with it a number of unwanted effects, most important of which is the development of tolerance (for the MOP receptor antagonism of the DOP receptor seems to reduce this, as shown in the Fichna et al. study). For the TRPV1 receptor, capsaicin used as an agonist is limited by pungency so an antagonist which, by definition, is devoid of action alone has a marked advantage. Switching off a painful signal – sensed by nociceptive afferents – by TRPV1 activation (inflammation, acidosis and raised temperatures) makes such good sense.

To end as I started: the isolation of orphan receptors and their methodical de-orphanization, genetic application(s) and integration of chemical synthesis is likely to provide many new pharmacological treasures. Hopefully, some of these will be of relevance to anaesthesia and anaesthetists.

References

1. Franks NP. Molecular targets underlying general anaesthesia. *Br J Pharmacol* 2006; 147 (Suppl. 1): S72–81.

2. Zaugg M, Lucchinetti E, Uecker M, Pasch T, Schaub MC. Anaesthetics and cardiac preconditioning. Part I. Signalling and cytoprotective mechanisms. *Br J Anaesth* 2003; **91**: 551–65.

3. Zaugg M, Lucchinetti E, Garcia C, Pasch T, Spahn DR, Schaub MC. Anaesthetics and cardiac preconditioning. Part II. Clinical implications. *Br J Anaesth* 2003; **91**: 566–76.

4. Preckel B, Weber NC, Sanders RD, Maze M, Schlack W. Molecular mechanisms transducing the anesthetic, analgesic, and organ-protective actions of xenon. *Anesthesiology* 2006; **105**: 187–97.

5. Sanders RD, Maze M. Xenon: from stranger to guardian. *Curr Opin Anaesthesiol* 2005; **18**: 405–11.

6. Soriano SG, Anand KJ, Rovnaghi CR, Hickey PR. Of mice and men: should we extrapolate rodent experimental data to the care of human neonates? *Anesthesiology* 2005; **102**: 866–8.

7. Sakurai T. The neural circuit of orexin (hypocretin): maintaining sleep and wakefulness. *Nature Reviews Neuroscience* 2007; **8**: 171–81.

8. Willie JT, Chemelli RM, Sinton CM, Tokita S, Williams SC, Kisanuki Y, Marcus JN, Lee C, Elmquist JK, Kohlmeier KA, Leonard CS, Richardson JA, Hammer RE, Yanagisawa M. Distinct narcolepsy syndromes in Orexin receptor-2 and Orexin null mice: molecular genetic dissection of Non-REM and REM sleep regulatory processes. *Neuron* 2003; **38**: 715–30.

9. Wessler I. Control of transmitter release from the motor nerve by presynaptic nicotinic and muscarinic autoreceptors. *Trends Pharmacol Sci* 1989; **10**: 110–14.

10. Faria M, Oliveira L, Timoteo MA, Lobo MG, Correia-De-Sa P. Blockade of neuronal facilitatory nicotinic receptors containing alpha 3 beta 2 subunits contribute to tetanic fade in the rat isolated diaphragm. *Synapse* 2003; **49**: 77–88.

11. Martyn J, Durieux ME. Succinylcholine: new insights into mechanisms of action of an old drug. *Anesthesiology* 2006; **104**: 633–4.

12. Mayer P, Hollt V. Pharmacogenetics of opioid receptors and addiction. *Pharmacogenetics and Genomics* 2006; **16**: 1–7.

13. Margas W, Zubkoff I, Schuler HG, Janicki PK, Ruiz-Velasco V. Modulation of Ca^{2+} channels by heterologously expressed wild-type and mutant human μ-opioid receptors (hMORs) containing the A118G single-nucleotide polymorphism. *J Neurophysiol* 2007; **97**: 1058–67.

14. Zollner C, Stein C. Opioids. *Handb Exp Pharmacol* 2007; **177**: 31–63.

15. Landau R. One size does not fit all. *Anesthesiology* 2006; **105**: 235–7.

16. Ananthan S. Opioid ligands with mixed μ/δ opioid receptor interactions: an emerging approach to novel analgesics. *The AAPS Journal* 2006; **8**: E118-E125.

17. Zhu Y, King MA, Schuller AG, Nitsche JF, Reidl M, Elde RP, Unterwald E, Pasternak GW, Pintar JE. Retention of supraspinal delta-like analgesia and loss of morphine tolerance in delta opioid receptor knockout mice. *Neuron* 1999; **24**: 243–52.

18. Freye E, Latasch L, Portoghese PS. The delta receptor is involved in sufentanil-induced respiratory depression – opioid subreceptors mediate different effects. *Eur J Anaesthesiol* 1992; **9**: 457–62.

19. Foxx-Orenstein AE, Jin JG, Grider JR. 5-HT$_4$ receptor agonists and delta-opioid receptor antagonists act synergistically to stimulate colonic propulsion. *Am J Physiol* 1998; **275**: G979–G983.

20. Szalasi A, Cortright DN, Blum CA, Eid SR. The vanilloid receptor TRPV**1**: 10 years from channel cloning to antagonist proof-of-concept. *Nature Reviews: Drug Discovery* 2007; **6**: 357–72.

21. Cortright DN, Szallasi A. Biochemical pharmacology of the vanilloid receptor TRPV1. An update. *Eur J Biochem* 2004; **271**: 1814–19.

22. Van Der Stelt M, Di Marzo V. Endovanilloids. Putative endogenous ligands of transient receptor potential vanilloid 1 channels. *Eur J Biochem* 2004; **271**: 1827–34.

23. Rami HK, Thompson M, Stemp G, Fell S, Jerman JC, Stevens AJ, Smart D, Sargent B, Sanderson D, Randall AD, Gunthorpe MJ, Davis JB. Discovery of SB-705498: a potent, selective and orally bioavailable TRPV1 antagonist suitable for clinical development. *Bioorg & Med Chem Lett* 2006; **16**: 3287–91.

24. Stein C, Schafer M, Machelska H. Attacking pain at its source: new perspectives on opioids. *Nat Med* 2003; **9**: 1003–8.

25. Mogil JS, Pasternak GW. The molecular and behavioral pharmacology of the orphanin FQ/nociceptin peptide and receptor family. *Pharmacol Rev* 2001; **53**: 381–415.

26. Zeilhofer HU, Calo G. Nociceptin/orphanin FQ and its receptor – potential targets for pain therapy? *J Pharmacol Exp Ther* 2003; **306**: 423–9.

27. Pavlov VA, Wang H, Czura CJ, Friedman SG, Tracey KJ. The cholinergic anti-inflammatory pathway: a missing link in neuroimmunomodulation. *Mol Med* 2003; **9**: 125–34.

28. Noera G, Lamarra M, Guarini S, Bertolini A. Survival rate after early treatment for acute type-A aortic dissection with ACTH-(1–24). *Lancet* 2001; **358**: 469–70.

29. Akira S, Takeda K. Toll-like receptor signaling. *Nature Reviews Immunol* 2004; **4**: 499–511.

30. Schwinn DA, Podgoreanu M. The new age of medical genomics. *Br J Anaesth* 2005; **95**: 119–21.

.

Part III

Monitoring and equipment

New technology applied to anaesthesia and critical care

TIM COOK

The following four chapters focus on aspects of developing technology applicable to the present, and potentially the future, for anaesthesiologists and intensivists.

One chapter examines the circumscribed but important topic of recent developments in aids for tracheal intubation, while the other three offer rather wider visions of how technology is transforming our working practices.

One notable feature of this section is that there is considerable shared ground in three of the four sections, with some papers applicable to more than one section. It is also notable that the chapter authors have sourced their material from some publications that many anaesthetists will not routinely open and, therefore, the material is broad based as well as up to date.

In this editorial I will not reflect greatly on the chapters themselves, as they stand on their own. Rather, I will offer some background on the topics covered by the chapters and comment on some of the wider issues the authors raise.

Simulation in anaesthesia and intensive care

Healthcare simulation is medical mimicry and ranges from, at its most simple, scenario and role play (a form of virtual simulation) to the use of complex, high-fidelity human patient simulators featuring physiological algorithms. Anaesthesia is one of the medical specialties most suited to the use of simulation, and it has been at the forefront of the introduction and subsequent development of healthcare simulation. This is, in part, due to the 'hands on' procedural nature of anaesthesia and also the rapidity of response required when physiological derangements occur in patients under an anaesthetist/intensivist's care. As such, it is a 'high-risk and low error-tolerant' specialty |1|.

The use of simulation in both training and evaluation is increasing and has become more popular for a variety of reasons. The most prominent reason is that simulators have become better: at the top end they are more visually and physically realistic and modelling of physiology is more accurate. However, they are a long way from such good mimicry as to be termed realistic. Therefore, performance of tasks still requires a degree of 'suspension of reality'. There are other reasons for simulation's popularity. Training time in many countries has become reduced and old-style 'apprenticeships' have disappeared from medicine. With shorter training periods, fewer procedures and clinical conditions are encountered so simulation allows an opportunity to fill these gaps. There is also an increasing acceptance that patients are to be cared for rather than practised on, so that new procedures, previously learnt on patients, are now more appropriately learnt, at least initially, using simulation. Pressures for this change are both from society, with patients demanding treatment from 'trained' staff, and the medical profession itself.

Organizations involved in standards and assessment of training are increasingly supporting simulation. The Royal College of Anaesthetists in the UK supports an increase in the availability and use of simulation by anaesthetists as part of continuous professional development |2| and incorporates use of simulators in its formal competency exams. The Australian and New Zealand College of Anaesthetists endorses the use of simulation in training and advocates completion of a college-developed simulation course in lieu of an otherwise mandatory 'Early management of severe trauma' course |3|. The Association of Paediatric Anaesthetists of Great Britain and Ireland suggests training and educational needs may be met by attendance at simulation courses, as an alternative to attachments to paediatric lists or secondment to specialist centres |4|. While currently falling short of mandating completion of such courses, in some areas this is likely, or indeed planned |1,5|.

Simulation is acknowledged to be enjoyable, to create a realistic (and anxiety-provoking) environment and can be demonstrated to improve compliance with protocol-based anaesthesia tasks and simple skills |6–9|. Simulation has been variously advocated for roles including education, professional examination, revalidation, retraining and assessment of fitness to practice. This has far-reaching implications, such as the validity of the assumption that 'simulator performance' equates to or is a surrogate for 'clinical performance'. After review of published research this assumption has been questioned |10|. The subject has developed since that publication and it is likely that progress has recently been made |11,12|. An interesting observation in the late 1990s was that older anaesthesiologists and those from the USA were less familiar with simulators and perhaps engaged less readily in simulation than their younger counterparts and those from Australia |6,13|. Whether such variation still exists is not known, but such findings have implications for use of simulation in assessment. Of note, it is plausible that assessment tools predominantly developed on trainees (as they are rather more likely to attend simulators during training than experienced colleagues) may not be equally applicable to other anaesthetists |2|. Issues such as assessment validity, inter and intra-rater variation |14| and whether the same tools can be used for all anaesthetists require more investigation |15|.

In simulation, skills may be divided into 'technical' and 'non-technical'. In some arenas the emphasis of simulation has been on technical skill acquisition through the use of simulators acting as patient substitutes, on which physical procedures and motor skills may be learnt, without harm to 'patient' or trainee. Physical/anatomical simulators may be accessed in the 'skills labs' many medical schools and hospitals now possess. These provide physical 'part task models' that enable practise of physical skills (e.g. central line insertion, epidural placement, percutaneous tracheostomy or other airway skills). These models are important learning devices and their range and quality has improved swiftly over the last few years. Some, such as epidural and mask ventilation simulators, feature computer technology that offers sophisticated operator feedback or allows modification of the difficulty of the task according to the experience of the learner |16|. Such models enable learning to occur at an appropriate pace, allow part-task learning as well as repetition and provide reproducible conditions in a risk-free environment.

More recently simulation has focused on the teaching of 'non-technical' skills. Simulation can provide a 'multisensory environment' in which non-technical skills may be taught, observed and evaluated. These non-technical skills include teambuilding, teamworking, situational awareness, communication and leadership |17|. It is recognized from previous work in aviation simulation, and more recently in medicine, that the ability to use technical skills efficiently under pressure is dependent on the possession of robust non-technical skills |18–21|.

For the more complex tasks and situations, more complex patient simulators are often used. They are ideally equipped to mimic critical patient events and environments that anaesthetists encounter infrequently but which require prompt action and minimal errors to ensure safe patient care. Simulators provide an environment in which rare and complex scenarios can be presented and individuals can role play safely as well as receiving feedback from observers, trainers and through video recordings of their performance. Remote observation of others' performances can also be educational. In this environment mistakes can be made and potentially learnt from, without consequence. This is the realm of 'crisis resource management' (CRM).

The term CRM is itself a mimicry of the aviation term 'crew resource management', also termed 'aircraft crew training'. Its origins lie in the 1970s when investigation of a series of high-profile aircraft crashes directed the attention of the aviation safety community away from aircraft hardware malfunctions: focusing instead on the human element and the role it plays in aviation safety. The crashes included a Lockheed L-1011 that crashed into a Florida swamp as the crew worked to repair a light bulb which had burned out; a Douglas DC-8 that ran out of fuel while the crew was troubleshooting a landing gear malfunction; and a DC-8 that flew into a mountain while the crew was distracted by attending to a minor electrical problem. Revolution in aircraft crew training was demanded.

In 1979 Ruffell Smith, of NASA's Ames Research Center, published a study titled 'A simulator study of the interaction of pilot workload with errors, vigilance, and decisions' |22|. His research suggested that crew performance was more closely associated with quality of crew communication than with either technical proficiency of individual pilots, increased physiological arousal or environmental workload. The importance of these behavioural factors was accepted: as was the sense in using simulators to train these techniques. Following on from this in June 1979, NASA sponsored a workshop titled 'Resource management on the flight deck' and the term 'crew resource management' was coined. Of note, much of the drive to improve understanding and standards of safety came from the pilots and flight crews themselves, rather than the airlines. For instance, the 'human factors group' formed as an independent voluntary group in 1990 and became part of the Royal Aeronautical Society in 1994, progressing to become a prominent industry advisor.

Anaesthesia non-technical skills are part of the broader term 'human factors', which impact on healthcare and safety. In the UK, recent interest in the impact of human factors in anaesthesia has been stimulated by, amongst other things, the death of a pilot's wife during routine anaesthesia |23|. Human factors training is starting to enter into undergraduate and postgraduate medical teaching. Simulators are likely to continue to play an important role in both training and research in this area. The papers chosen by Glavin (Chapter 11) present an overview of the progress and remaining challenges in simulation, as applied to anaesthesia and intensive care medicine.

Equipment for cardiopulmonary resuscitation

The chapter on equipment for cardiopulmonary resuscitation forms something of a bridge between those describing simulation and the expanding role of computers in our specialties. Much of resuscitation training is, of course, performed in multiprofessional scenario-based environments, utilizing medium- and high-fidelity simulators. Glavin refers to one small study in his chapter, on simulation, that might equally fit in Soar's, on resuscitation equipment (Chapter 9). In this study, we made an attempt to evaluate the fidelity of four medium-complexity manikins designed for teaching airway management and, therefore, frequently used in resuscitation training |24|. Much emphasis is placed on airway management in life support courses, but often little attention is paid to the manikins used to support this training. In particular, issues of fidelity exist: how well do the manikins simulate the tasks they wish to mimic? Several supraglottic airways are now recommended for airway maintenance during cardiac arrest and training needs are changing |25,26|. We studied four manikins, each designed for simulation of both tracheal intubation and supraglottic airway insertion. As the studies were not restricted to determining the manikins' utility for resuscitation but also for difficult airway management, we studied, in addition to classic laryngeal mask airways, newer single-use laryngeal masks |27|; a wide variety of supraglottic airways |28|; and advanced airway management techniques |29|. We found that no single simulator was suitable for teaching all skills. Teaching a wide range of techniques requires purchase of at least two manikin types. This is consistent with previous research on procedural skills |30|. Rather disappointing was that despite their proposed uses (intubation and insertion of supraglottic airways), several of the devices fell well short of good mimicry, in particular when inserting several types of laryngeal mask airway.

Soar's chapter describes new devices designed and marketed to improve prevention and management of cardiac arrest, ranging from the simple and inexpensive to the sophisticated and very expensive. Some studies offer an insight into developing technology that requires further development (e.g. transthoracic impedance monitoring of efficacy of ventilation and cardiac output). In contrast, many of the studies examine 'developed' devices that have been marketed for several years without full evaluation. Of note, some of the studies now emerging are supportive of the new equipment (e.g. a simple device for monitoring adequacy of chest compression) while some offer evidence that the new devices are less effective than has been assumed (e.g. mechanical chest compressors), offering little robust evidence of benefit over standard practices. Fortunately, none of the devices evaluated in Soar's chapter appears to cause harm. All such studies should be welcomed, as without them we are at risk of being influenced by the marketing departments of manufacturing companies more than is advisable.

New technology is often supported by sound logical reasons as to why its use should be beneficial. There is also an element to which new technology is intrinsically appealing, even seductive. However, new technology should never be assumed to be beneficial without evidence. The introduction of new equipment into medical practice remains something of a quagmire. Statutory responsibility in the UK for the introduction of new medical devices lies with the Secretary of Health, and this is delegated to the Medicines and Healthcare products Regulatory Agency (MHRA) |31|. Since harmonization of European law, demonstration of compliance with the 'essential requirements' of several European 'medical device directives' allows a manufacturer to affix the CE mark to a product |32|, after which the device may be marketed throughout Europe without the need to satisfy other local, national or international standards. It remains generally true that the process of CE marking demands demonstration of compliance with standards of consistency of manufacturing quality and use of safe materials, rather than a measure of whether the device is 'fit for purpose' |33|. While the MHRA operates a post-marketing vigilance system |34| that should allow identification of ineffective devices (and the MHRA has the authority to demand their withdrawal), it is not clear that this system achieves that end, perhaps focusing more on the dangers of poorly manufactured equipment over efficacy. Outside of Europe, the Food and Drugs Administration (FDA) of the USA is generally more likely to require manufacturers to demonstrate, through clinical trials, the efficacy of devices. However, the fact remains that, unlike drugs, much medical equipment is 'introduced first and evaluated after'.

For those who do wish to investigate the effectiveness and safety of new devices there are barriers. First, research involving equipment before it is CE marked requires not only special arrangements for patient insurance and hospital indemnity (usually funded by the manufacturer) but must also be approved by the MHRA. At present, 80% of such research is declined. Second, the European Clinical Trials directive, while having a generally complicating effect on the pursuit of all research |35| has had a particularly deleterious effect on research in resuscitation (and other areas with mentally incompetent patients) |36|.

Despite the impediments, Soar's chapter demonstrates that research on device performance continues to be performed. In reality, both moral and economic pressures mean that very few manufacturers would wish to market a device that does not do the job it is designed for: it is not in their long-term interests. Clinicians and responsible manufacturers can, therefore, work together to improve the quality of the equipment we use and increase the likelihood of introduction of innovative technologies. In certain areas, however, it does no harm to retain a healthy scepticism.

There is also an overlap between Soar's chapter and Verma's chapter on developments in computers for anaesthesia and intensive care (Chapter 10). Computerization of patient monitoring offers significant hopes of early detection (and, therefore, earlier intervention) in the physiological deterioration that ultimately leads to cardiac arrest and the need for cardiopulmonary resuscitation. This topic is considered below.

Computers in anaesthesia and intensive care

Moore's law, describing the rate at which computer technology evolves, is widely misquoted. In 1965, in an article about microchip technology |37|, Gordon Moore, Intel's founder, observed that 'The complexity for minimum component costs has increased at a rate of roughly a factor of two per year'. This statement morphed in 1975 to 'the number of transistors on an integrated circuit for minimum component cost doubles every 24 months'. As the number of components on a computer chip is closely related to power, 'Moore's law' is more popularly quoted as 'the power of computers doubles every two years' (… or year … or 18 months, according to the varied sources). Subsequently, the rate of progress has been found to lie approximately between these limits and so the 'law' is now frequently quoted with doubling every 18 months |38|. Whichever version of Moore's law we adopt, the reality is that, at present, computer power and speed continues to progress at an exponential rate. There are similar laws for computer data storage, where the interval for doubling of capacity is approximately 1 year: Kryder's law states that 'magnetic disk storage density doubles annually' |39|.

Processing speed and storage capacity are the fundamental prerequisites for realizing the massive potential that computers have for revolutionizing the way we handle data in medicine. Medicine is complex and clinical decisions often require rapid assimilation and processing of vast amounts of data. Can computers help us with these complex tasks? Previously, computers have largely been labour-saving devices in medicine, but, at last, technology offers the potential to store, analyse and interpret data in ways humans cannot manage.

In the UK the largest technological challenge that has recently been undertaken is the attempt to 'computerize' the National Health Service (NHS) |40|. This laudable plan was initiated by the government's NHS Information Authority (now Connecting for Health [CfH]) in 1998 and led to the launch of the National

Programme for Information Technology (NPfIT) in 2000. The programme aims to create a fully digitized NHS and is the biggest non-military IT project in the world. This programme includes, but is not restricted to, development of electronic patient records (EPRs), electronic radiology (picture archiving and communication system [PACS]), electronic prescribing service (EPS) and an internal encrypted NHS communication system (NHSmail). These developments will require, first, harmonization of medical terminology and clinical coding and, second, a considerable increase in the capacity of the NHS to transfer information. These needs are supported by new terminology and classification services and by provision of a new network, 'the National Network for the NHS' (N3), designed to cope with immediate and future broadband capacity. The EPR will incorporate not only a full chronological record of NHS care but also a 'summary care record' (termed a 'spine'). Provision of a central database is designed to allow storage and sharing of data so that any patient's summary data (or full EPR) is instantly and securely available to any appropriate healthcare worker, anywhere in the UK. Despite major criticisms of the process, scope, timescale and mushrooming budget of the program (initially £1 billion, now above £12 billion, projected to exceed £20 billion) it still has the potential to genuinely revolutionize a nation's healthcare. Data transfer, reliability of and access to patient information and collection of national and local statistics for benchmarking, comparative audit and research are all exciting, if daunting, prospects.

Simple tasks perhaps illustrate the potential of the system as readily as complex ones. Consider prescription of medicines. With e-prescribing there is the capacity for 'smart alerts' and system integration. When a prescription is written a smart system can analyse the following: patient allergy to this or related drugs, relative contraindications to the drug based on patient diagnosis, suitability of dose according to patient weight, duplication of drugs or drug classes, and potential for pharmacokinetic or pharmacodynamic drug interactions. If e-prescribing is integrated to other hospital IT systems, other issues such as suitability of drug and dose according to age, diagnosis, renal or other organ function might also be accessible. Linkage to an electronic library offers the potential for immediate access to further generic or specific information as required. The potential to minimize drug prescription errors and complications from drug administration is clearly considerable.

At last NPfIT is starting to deliver. As of September 2007, PACS was installed in 75% of UK hospitals, EPS was being used for 15% of all prescriptions, a quarter of a million employees were registered with NHSmail and 99% of GP surgeries were connected to 'N3' |41|.

As well as creating benefits, such technological advances are accompanied by new problems and threats to safe and confidential healthcare. Storage and transfer of patient-specific data immediately raises considerable issues of data security: restrictions to access, tracking who has accessed and altered data, and protection from unapproved access and alteration. There are also issues around data reliability and back-up of both data and the data management systems. Hospitals with patient archiving and cataloguing systems and other forms of digital patient records are already encountering these issues. The ability of many portable devices to transfer data wirelessly also raises ethical problems and many hospitals have already identified issues for example confidentiality and data protection issues, relating to mobile phones and personal digital assistants (PDAs) with the capacity to capture and send photographs, written or audio documents. Mobile communication devices may also lead to problems as a result of radiowave interference with medical electronic equipment: a problem that exists but is often exaggerated, as discussed in Verma's chapter.

Verma reviews a wide spectrum of emerging technologies in his chapter. This includes the use of computers for data capture, data storage, paper-free medical record systems, 'digital theatres' and storage of educational resources for immediate access. These developments offer an opportunity for increased efficiency and reliability of tasks already routinely performed in medicine and can clearly offer benefit to patients. They rely largely on increases in computer storage capacity.

The increasing ability to transfer large amounts of data without corruption or loss, over vast distances and through both fixed and wireless systems offers the prospect of increased integration of data from multiple healthcare sources and improved access to relevant data for healthcare workers. It also offers the genuine prospect of allowing global access to expert healthcare via remote e-medicine. Here, as elsewhere, the technology is but one of the challenges.

Computers also offer the potential to revolutionize the way patients are monitored, and what is done with that data. Two high-profile UK documents recently focused on the plight of acutely ill patients. The first of these is the National Patient Safety Agency (NPSA) document *Safer care for the acutely ill patient: learning from serious incidents* |42|. This identifies the two greatest priorities in acute patient care as 'deterioration (patient deterioration not recognised and not acted upon)' and 'resuscitation'. The document is a report of the conclusions of an expert panel review of over 1800 serious incidents and deaths, reported to the NHS National Reporting and Learning System (NRLS) in 2005. The reviewers concluded that over 500 potentially avoidable deaths occurred. Sixty-four deaths were considered to be due to failure to detect or respond to patient deterioration. This is not a new finding |43|. Of six key recommendations made in this document, it is plausible that three (a, better recognition of patients at risk of, or who have deteriorated; b, appropriate monitoring of vital signs, accurate interpretation of clinical findings; and c, calling for help early) might be resolved with improved technology.

The first requirement for responding to deterioration is to detect it, and this requires monitoring. The NPSA document states, 'First, it often takes busy healthcare staff too long to recognise patients who are clinically or physiologically deteriorating'. It cites examples where vital sign monitoring was not done at all, lack of recognition of the importance of worsening condition and delay in responding to deteriorating vital signs. It is unlikely that this is a problem unique to the UK: indeed, the writer of the foreword states, 'These problems are not unique to the

NHS; indeed, they are global. I know that in my own health system within the USA, the same shortcomings exist' |**42**|.

Physiological variables are recorded in most hospitals as 'observations'. Marked or prolonged deviation from normality is usually an indicator of severity of illness and such deviations can generally be detected both before the need for admission to critical care areas and before cardiac arrest |**44,45**|. In most hospital areas 'vital signs' or 'observation' are recorded intermittently onto paper, often by inexperienced healthcare staff. The data are available only where they are recorded; in practice, the information is often hard to find and may be lost. It is recognized that this process is flawed, with observations frequently not planned, omitted or incorrectly recorded |**43,44,46**|.

The second requirement for managing patients who deteriorate is to ensure deteriorations in patient physiology, once detected, are acted on. There is evidence that, either through error or lack of understanding, even when they are recorded, abnormal observations are frequently not acted upon |**44,46,47**|. Concerns have been raised that these problems may contribute to substandard care of patients |**48,49**| and the NPSA document endorses this view, stating 'the right people to do the right things are not always available'.

A companion document to the NPSA's was published by the National Institute for Health and Clinical Excellence (NICE) in July 2007: *Acutely ill patients in hospital. Recognition of and response to acute illness in adults in hospital* |**50**|. This document emphasizes the importance of systems that respond to abnormal findings and encourages their use. These are physiological track and trigger systems (PTTSs) |**45**| and require a monitoring system to detect physiological abnormality and a mechanism to respond to such occurrences. In track and trigger systems physiological variables are measured and deviations from population norms are recorded or converted into scores. Individual scores may be used or summed to create a score (early warning score [EWS]) that increases with worsening physiological deterioration. Scores of individual variables may be weighted, often arbitrarily, in deriving the summed score. When an individual or summed score reaches a certain level (the 'call out criteria') the system is 'triggered'. Ward staff are then required to take action: be it calling senior medical staff or placing an alert to a response team. The response team is variously branded a 'medical emergency team', 'patient at risk team' or 'rapid response team'. The NICE document strongly recommends widespread training in the use of PTTSs and their routine adoption.

A recent systematic review of PTTSs found a total of 25 different PTTSs, with huge inconsistency in the variables monitored (ranging from 4 to 17) and the weighting applied to derive scores |**51**|. In addition, there was great variation in the trigger levels, the response required of the ward staff, and the type of response team (where one existed). Only one of the 25 systems had been developed using robust methods: determining which variables predicted poor outcome and establishing which indices could then be removed without reducing the predictive power of the system |**46**|. Overall, the ability of the PTTS to detect rapid physiological deterioration could not be determined with confidence nor could the best system be identified.

Intervention studies have failed to demonstrate improved outcome when a PTTS is introduced |**52,53**|. Although a recent systematic review suggested that patient outcomes are improved (reduction in mortality, cardiac arrest rates and length of stay) by PTTSs, the evidence on which this was concluded was not considered robust |**54**|.

Among proposed reasons for the failure of such systems to improve patient outcomes are errors in physiological measurements, failure to correctly calculate the EWS |**55**| and delays in responding to the triggers |**52,56**|.

Accepting that routine paper-based recording of observations may introduce errors of measurement, recording and transcription there is no reason to think the EWS recording and calculation is immune. There is good evidence that EWS calculation may be a 'system weakness'. EWS calculation adds complexity to recording observations. Error in EWS calculation appears to vary, depending on who measures and records the data and which scoring system is used: with error rate in score calculation as high as 23% for some systems |**52,57,58**|. Error increases as the complexity of the scoring system rises.

So the evidence states that the ritual of vital signs monitoring is old and widely abused. Early warning scores and physiological track and trigger systems have had lesser impacts than anticipated. Can computers help?

First they may help in data capture, data analysis and data distribution.

At its simplest, computers may reduce EWS miscalculations. One study comparing EWS calculation when performed manually or with a PDA found that in addition to saving time, use of a PDA reduced both score miscalculation and incorrect conclusions on required actions, three-fold. Paper-based error increased as the complexity of the scoring system rose |**58**|.

The process would be improved if it were possible to ensure that the data, at least when abnormal or when 'calling criteria' were met, could reach the relevant medical staff as soon at they were collected: whether they are present or not. Such systems are under development. In one such system (described in Soar's chapter, but equally applicable to Verma's) vital signs are recorded directly onto a PDA |**59**|. Alerts can be set to remind nursing staff that observations are due. Once the data are entered, the software can compare them against predefined limits such as an EWS (which the PDA calculates automatically). Other triggers may be added if desired. When a trigger is reached, the PDA sets off an alert. By linkage with the hospital local area network (LAN), the alert can be transmitted direct to appropriate medical personnel, either in the hospital or outside it. For those outside the limit of a local network the system can be linked to a mobile phone SMS service. The potential benefits of alerting appropriate medical staff almost instantaneously are obvious, enabling doctors and other healthcare workers the 'freedom to roam' in the knowledge that patient deteriorations will be communicated to them electronically as soon as they occur. Other potential benefits include access to patients' observations elsewhere in the hospital, reliable storage of the data, increased ease of tracking data trends, transfer of data when patients move locations and the possibility of refining the system to improve the quality of the data collected. Integration of the 'vital signs' with other hospital systems such as pathology results could lead to more far-reaching benefit.

The above system offers the ability to collect, store and analyse intermittently collected data as well as disseminating it rapidly. Its limitations are that it records only intermittent data, that it relies on the patient remaining where he or she can be observed and that the nurse must both remember to enter the data and do this correctly. Other developments offer the possibility of collecting continuous physiological data from a patient leading to lesser patient restrictions and reduced needs for nursing care. It is recognized that many patients on normal wards suffer major physiological abnormalities prior to ICU admission and that these are often not detected |60|. At present, most patients on wards have infrequent, intermittent monitoring with the likelihood that, even without omission of observations, deterioration may occur for considerable periods before it is recognized. Continuous physiological monitoring occurs only in operating theatres and in critical care wards and this is by means of wire-based monitors attached to bedside monitors. Increased miniaturization and decreased cost now make it feasible for wireless monitoring to be incorporated into patient garments, allowing real-time monitoring of respiratory rate and pattern, electrocardiograph, pulse oximetry and skin temperature. Blood pressure monitoring remains more of a problem, but developments in near-patient monitoring may soon also allow measurement of transcutaneous carbon dioxide, oxygen and even monitoring of other metabolic variables such as blood glucose |61|. These continuous monitors offer several possibilities for inpatients. First, they might increase the frequency and reliability with which 'patient observations' are performed and documented. Second, nursing staff can be freed up for other tasks. Third, the patient may have greater freedom of movement while still benefiting from improved, continuous monitoring of physiological status: a move from monitoring beds to monitoring patients.

Continuous remote wireless monitoring is starting to be trialled, with largely positive results. There are a huge number of potential applications. In critical care remote monitoring would enable improved access to the patient and make patient transfers far less laborious and potentially safer. On the rare occasions that it is desirable that a patient is approached as little as possible (e.g. highly contagious conditions or severe immunosuppression) this technology might provide a level of monitoring not otherwise easily achieved. It might also reduce the need for 'traffic' into and out of a patient's room, with potential infection control benefits for all patients requiring isolation. Hospital-to-hospital transfers might be improved |62|. On wards a large group who could benefit are those recently discharged from critical care areas and those who are identified as at high risk of deterioration. However, there is the exciting potential to monitor all hospitalized patients |63|. In the community there is the potential to allow some patients home from hospital, if monitored, sooner than at present |64|. Other community-based patients considered at risk of deterioration may be included (e.g. patients with risks of anaphylaxis, acute severe asthma, brittle diabetes, arrhythmias or silent ischaemia) |**65,66**|. Widespread use of such systems might shed light on a number of diseases, for instance informing us of the physiological changes that occur prior to cardiac arrest in the community. The concept also has potential for wider quasi-medical applications: high-performance athletes might benefit from monitoring. There is also likely to be interest from the pharmaceutical industry for use during drug development. At present, protracted, costly trials are required to demonstrate safety of drugs before they can be brought to market. Remote monitoring could provide robust verifiable data substantially quicker, while reducing the costs for the investigators and the risk to enrolled patients. The technology has obvious potential in genuinely remote sites for use in telemedicine. In the parts of the world where infectious disease outbreaks are common such systems offer benefit to patients, but also in disease profiling, both in the community and within hospitals. For the military and other organizations, such systems offer the potential to monitor personnel exposed to hazardous environments |**67**|. The sky is the limit, and beyond, for such applications are mooted for use in space |**68**| and mock-ups have already been used to test their capabilities |**69**|. Indeed, in many of these areas clinical trials are already planned and a journal published by the Institute of Electrical and Electronics Engineers ('IEEE transactions on information technology in biomedicine') reports considerable research into these developments.

Once collected, the data can be used in a number of ways. The most basic step is to store it, while the next level of sophistication is to perform simple analysis (e.g. calculation of EWS). However, the data might be made more patient specific through integration with data in hospital IT systems. Instead of triggers being restricted to a small set of physiological variables referenced against 'population norms', integration of the data with other systems would allow 'triggers' that were modified according to known patient factors such as age, initial physiology and diagnosis. Further variables extracted from the EPR and pathology results might produce a more sophisticated and personalized track and trigger system than one based solely on physiological variables and with limits set according to population norms. Finally, the information (however integrated or analysed) could then be instantly disseminated to anyone within (or outside) the hospital who needs access to it.

Such systems are starting to be developed. One such system uses application of a 'logic module' to examine trends in physiological data. This system was compared with more traditional data analysis, based on single variables rather than absolute values, to initiate triggers. Early results suggest this 'logic module' may increase the ability to detect clinically important changes (increased positive predictive values) |**70**|.

Another system: the 'BioSign' (Oxford Biosignals, Oxford, UK) tracks five physiological variables with heart rate, respiratory rate, oxygen saturation and temperature all recorded every 5 min and blood pressure recorded every 30 min |**71**|.

The five variables are combined (fused) into a single measure, termed the 'patient status index' (PSI). The system incorporates a data set of vital signs derived from over 3000 hours of monitoring of high-risk patients: with heart failure or following myocardial infarction or acute respiratory problems or awaiting surgery for hip fracture. These data have been normalized (i.e. transformed so each variable is expressed over the same range) and then used to create a 'training data set'. The process is described as like a five-dimensional histogram of measurement distribution. Probability density is estimated after data fusion and pattern recognition uses Parzen windows. Once the system data set is created, patient data can be compared with this using a 'probabilistic model' to determine the likelihood that the patients data came from the same population (i.e. are 'normal') or to what extent they deviate. Triggering occurs when the PSI falls outside the 'envelope of normality'. This approximates to one variable deviating from 'normality' for 80% of a 5-min time window, by at least three standard deviations (type A alert), but importantly may also be caused by two or more variables deviating simultaneously to lesser degrees (type B alert). The process works in real time and can be incorporated into existing patient monitors. Processes are built in to detect and exclude artefactual data and to minimize the effects of missing data.

The system has been studied in a trial in which patients were randomized to BioSign monitoring or standard care |**72**|. Investigators followed 402 high-risk medical and surgical patients for 72 h on general wards. The patients were randomized equally to remote five-channel 'BioSign' monitoring or to 'standard care' (with monitoring not dictated). In the BioSign group, although data capture was successful for 84% of the time period, suggesting that the system worked, continuous monitoring for the full period was achieved in only 16% of patients suggesting that considerable improvements might be achieved. 'Abnormal physiology' (alterts) was detected by BioSign once in approximately every 7 h of monitoring. When reviewed 'offline', BioSign-generated alerts were deemed to represent 'severe physiological abnormalities' with 95% reliability (true positives). A small number of false positives arose due to failure to reject artefactual data during movement. Use of the PSI detected deterioration before 'single-channel monitoring'. Type A alerts led to BioSign triggering a modest time before single-channel monitoring (0.1–5 min) while type B alerts preceded single-channel alerts by up to several hours. Despite this there were no differences in outcomes (alerts, adverse events or mortality) between the two groups of patients. The hospital where the study was performed did not have a 'rapid response team' and failure to respond to triggers may have been an issue in the study. The response from one commentator to this study was highly positive, stating 'There is no doubt in many of our minds that universal continuous monitoring for hospital patients will occur sooner rather than later' |**56**|.

Further developments might include inclusion of additional physiological data already used in many EWS (e.g. conscious level and urine output). There is also potential to integrate a system such as BioSign with other hospital-based IT systems (e.g. laboratory results, diagnosis, premorbid conditions). Such developments offer the possibility of developing more sophisticated track and trigger systems. By integrating with other systems, 'smart triggers' might also be incorporated, for instance taking elements of established scoring systems, such as APACHE or diagnostic tools (e.g. definitions of sepsis, severe sepsis and septic shock). 'Intelligent' monitors might not only recognize these conditions and alert the healthcare staff far earlier than at present, but when linked to PDAs and other computers they may also provide immediate access to evidence-based data advising or assisting the healthcare staff in choosing appropriate treatment and then monitoring the progress of such treatment. This not a pipedream and already monitors exist with some of these elements (www.medical.philips.com/uk), for instance the ability to trigger in response to physiological deterioration and in doing so activate a 'carebundle' or 'protocolwatch' based on the surviving sepsis guidelines |73|. As well as continuing to monitor the patient, the system prompts clinicians to search out further septic indicators and guides subsequent treatment with a combination of smart-monitoring and protocol-based reminders, all delivered while indicating time elapsed since the bundle was triggered. Such a system is unproven, but guideline-based care generally improves outcome and more of such systems can be expected.

Perhaps there is still more we could anticipate. Computers have the capacity to recognize or analyse patterns and trends in data that humans cannot detect. By detecting patterns or changes, measures such as heart rate variability (RR interval) or corrected QT duration, or indeed cardiopulmonary interactions, monitors might detect changes in autonomic nervous system activity or other predictors of outcome. If sufficiently large data sets are built up, these might be interrogated to determine whether such measures, or others, do reflect increased patient risk. Computer processing power could, thus, be harnessed to develop new 'risk scores'. For individual patients, systems that learn patient norms might be used to develop a real-time patient-specific trigger system. In such ways smart monitoring may advance from being labour-saving to genuinely achieving tasks that humans currently cannot.

Novel intubation equipment

Finally, consider the rather more circumscribed topic of devices designed to assist with tracheal intubation. Lam and Hagberg (Chapter 12) offer a very up-to-date overview of the new rigid optical devices much reported in the literature. The new 'scopes' are rigid fibreoptic devices that aim to allow the intubator a view of the larynx when this is either difficult or impossible with routine direct laryngoscopy. Most, but not all, use fibreoptic technology.

They can be classified into three groups. The first group comprises bladed devices based on conventional laryngoscopes: an older group of Bullard, Wuscope, Upsherscope and a newer group including the McGrath, Glidescope and Macintosh videolaryngoscope. Broadly, this group might also include simpler modifications of the Macintosh blade such as the McCoy, McMorrow and flexiblade laryngoscope blades. The second group are the fibreoptic stylets, which are rigid optical endoscopes designed to be placed within the tracheal tube. Included in this group are the Shikani Optical Stylet (SOS) and Bonfils, with more recent additions of the Sensascope and FTS stylet. Third are devices that act both as fibreoptic blades and conduits through which the tracheal tube is passed. These conduit devices include the C-Trach LMA. The Airtraq and Pentax AWS have elements of both blade and conduit groups.

Many of these devices benefit from improvements in the quality, miniaturization and reduced cost of cameras, fibreoptic bundles and monitors. There is now an impressive array of slightly dissimilar videolaryngoscopes available to the anaesthesiologist, intensivist and emergency physician, but as the light available from these devices becomes ever stronger and clearer the answers to two questions remain hidden: do these devices actually make intubation easier and, if so, which are the best of the devices: the one or ones worth purchasing?

For review of this chapter I will intentionally step away from the technological issues and examine in more detail the methodological problems that bedevil this area of study.

Unfortunately, many of the data that have been published in this area (and are used to market these devices) do not answer the above questions. There are several reasons for this. First, the area for which these devices are designed ('patients in whom tracheal intubation is difficult') is an intrinsically difficult one to study. These patients are relatively uncommon and, worse, they are difficult to predict. The vast majority of the data on these devices are derived from study of unselected patients undergoing routine tracheal intubation. Where selection has taken place it is most frequently to exclude those patients with predicted difficult intubation.

Consider what we mean by 'difficult intubation'. There are numerous definitions |74| but the commonest definition used is that of 'all Cormack and Lehane grade 3 and 4 cases' |75|. In prospective studies of largely unselected patients such difficult laryngoscopies occur in between 5% |76| and less than 1% of cases |77,78|. But are these awkward laryngoscopies actually synonymous with 'difficult intubation'? In practice, over 90% of grade 3 laryngoscopic views require no more than the gum elastic bougie to achieve intubation |76|, implying that only around 10% of these cases are genuinely difficult. So, in studies of unselected elective cases (especially where predicted difficult cases are excluded from study) we can predict that the larynx will be visible in 95–99% of intubations and, of the 1–5% in which the larynx cannot be seen, intubation will be achieved without great difficulty in 90%. So, ability to view the larynx of well above 95% of cases and achieve intubation in above 98% of cases might be anticipated to be the norm, or benchmark, in such studies. Few of the devices mentioned above achieve such results.

More robust data should come from studies in which researchers study patients with 'difficult airways'. However, here we encounter the well-recognized problem of identifying these patients prior to study |79|. Although several prospective tests are widely used, they have very poor sensitivity and positive predictive value |80|. The most widely used test is the modified Mallampati test |81,82| but, even with this test, prediction is poor. Various studies report a Mallampati class 3–4 is associated with a Cormack and Lehane grade 3–4 laryngoscopy as infrequently as 3–8% |83|. A recent meta-analysis of these preoperative bedside tests reported that even when the most effective two tests are combined (modified Mallampati 3–4 and thyromental distance <6 cm), their combined presence only increases the 'pooled likelihood ratio' of a grade 3 laryngoscopy 10-fold |84|. So, the presence of both factors in an otherwise normal patient might lead to an expectation of a grade 3 laryngoscopy in 10–50% of patients, of whom only one-tenth will actually be 'difficult to intubate', i.e. 1–5%. This obviously has implications for studies that recruit patients as 'difficult patients' on the basis of a modified Mallampati class 3–4: we should anticipate that as few as 10% will have a grade 3 or 4 laryngoscopy and only around 1–5% of patients will actually be difficult to intubate. Results with the new intubation devices should be interpreted against this background.

Most of the published studies on these new devices are case series, but, despite this, fewer than 15% of the data are from patients who are 'predicted difficult to intubate', and less than 10% of the studies compare the device either with a Macintosh 3 blade or with other novel intubation devices |85|.

There are other practical difficulties with studies. In many studies the ability to see the larynx is used as an endpoint rather than ease of intubation or intubation success. Despite good visualization of the larynx, tracheal tube placement may be more difficult with the newer devices than with direct laryngoscopy: because of the indirect nature of the view, unfamiliarity with tube manipulation while observing a monitor, or because the intubating device restricts tube manipulation. So, more relevant endpoints for these studies include measures of intubation ease (rather than view at laryngoscopy), such as time to intubation and rates of intubation failure: few report these. Finally, most devices requiring new skills have a learning curve of at least 20 cases. Not all researchers achieve this learning curve before collecting data on device performance and this may bias against the new equipment both in case series and in comparative studies.

Overall, there is a genuine lack of robust data on these devices. For those wishing to consider purchasing the devices this lack of evidence is compounded by their high unit cost and difficulties gaining appropriately long trial periods in which they can rise up the learning curve and get experience in genuinely difficult cases.

Better trial design is needed. Manikin data are not transferable to humans, cohort studies rarely offer more than 'proof of concept' and randomized controlled trials in unselected patients are unlikely to provide useful information about effectiveness in difficult patients. A different approach to study of these devices is required and may include focused trials in genuinely difficult patients or collection of data on multiple uses by means of multicentre or international databases. It is likely that some of these devices do offer genuine benefit and use is likely to increase in the next decade. On the basis of the present data, it is not clear which.

References

1. Eich C, Timmermann A, Russo SG, Nickel EA, McFadzean J, Rowney D, Schwarz SKW. Simulator based training in paediatric anaesthesia and emergency medicine – thrills skills and attitudes. *Br J Anaesth* 2007; **98**: 417–19.

2. Bruce RCH, McLeod, Smith GB. A survey of UK anaesthetic trainee attitudes towards simulator based training experience. Royal College of Anaesthetists: *Bulletin* 2005; **34**: 1722–3

3. http://www.anzca.edu.au/publications/reports/amcsub/rprt_education.htm (accessed September 2007).

4. http://www.rcoa.ac.uk/docs/Paeds.pdf. (accessed September 2007).

5. Molyneux M, Lauder G. A national collaborative simulation project: paediatric anaesthetic emergencies. *Paed Anaes* 2006; **16**: 1302.

6. Kurrek MM, Fish KJ. Anaesthesia crisis resource management training: an intimidating concept, a rewarding experience. *Can J Anaesth* 1996; **43**: 430–4.

7. Cleave-Hogg D, Morgan PJ. Experiential learning in an anaesthesia simulation centre: analysis of students' comments. *Med Teach* 2002; **24**: 23–6.

8. Chopra V, Gesink BJ, de Jong J, Bovill JG, Spierdijk J, Brand R. Does training on an anaesthesia simulator lead to improvement in performance? *Br J Anaesth* 1994; **73**: 293–7.

9. Ashurst N, Rout CC, Rocke DA, Gouws E. Use of a mechanical simulator for training in applying cricoid pressure. *Br J Anaesth* 1996; **77**: 468–72.

10. Byrne A, Greaves J. Assessment instruments used during anaesthetic simulation: a review of published studies. *Br J Anaesth* 2001; **86**: 445–50.

11. Fletcher G, Flin R, McGeorge P, Glavin R, Maran N, Patey R. Anaesthetists' Non-Technical skills (ANTS): evaluation of a behavioural marker system. *Br J Anaesth* 2003; **90**: 580–8.

12. Forrest FT, Taylor MA, Postlethwaite K, Aspinall R. Use of a high fidelity simulator to develop testing of the technical performance of novice anaesthetists. *Br J Anaesth* 2002; **88**: 338–41.

13. Riley R, Wilks D, Freeman J. Anaesthetists' attitudes toward an anaesthesia simulator. A comparative survey: USA and Australia. *An Int Care* 1997; **25**: 514–19.

14. Weller JM, Bloch M, Young S, Maze M, Oyesola S, Wyner J, Dob D, Haire K, Durbridge J, Walker T, Newble D. Evaluation of high fidelity patient simulator in assessment of performance of anaesthetists. *Br J Anaesth* 2003; **90**: 43–7.

15. Forrest F, Haslam M, Wilford A. Anaesthetic trainees: are we ready to assess competence? *Bulletin of the Royal College of Anaesthetists* 2003; **22**: 1084–7.

16. Sudhir G, Stacey WRX, Hampson J, Mecklenburgh J. Evaluation of the Basic Airway Model, a novel mask ventilation training manikin. *Anaesthesia* 2007; **62**: 944–7.

17. Issenberg BS, Mcgaghie WC, Petrusa ER, Gordon DL, Salese RS. Features and use of high-fidelity medical simulations that lead to effective learning: a BEBE systematic review. *Med Teach* 2005; **27**: 10–28.

18. Gaba DM. What makes a good anaesthesiologist? *Anesthesiology* 2004; **101**: 1061–3.

19. Gaba DM, Singer SJ, Sinaiko AD, Bowen JD, Ciavarelli AP. Differences in safety climate between hospital personnel and naval aviators. *Hum Factors* 2003; **45**: 173–85.

20. Reader T, Flin R, Lauche K, Cuthbertson BH. Non-technical skills in the intensive care unit. *Br J Anaesth* 2006; **96**: 551–9.

21. Mishra A, Catchpole K, Dale T, McCulloch P. The influence of non-technical performance on technical outcome in laparoscopic cholecystectomy. *Surg Endosc* 2007; **21**: [electronic publication ahead of print May 2007; doi 10.1007/s00464–007–9346–1].

22. Ruffell Smith HP. A simulator study of the interaction of pilot workload with errors, vigilance, and decisions. (NASA Technical Memorandum 78482). Moffett Field, CA: NASA-Ames Research Center; 1979, pp. 1–54.

23. When surgery goes wrong: weighing up the risks. *The Independent*, 14 November 2006. http://news.independent.co.uk/health/article1982332.ece (accessed September 2007).

24. Silsby J, Jordan G, Bayley G, Cook TM. Evaluation of four airway training manikins as simulators for insertion of the LMA classic. *Anaesthesia* 2006; **61**: 576–9.

25. European Resuscitation Council Guidelines for Resuscitation **2005**: Section **4**: Adult Advanced Life Support. *Resuscitation* 2005; **67**: S39–86.

26. Cook TM, Hommers C. New airways for resuscitation? *Resuscitation* 2006; **69**: 371–87.

27. Cook TM, Green C, McGrath J, Srivastava R. A comparison of four different advanced airway mannequins for single use LMA insertion. *Anaesthesia* 2007; **62**: 713–18.

28. Jackson KM, Cook TM. A comparison of four different advanced airway mannequins for SAD insertion. *Anaesthesia* 2007; **62**: 388–93.

29. Cook TM, Bayley G, Jordan G, Silsby J. A comparison of four different advanced airway mannequins for training DAS guidelines. *Anaesthesia* 2007; **62**: 708–12.

30. Parry K, Owen H. Small simulators for teaching procedural skills in a difficult airway algorithm. *Anaesthesia and Intensive Care* 2004; **32**: 401–9.

31. http://www.mhra.gov.uk/home/idcplg?IdcService=SS_GET_PAGE&nodeId=48 (accessed September 2007).

32. http://ec.europa.eu/enterprise/medical_devices/index_en.htm (accessed September 2007).

33. Cook TM. Spoilt for choice? New supraglottic airways. *Anaesthesia* 2003; **58**: 107–10.

34. http://www.mhra.gov.uk/home/idcplg?IdcService=SS_GET_PAGE&nodeId=197 (accessed September 2007).

35. Hall JE, Diaz-Navarro C. Living with the European Clinical Trials Directive: one year on. *Anaesthesia* 2005; **60**: 949–51.

36. Druml C. Informed consent of incapable (ICU) patients in Europe: existing laws and the EU Directive. *Curr Opin Crit Care* 2004; **10**: 570–3.

37. Moore GE. Cramming more components onto integrated circuits. *Electronics* 1965; **8**: 114–17.

38. http://www.ieee.org/portal/cms_docs_societies/sscs/PrintEditions/200609.pdf (accessed September 2007).

39. http://www.sciam.com/article.cfm?articleID=000B0C22–0805–12D8-BDFD83414B7 F0000&ref=sciam&chanID=sa006 (accessed September 2007).

40. http://www.connectingforhealth.nhs.uk/(accessed September 2007).

41. http://www.connectingforhealth.nhs.uk/newsroom/latest/factsandfigures/deployment (accessed September 2007).

42. The fifth report from the Patient Safety Observatory. Safer care for the acutely ill patient: learning from serious incidents. NPSA 2007.

43. Cullinane M, *et al*. An Acute Problem? A report of the National Confidential Enquiry into Patient Outcome and Death. London 2005. Available at: www.ncepod.org.uk/2005. htm (accessed September 2007).

44. Kause J, Smith G, Prytherch D, Parr M, Flabouris A, Hillman K; Intensive Care Society (UK). Australian and New Zealand Intensive Care Society Clinical Trials Group. A comparison of antecedents to cardiac arrests, deaths and emergency intensive care admissions in Australia and New Zealand, and the United Kingdom – the ACADEMIA study. *Resuscitation* 2004; **62**: 275–82.

45. Goldhill DR, Worthington L, Mulcahy A, Tarling M, Sumner A. The patient-at-risk team: identifying and managing seriously ill ward patients. *Anaesthesia* 1999; **54**: 853–60.

46. Hodgetts TJ, Kenward G, Vlachonikolis IG, Payne S, Castle N. The identification of risk factors for cardiac arrest and formulation of activation criteria to alert a medical emergency team. *Resuscitation* 2002; **54**: 125–31.

47. Hodgetts TJ, Kenward G, Vlackonikolis I, Payne S, Castle N, Crouch R, Ineson N, Shaikh L. Incidence, location and reasons for avoidable in-hospital cardiac arrest in a district general hospital. *Resuscitation* 2002; **54**: 115–23.

48. McQuillan P, Pilkington S, Allan A, *et al*. Confidential enquiry into quality of care before admission to intensive care. *Br Med J* 1998; **316**: 1853–8.

49. McGloin H, Adam SK, Singer M. Unexpected deaths and referrals to intensive care of patients on general wards. Are some cases potentially avoidable? *J R Coll Physicians London* 1999; **33**: 255–9.

50. The National Institute for Health and Clinical Excellence (NICE). *Acutely ill patients in hospital. Recognition of and response to acute illness in adults in hospital. NICE clinical guideline 50*. NICE July 2007. Available at: http://guidance.nice.org.uk/CG50 (accessed September 2007).

51. Gao H, McDonnell A, Harrison DA, Moore T, Adam S, Daly K, Esmonde L, Goldhill DR, Parry GJ, Rashidian A, Subbe CP, Harvey S. Systematic review and evaluation of physiological track and trigger warning systems for identifying at-risk patients on the ward. *Intensive Care Medicine* 2007; **33**: 667–79.

52. Hillman K, Chen J, Cretikos M, Bellomo R, Brown D, Doig G, Finfer S, Flabouris A; MERIT study investigators. Introduction of the Medical Emergency Team (MET) system: a cluster randomised controlled trial. *Lancet* 2005; **365**: 2091–7.

53. Subbe CP, Davies RG, Williams E, Rutherford P, Gemmell L. Effect of introducing the modified Early warning Score on clinical outcomes, cardio-pulmonary arrests and intensive care utilisation in acute medical admissions. *Anaesthesia* 2003; **58**: 797–802.

54. Esmonde L, McDonnell A, Ball C, Waskett C, Morgan R, Rashidian A, Bray K, Adam S, Harvey S. Investigating the effectiveness of Critical Care Outreach Services: a systematic review. *Intensive Care Medicine* 2006; **23**: 1713–21.

55. Institute for Healthcare Improvement. The MERIT trial of medical emergency teams in Australia: an analysis of the findings and implications for the 100,000 lives campaign. Available at: http://www.ihi.org/NR/rdonlyres/F3401FEF-2179–4403–8F67-B9255C57E207/0/LancetAnalysis81505.pdf (accessed September 2007).

56. Hillman K. What is it vital to measure? *Anaesthesia* 2006; **61**: 1027–30.

57. Christian P, Subbe CP, Gao H, Harrison DA. Reproducibility of physiological track-and-trigger warning systems for identifying at-risk patients on the ward. *Intensive Care Med* 207; **33**: 619–24.

58. Prytherch D, Smith GB, Schmidt P, Featherstone PI, Stewart K, Knight D, Higgins B. Calculating early warning scores – a classroom comparison of pen and paper and hand-held computer methods. *Resuscitation* 2006; **70**: 173–8.

59. Smith GB, Prytherch DR, Schmidt P, Featherstone PI, Knight D, Clements G, Mohammed MA. Hospital-wide physiological surveillance – A new approach to the early identification and management of the sick patient. *Resuscitation* 2006; **71**: 19–28.

60. Hillman KM, Bristow PJ, Chey T, Daffurn K, Jacques T, Norman SL, Bishop GF, Simmons G. Duration of life-threatening antecedents prior to intensive care admission. *Intensive Care Med* 2002; **28**: 1629–34.

61. Piper HG, Alexander JL, Shukla A, Pigula F, Costello JM, Laussen PC, Jaksic T, Agus MS. Real-time continuous glucose monitoring in pediatric patients during and after cardiac surgery. *Pediatrics* 2006; **118**: 1176–84.

62. Lin YH, Jan IC, Ko PC, Chen YY, Wong JM, Jan GJ. A wireless PDA-based physiological monitoring system for patient transport. *IEEE Trans Inf Technol Biomed* 2004; **8**: 439–47.

63. Anliker U, Ward JA, Lukowicz P, Tröster G, Dolveck F, Baer M, Keita F, Schenker EB, Catarsi F, Coluccini L, Belardinelli A, Shklarski D, Alon M, Hirt E, Schmid R, Vuskovic M. AMON: a wearable multiparameter medical monitoring and alert system. *IEEE Trans Inf Technol Biomed* 2004; **8**: 415–27.

64. Aziz O, Atallah L, Lo B, Elhelw M, Wang L, Yang GZ, Darzi A. A pervasive body sensor network for measuring postoperative recovery at home. *Surg Innov* 2007; **14**: 83–90.

65. Yao J, Schmitz R, Warren S. A wearable point-of-care system for home use that incorporates plug-and-play and wireless standards. *IEEE Trans Inf Technol Biomed* 2005; **9**: 363–71.

66. Piccini L, Parini S, Maggi L, Andreoni G. A Wearable Home BCI system: preliminary results with SSVEP protocol. *Conf Proc IEEE Eng Med Biol Soc* 2005; **5**: 5384–7.

67. Montgomery K, Mundt C, Thonier G, Tellier A, Udoh U, Barker V, Ricks R, Giovangrandi L, Davies P, Cagle Y, Swain J, Hines J, Kovacs G. Lifeguard – a personal physiological monitor for extreme environments. *Conf Proc IEEE Eng Med Biol Soc* 2004; **3**: 2192–5.

68. Mundt CW, Montgomery KN, Udoh UE, Barker VN, Thonier GC, Tellier AM, Ricks RD, Darling RB, Cagle YD, Cabrol NA, Ruoss SJ, Swain JL, Hines JW, Kovacs GT. A multiparameter wearable physiologic monitoring system for space and terrestrial applications. *IEEE Trans Inf Technol Biomed* 2005; **9**: 382–9.

69. Harnett BM, Doarn CR, Russell KM, Kapoor V, Merriam NR, Merrell RC. Wireless telemetry and Internet technologies for medical management: a Martian analogy. *Aviat Space Environ Med* 2001; **72**: 1125–31.

70. Schoenenberg R, Sands DZ, Safran C. Making ICU alarms meaningful: an analysis of traditional versus trend based algorithms. *Proc AMIA Symp* **1999**: 379–83.

71. Tarassenko L, Hann A, Young D. Integrated monitoring and analysis for early warning of patient deterioration. *Br J Anaesth* 2006; **97**: 64–8.

72. Watkinson PJ, Barber VS, Price JD, Hann A, Tarassenko L, Young JD. A randomised controlled trial of the effect of continuous electronic physiological monitoring on the adverse event rate in high risk medical and surgical patients. *Anaesthesia* 2006; **61**: 1031–9.

73. Dellinger RP, Carlet JM, Masur H, Gerlach H, Calandra T, Cohen J, Gea-Banacloche J, Keh D, Marshall JC, Parker MM, Ramsay G, Zimmerman JL, Vincent JL, Levy MM; Surviving Sepsis Campaign Management Guidelines Committee. Surviving Sepsis Campaign guidelines for management of severe sepsis and septic shock. *Crit Care Med* 2004; **32**: 858–73

74. Rose DK, Cohen MM. The incidence of airway problems depends on the definition used. *Can J Anaesth* 1996; **43**: 30–4.

75. Cormack and Lehane. Difficult intubation in obstetrics. *Anaesthesia* 1984; **39**: 1105–11.

76. Cook TM. A new practical classification of laryngeal view. *Anaesthesia* 2000; **55**: 274–9.

77. Williams KN, Carli F, Cormack RS. Unexpected, difficult laryngoscopy: a prospective survey in routine general surgery. *Br J Anaesth* 1991; **66**: 38–44.

78. Bellhouse CP, Dore C. Criteria for estimating likelihood of difficulty of endotracheal intubation with the Macintosh laryngoscope. *Anaesth Intensive Care* 1988; **16**: 329–37.

79. Wilson ME. Predicting difficult intubation. *Br J Anaesth* 1993; **71**: 333–4.

80. Yentis SM. Predicting difficult intubation – worthwhile exercise or pointless ritual? *Anaesthesia* 2002; **57**: 105–9.

81. Mallampati SR, Gatt SP, Gugino LD. A clinical sign to predict difficult tracheal intubation: a prospective study. *Can Anaest Soc J* 1995; **32**: 429–34.

82. Samsoon GL, Young JR. Difficult tracheal intubation: a retrospective study. *Anaesthesia* 1987; **42**: 487–90.

83. Cattano D, *et al.* Risk factors assessment of the difficult airway: an Italian survey of 1956 patients. *Anesth & Analg* 2004; **99**: 1774–9.

84. Shiga T, Wajima Z, Inoue T, Sakamoto A. Predicting difficult intubation in apparently normal patients. A metaanalysis of bedside screening test performance. *Anaesthesiology* 2005; **103**: 429–37.

85. Mihai R, Blair E, Kay H, Cook TM. Quantitative review and meta-analysis of performance of non-standard laryngoscopes and rigid fibreoptic intubation aids. *Anaesthesia* 2008; in press.

Declaration of interest

Dr Cook has received honoraria from Intavent Orthofix and the LMA company, distributors of Laryngeal Mask Airways (Classic LMA, Unique LMA, Intubating LMA and ProSeal LMA) for lecturing. He has also received free or reduced-price equipment from other manufacturers of airway equipment, for research.

9

Equipment for cardiopulmonary resuscitation

JASMEET SOAR

Introduction

Survival from cardiac arrest depends on the sequence that makes up the chain of survival (Fig. 9.1) |1|. For the best chance of survival all four links in the chain must be strong. New guidelines for cardiopulmonary resuscitation (CPR) introduced in 2005 emphasize the importance of good-quality chest compressions with minimal interruption |2|.

The item of equipment that saves most lives remains the defibrillator |3|. Even well-trained resuscitation teams deliver suboptimal CPR in the clinical setting |4,5|. Many of the new CPR devices have been developed to improve the delivery of CPR by rescuers by either prompting rescuers to perform tasks (e.g. feedback on compression rate and depth) or doing the task instead of the rescuer (e.g. mechanical chest compressions, rhythm analysis).

Surprisingly, many of the devices manufactured for CPR are sold without any formal evaluation of their overall efficacy. This remains common for medical devices, with formal studies only taking place after they are commercially available.

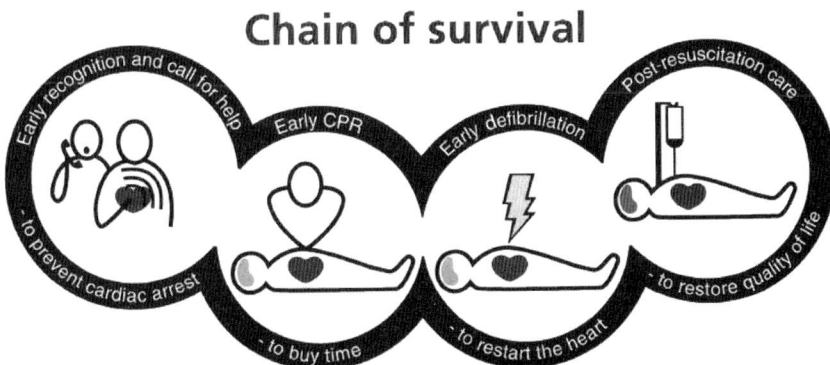

Fig. 9.1 Chain of survival. Reproduced with permission from the Resuscitation Council UK.

The primary endpoint for most device studies is how well they perform the task they were designed for (e.g. depth of chest compression). Patient-focused endpoints are more important, however. The main endpoints used for CPR research are return of spontaneous circulation (ROSC), survival to hospital admission for out-of-hospital cardiac arrests, and survival to hospital discharge. Few studies give long-term survival and neurological outcomes.

Early recognition to prevent cardiac arrest

Patients who have a cardiac arrest or unanticipated intensive care unit (ICU) admission often have evidence of an unrecognized, or untreated, deterioration. The ACADEMIA study showed antecedents in 79% of cardiac arrests, 55% of deaths and 54% of unanticipated ICU admissions [6]. Devices that enable early recognition and trigger a response might prevent some cardiac arrests, deaths and unanticipated ICU admissions.

Hospital-wide physiological surveillance – a new approach to the early identification and management of the sick patient

Smith GB, Prytherch DR, Schmidt P, et al. Resuscitation 2006; **71**: 19–28

BACKGROUND. Hospital patients who suffer cardiac arrest or have unplanned ICU admission often have premonitory abnormalities in vital signs. Sometimes the deterioration is well documented, though there is little evidence of intervention. In other cases, monitoring and recording of vital signs is infrequent or incomplete. Many hospitals use 'track and trigger' systems to enable early identification of high-risk patients and calling of a resuscitation team (e.g. medical emergency team). Even when track and trigger systems are used, the recording of vital signs and team activation can be suboptimal. The collaborators between a public hospital and a commercial company describe a system for collecting routine vital signs data at the bedside using standard personal digital assistants (PDAs). Nursing staff are reminded to do patient observations by the PDA. The PDAs are linked by a wireless local area network (W-LAN) to the hospital's intranet system, where raw and derived data are integrated with other patient information; for example, name, hospital number and laboratory results. It is possible for raw physiology data, early warning scores (EWSs), vital signs charts and oxygen therapy records to be made instantaneously available to any member of the clinical team via the W-LAN or hospital intranet. Early contact with members of the patient's primary clinical team or resuscitation team can be made through an automated alerting system, triggered by the EWS data.

INTERPRETATION. The ability to measure physiological data at the bedside, and to make these available to anyone with access rights at any time and in any place, should be beneficial. Analysis of the raw physiological data and patient outcomes will also make it possible to validate existing and future 'track and trigger' systems.

Comment

Many in-hospital cardiac arrests are preventable. This team has shown that it is feasible to use an electronic observation system to improve the reliability of the process of patient vital sign charting and to alert staff to patient deterioration. Most doctors know from personal experience that standard techniques are often poor. This group describe their system in detail and have collected large amounts of physiological data but have not yet published this nor shown that this will lead to decreased morbidity and mortality in ward patients.

Improving the quality of CPR

Good-quality chest compression with minimal interruption and delays before defibrillation are likely to improve survival from cardiac arrest |7|. In reality, manual chest compression quality is poor in both in-hospital and out-of-hospital settings, even when performed by professional rescuers |4,5|. Devices have been developed to improve chest compression quality. These include feedback devices that prompt the rescuer to give chest compressions at the correct depth and rate |8|. Measuring changes in transthoracic bioimpedance through the defibrillator pads may be useful to assess ventilation and cardiac output.

CPREzy™ improves performance of external chest compressions in simulated cardiac arrest

Beckers SK, Skorning MH, Fries M, *et al. Resuscitation* 2007; **72**: 100–7

BACKGROUND. The CPRezy (Fig. 9.2) is a portable device that is placed on the victim's sternum and compressed during chest compression. Chest compression rate is guided by a metronome bleeping at 100/min. A series of lights illuminate with each compression and turn off with complete release. The correct depth for compression is indicated by a sequence of lights that change with depth of compression. The depth for differing body weights and sizes is shown next to the lights. A total of 202 first-year medical students were randomized and asked to perform 5 min of single-rescuer CPR on a manikin. The manufacturer of the CPREzy devices, Health Affairs Limited UK, loaned the devices to the investigators. Group 1 ($n = 111$) was taught standard chest compressions, followed by compressions with the CPREzy and was tested in CPR with the CPREzy. Group 2 ($n = 91$) was taught and tested on standard compressions only. One week later each group was divided: group 1A was tested using the CPREzy; group 1B was tested in standard compressions. Group 2A was taught and tested with the CPREzy; group 2B was tested using standard CPR again. Initial chest compression quality was better with CPREzy (group 1 correct rate: 93.7% vs. group 2, 19.8%, $P < 0.01$; depth: 71.2% vs. 34.1%, $P < 0.01$). At the assessment one week later the group tested with CPREzy (2A; $n = 36$) improved significantly in correct compression rate (19.8% vs. 88.9%, $P \leq 0.01$) and compression depth (34.1% vs. 75.0%, $P \leq 0.02$).

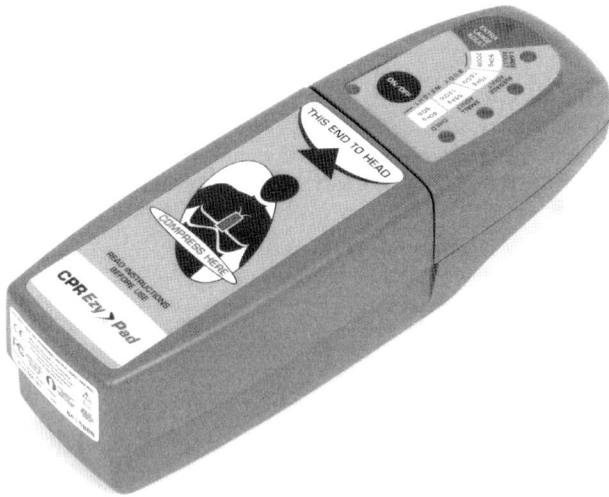

Fig. 9.2 CPREzy. Reproduced with permission from Health Affairs.

INTERPRETATION. The CPREzy can guide rescuers to deliver good quality chest compressions during CPR on a manikin.

Comment

The CPREzy has been shown to be effective at improving chest compression quality only in manikin studies. This is one of a number of studies that has shown this. It is reusable and relatively simple to use. Human studies are needed to assess whether the feedback results in correct chest compression depth (40–50 mm) in real patients. Ideally, if it were to be used, the CPREzy should be kept with a defibrillator. Many new defibrillators, however, already incorporate feedback on chest compression rate and depth to guide rescuers. This study also confirms that even after training, most rescuers do poor-quality chest compressions.

CPR quality improvement during in-hospital cardiac arrest using a real-time audiovisual feedback system

Abella BS, Edelson DP, Kim S, *et al. Resuscitation* 2007; **73**: 54–61

BACKGROUND. The authors tested whether real-time feedback improves the performance of chest compressions and ventilations during in-hospital cardiac arrest. A defibrillator with CPR-sensing and feedback capabilities was used during in-hospital cardiac arrests from December 2004 to December 2005. The defibrillator detected chest compressions via a pad placed between the rescuer's hands and the patient's sternum. The pad contains a force detector and accelerometer that enable calculation of chest compression rate and depth. The defibrillator gave verbal prompts to rescuers during CPR to correct any deficiencies in measured chest compression and ventilation quality. Ventilation rate and volume were measured with defibrillation pads through changes in thoracic impedance. This study included a commercial partner (Laerdal, Stavanger, Norway) who developed the quality feedback system with physicians working in the USA and Norway. Chest compression and ventilation characteristics were recorded and quantified for the first 5 min of resuscitation and compared with a baseline cohort of arrest episodes without feedback, from December 2002 to April 2004. Data from 55 resuscitation episodes in the baseline pre-intervention group were compared with 101 resuscitations in the feedback intervention group. Mean values of CPR variables numerically improved in the feedback group with a statistically significant narrowing of CPR variable distributions, including chest compression rate (104 ± 18 to 100 ± 13/min; test of means, $P = 0.16$; test of variance, $P = 0.003$) and ventilation rate (20 ± 10 to 18 ± 8/min; test of means, $P = 0.12$; test of variance, $P = 0.04$). There were no statistically significant differences between the groups in either ROSC or survival to hospital discharge.

INTERPRETATION. Feedback during CPR improved chest compression quality by a small amount and did not improve survival to discharge.

Comment

In theory, feedback during CPR should improve chest compression quality. The lack of improvement with feedback in this study is likely to have been caused by both machine and rescuer factors. When and how feedback is given during CPR probably needs to be optimized. Also, rescuers must respond to the feedback. It is not clear how teamworking and noise factors contributed to this. Only the first 5 min of CPR were studied. There may have been greater benefit with feedback after this initial period as rescuers become more tired and chest compression quality worsens. This study used a historical control group and the number of patients is too small to make firm conclusions about survival. This study was conducted before the current CPR guidelines, which have a much greater emphasis on chest compression quality, were implemented.

Thoracic impedance changes measured via defibrillator pads can monitor signs of circulation

Losert H, Risdal M, Sterz F, et al. Resuscitation 2007; **73**: 221–8

BACKGROUND. To investigate the potential for finding an alternative for the 'pulse check' during CPR, the use of thoracic impedance measured via the defibrillator pads for circulation assessment during CPR was studied. Transthoracic impedance, ECG and arterial pressures were recorded on 69 patients, with a resulting data set of 434 segments. A low, but significant, correlation coefficient (0.3) was found between blood pressure and transthoracic impedance changes.

By dividing the data set into groups with sufficient and insufficient circulation and using a neural network, trends in features of the impedance wave form showed a discriminative potential for the two groups. The classifier achieved a sensitivity of 90% for recognizing insufficient circulation with a specificity of 82%.

INTERPRETATION. Circulation-related information found in the impedance signal may be used for circulatory assessment.

Comment

This is an early study looking at monitoring cardiac output through defibrillator pads. Defibrillators that can monitor cardiac output via the defibrillation pads by measuring beat-to-beat variation in the transthoracic impedance signal would be useful if they can be incorporated into automated external defibrillators (AEDs). This would help rescuers confirm cardiac arrest and start CPR earlier. This is important when patients have pulseless electrical activity and the AED does not recommend a shock. This is emerging technology and needs further development.

Advanced cardiac life support before and after tracheal intubation – direct measurements of quality

Kramer-Johansen J, Wik L, Steen PA. *Resuscitation* 2006; **68**: 61–9

BACKGROUND. Tracheal intubation should improve the quality of CPR by enabling adequate ventilation without pauses in external chest compressions. Out-of-hospital cardiac arrests were sampled in this non-randomized, observational study of advanced cardiac life support in three ambulance services (Akershus, London and Stockholm). Defibrillators registered all chest compressions via an extra chest pad with an accelerometer mounted over the lower part of sternum and ventilations from changes in transthoracic impedance between the standard defibrillator pads. The quality of CPR was analysed offline for 119 cardiac arrests. Numbers and differences are given as mean ± standard deviation (SD) and differences as mean and 95% confidence intervals. Chest compressions were not given in cardiac arrest for 61 ± 20% of the time before tracheal intubation compared with 41 ± 18% after tracheal intubation (difference: 20% [16–24%]). Compressions and ventilations per minute increased from 47 ± 25 to 71 ± 23 (difference: 24 [19, 29]) and 5.6 ± 3.7 to 14 ± 5.0 (difference: 8.7 [7.6, 9.8]), respectively. Four cases of unrecognized oesophageal intubation (3%) were suspected from the disappearance of ventilation-induced changes in thoracic impedance after intubation.

INTERPRETATION. The quality of CPR improves after tracheal intubation. Online analysis of thoracic impedance might be a practicable aid to avoid unrecognized oesophageal intubation.

Comment

This paper shows that tracheal intubation enables improvement in quality of CPR. The study does not have sufficient power to determine whether this improves patient outcomes. Ventilation was monitored by measuring changes in transthoracic impedance through the defibrillator pads.

The study had an unexpected and potentially even more beneficial outcome: the possibility that transthoracic impedance may be used to identify oesophageal intubation. Oesophageal intubation at cardiac arrest is likely to be underdiagnosed. Detection of oesophageal intubation can be achieved with capnography, fibreoptic inspection of tube position or use of an oesophageal detector device |**9**|. Capnography is of limited use during cardiac arrest and fibrescopes remain too expensive for this to be routinely practical. There are still not enough data to identify the optimal method for confirming tube placement during cardiac arrest and all devices should be considered adjuncts to other confirmatory techniques. There are no data quantifying the capability for any of these devices to monitor tube position after initial placement during CPR. During lung ventilation transthoracic impedence increases with an increase in cross-sectional area of the chest. If ventilation via a 'tracheal tube' fails to alter transthoracic impedance, this will just be another pointer to recheck tracheal tube position. Further research is needed in this area.

Mechanical chest compressions

Manual (external) chest compression causes rescuer fatigue within a few minutes of starting |**10**|. Chest compressions are also difficult while transporting patients |**11**|. This has led to the use of mechanical chest compression devices. These devices have been available since the 1960s |**12**|. The Lund University cardiac arrest system (LUCAS™) and a load-distributing band (AutoPulse®) system are the most popular devices currently used (Fig. 9.3). The LUCAS™ (Jolife, Sweden) is a gas-driven sternal compression device incorporating a suction cup that actively re-expands the chest during chest decompression |**13**|. Active re-expansion generates a negative intrathoracic pressure and increases venous return to the heart. This increases cardiac output and subsequent coronary and cerebral perfusion pressure during the following chest compression phase. The AutoPulse® (Zoll, USA) is an automated device that uses a load-distributing band (LDB) that is applied around the front of the chest and is attached to a backboard that the patient lies on |**14**|. Rather than compressing the sternum, the LDB compresses across the entire chest and there is no active decompression phase.

(a)   (b)

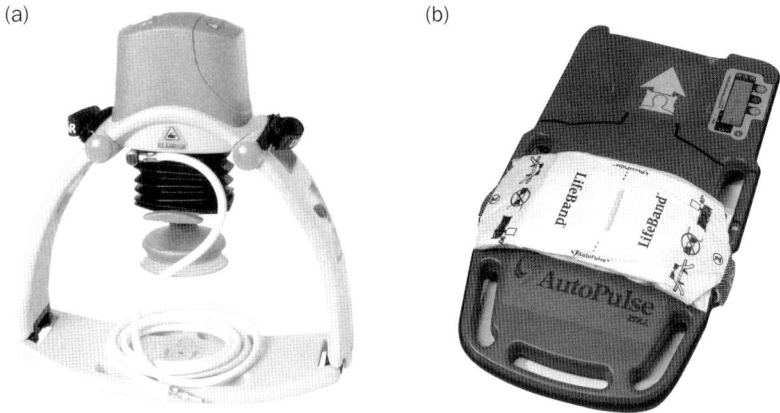

Fig. 9.3 (a) The LUCAS™ device (reproduced with permission from Jolife, Lund, Sweden); (b) AutoPulse® (reproduced with permission from ZOLL Medical Corporation, Chelmsford MA, USA).

Clinical consequences of the introduction of mechanical chest compression in the EMS system for treatment of out-of-hospital cardiac arrest – a pilot study

Axelsson C, Nestin J, Svensson L, et al. Resuscitation 2006; **71**: 47–55

BACKGROUND. This study evaluated the outcome among patients suffering from witnessed out-of-hospital cardiac arrest after the introduction of the LUCAS™ device compared with standard CPR (SCPR) in two emergency medical service (EMS) systems. Exclusion criteria were age less than 18 years and cardiac arrest caused by trauma, pregnancy, hypothermia, intoxication, hanging and drowning or ROSC prior to the arrival of the advanced life support (ALS) unit. Two LUCAS™ devices were allocated during 6-month periods between four ALS units for a period of 2 years (cluster randomization). In all, 328 patients fulfilled the criteria for participation and 159 were allocated to the LUCAS™ group (the device was used in 66% of cases) and 169 to the SCPR group. In the LUCAS™ group, 51% had ROSC (primary endpoint) vs. 51% in the SCPR group. The corresponding values for hospital admission alive (secondary endpoint) were 38% and 37% (not significant). In the subset of patients in whom the device was used, the percentage who had ROSC was 49% vs. 50% in a control group matched for age, initial rhythm, aetiology, bystander-/crew-witnessed status and delay to CPR. The percentage of patients discharged alive from hospital was 8% vs. 10% (not significant) for all patients and 2% vs. 4%, respectively (not significant) for the patients in the LUCAS™ and matched cohort subsets.

INTERPRETATION. In this study, mechanical CPR with the LUCAS™ device did not improve ROSC or survival to discharge in patients who had a witnessed out-of-hospital cardiac arrest.

Comment

This is the first attempt at studying the clinical effectiveness of the LUCAS™ device. There is no randomization in this study. The LUCAS™ device, if correctly applied, seems to provide high-quality chest compressions. The downside seems to be the time taken for it to be brought to the patient, set up and started. The median delay from collapse to using the LUCAS™ device was 18 min. One-third of the patients allocated the LUCAS™ did not have it used on them, often because they had already been resuscitated before the device could be applied. The authors do not comment on whether patients having mechanical chest compressions suffer more injuries, or less, than those who have standard CPR. This has been highlighted as a potential problem with the LUCAS™ device [15]. Despite the lack of good studies of efficacy, the LUCAS™ device has become popular in the pre-hospital setting. A recent paper has highlighted another potential problem with the LUCAS™. The LUCAS™ is driven by over 70 l/min oxygen, which increases ambient oxygen concentrations [16]. This may increase fire risk in the presence of sparks and inflammable materials, such as may occur during attempted defibrillation.

Mechanical chest compressions with a load-distributing band

There are two studies, with contradictory results, comparing manual chest compressions with mechanical chest compressions using a LDB (AutoPulse®).

Use of an automated, load-distributing band chest compression device for out-of-hospital cardiac arrest resuscitation

Ong ME, Ornato JP, Edwards DP, et al. JAMA 2006; **295**: 2629–37

BACKGROUND. The resuscitation outcomes before and after an urban emergency medical services (EMS) system switched from manual cardiopulmonary resuscitation (CPR) to load-distributing band (LDB) CPR were compared. This was a phased, observational cohort evaluation with intention-to-treat analysis of 783 adults with out-of-hospital, non-traumatic cardiac arrest. A total of 499 patients were included in the manual CPR phase (1 January 2001 to 31 March 2003) and 284 patients in the LDB-CPR phase (20 December 2003 to 31 March 2005). The LDB device was applied in 210 patients. The main outcome measures were return of spontaneous circulation (ROSC), with secondary outcome measures of survival to hospital admission and hospital discharge, and neurological outcome at discharge. Patients in the manual CPR and LDB-CPR phases were comparable, except for a faster response time interval (mean difference, 26 s) and more EMS-witnessed arrests (18.7% vs. 12.6%) with LDB. Rates for ROSC and survival were increased with LDB-CPR compared with manual CPR (for ROSC, 34.5%; 95% confidence interval [CI] 29.2–40.3% vs. 20.2%; 95% CI 16.9–24.0%; adjusted odds ratio [OR], 1.94; 95% CI 1.38–2.72; for survival to hospital admission, 20.9%; 95% CI 16.6–26.1% vs. 11.1%; 95% CI 8.6-14.2%; adjusted OR, 1.88; 95% CI 1.23–2.86; and for survival to hospital discharge, 9.7%; 95% CI 6.7–13.8% vs. 2.9%; 95% CI 1.7–4.8%; adjusted OR 2.27; 95% CI 1.11–4.77). In secondary analysis of the 210 patients in whom the LDB device was applied, 38 patients (18.1%) survived to hospital admission (95% CI 13.4–23.9%) and 12 patients (5.7%) survived to hospital discharge (95% CI 3.0–9.3%). Among patients in both groups who survived to hospital discharge, there was no significant difference in cerebral performance category ($P = 0.36$) or overall performance category ($P = 0.40$). The number needed to treat for the adjusted outcome survival to discharge was 15 (95% CI 9–33).

INTERPRETATION. Compared with resuscitation using manual CPR, a resuscitation strategy using LDB-CPR on EMS ambulances is associated with improved survival to hospital discharge in adults with out-of-hospital non-traumatic cardiac arrest.

Manual chest compression versus use of an automated chest compression device during resuscitation following out-of-hospital cardiac arrest. A randomized trial

Hallstrom A, Rea TD, Sayre MR, et al. JAMA 2006; **295**: 2620–8

BACKGROUND. Outcomes following out-of-hospital cardiac arrest were compared between standard emergency medical services (EMS) care with manual CPR or with an automated LDB-CPR device (AutoPulse®). This is a multicentre, randomized trial of patients experiencing out-of-hospital cardiac arrest in the United States and Canada. Standard EMS care for cardiac arrest with an LDB-CPR device ($n = 554$) or manual CPR ($n = 517$). The primary endpoint was survival to 4 h after the emergency call. Secondary endpoints were survival to hospital discharge and neurological status among survivors. Following the first planned interim monitoring conducted by an independent data and safety monitoring board, study enrolment was terminated. No difference existed in the primary endpoint of survival to 4 h between the manual CPR group and the LDB-CPR group overall ($n = 1071$; 29.5% vs. 28.5%; $P = 0.74$). The primary study population excluded patients who had a cardiac arrest after the EMS had arrived, those who had a non-cardiac cause of cardiac arrest, or had been attended by another advanced life support EMS crew for more than 90 s before the study crew arrived on scene. There was no difference between manual CPR and LDB-CPR for this primary study population ($n = 767$; 24.7% vs. 26.4%, respectively; $P = 0.62$). However, among the primary population, survival to hospital discharge was 9.9% in the manual CPR group and 5.8% in the LDB-CPR group ($P = 0.06$, adjusted for covariates and clustering). A good neurological outcome (cerebral performance category of 1 or 2) at hospital discharge was recorded in 7.5% of patients in the manual CPR group and in 3.1% of the LDB-CPR group ($P = 0.006$).

Table 9.1 Comparison of contradictory LDB-CPR studies

	Hallstrom et al. (2006)	Ong et al. (2006)
Design	Prospective, cluster randomization	Retrospective, before and after study
Setting	Five EMS systems in USA, Canada	Single EMS system in USA
Study population	Out-of-hospital cardiac arrest of presumed cardiac origin	
Intervention	LDB-CPR vs. manual CPR	
EMS response time	LDB-CPR 5.6 min Manual CPR 5.7 min	LDB-CPR 4.6 min Manual CPR 4.6 min
Mean time to LDB-CPR	11.9 min	Not measured
Patients with VF/VT	LDB-CPR 31% Manual CPR 32%	LDB-CPR 24% Manual CPR 21%
Primary outcome	Survival to 4 h LDB-CPR 26% Manual CPR 25%	ROSC LDB-CPR 35% Manual CPR 20%
Secondary outcomes	Survival to hospital discharge LDB-CPR 6% Manual CPR 10% Good neurological outcome (CPC score of 1 or 2) LDB-CPR 3% Manual CPR 8%	Survival to hospital discharge LDB-CPR 10% Manual CPR 3% Good neurological outcome (CPC score of 1 or 2) LDB-CPR 6% Manual CPR 2%

Table 9.1 Comparison of contradictory LDB-CPR studies (continued)

	Hallstrom et al. (2006)	Ong et al. (2006)
Potential confounders	Heterogeneity of treatment sites	Quicker advanced life support and more witnessed arrests in LDB-CPR
	Slower time to first shock in manual CPR group	Use of therapeutic hypothermia after resuscitation during LDB-CPR phase
	Enrolment bias	Quality of CPR in manual CPR group not assessed and controlled
	Quality of CPR in manual CPR group not assessed and controlled	
Conflicts of interest/study funding	Funded by Zoll, manufacturer of the AutoPulse®. Zoll did not influence design or conduct of study. Zoll was able to comment on manuscript but not have final say on published paper	One of the authors is a paid science advisor to Zoll, manufacturer of the AutoPulse®. This author did not take part in data acquisition or analysis. The AutoPulse® devices were loaned by Zoll for the study. These, plus additional devices, were purchased by the EMS at the end of the study

LDB-CPR, Load distributing band cardiopulmonary resuscitation; EMS, emergency medical system; VF/VT, ventricular fibrillation/pulseless ventricular tachycardia; ROSC, restoration of spontaneous circulation; CPC, cerebral performance category. Adapted from Lewis RJ, Niemann JT. JAMA 2006; **295**: 2661–4.

INTERPRETATION. Use of an automated LDB-CPR device as implemented in this study was associated with worse neurological outcomes. LDB-CPR was also associated with a worse survival than manual CPR, although this was not statistically significant.

Comment

These two studies published at the same time give contradictory results. The key differences between the papers are summarized in Table 9.1 |**17**|. Despite the higher level study by Hallstrom and colleagues showing no benefit and potential harm from LDB-CPR, there has been wide adoption of LDB-CPR. The manufacturer's annual report for 2005 states that 160 hospitals and ambulance services were using the AutoPulse®. This may be due to marketing material and the enthusiasm of the early adopters of the device. As for the LUCAS™, the downside of any manual compression device such as the LDB is the delay in getting it to the patient, and the likelihood that the best survivors are usually resuscitated before the device arrives.

Enhancing organ flow during CPR

The impedance threshold valve (ITV) is a valve that limits air entry into the lungs during chest recoil between chest compressions; this decreases intrathoracic pressure and increases venous return to the heart |**18**|. When used with a cuffed tracheal tube and active compression–decompression, the ITV is thought to act synergistically to enhance venous return during active decompression. This will then increase organ perfusion during the subsequent chest compression.

The impedance threshold valve for adult cardiopulmonary resuscitation: a review of the literature

Pirracchio R, Payen D, Plaisance P. *Curr Opin Crit Care* 2007; **13**: 280–6

BACKGROUND. Heart–lung interaction is important in the understanding of blood flow during CPR. The impedance threshold valve is a device which has been created to increase venous return by occluding the airway during the decompression phase of CPR. During clinical evaluation when used in conjunction with active compression/decompression CPR, addition of the impedance valve resulted in a sustained increase in systolic and diastolic pressures as well as improvement of vital organ blood flow. There are three clinical studies comparing the ITV with standard CPR |19–21|, none of which has survival to hospital discharge as an endpoint. Pirrallo *et al.* |21| reported significant haemodynamic improvements with the use of the ITV in comparison with standard CPR with a sham valve (systolic blood pressure 43 mmHg for standard CPR compared with 85 mmHg for ITV, $P < 0.05$), without any adverse effect. Aufderheide *et al.* |20| compared on-scene standard CPR with an ITV or with a sham valve (116 patients sham valve, 114 patients ITV). Patients presenting with pulseless electrical activity had ICU admission and 24-h survival rates of 20% and 12% in the sham group (*n* = 25) compared with 52% and 30% in the active ITV groups (*n* = 27; *P* = 0.018 and *P* = 0.12 respectively). Thayne et al. |19| showed that for out-of-hospital non-traumatic arrests, compared with historical controls, patients treated with the ITV had a significantly greater survival rate: 22% compared with 34% (*P* < 0.01).

INTERPRETATION. Animal and human data show that increased preload by a decrease in the intrathoracic pressure in the decompression phase improves overall blood flow during CPR that may confer survival benefit.

Comment

There are currently no good studies with long-term survival as an endpoint for the ITV. A multicentre study to determine whether performing active compression/decompression cardiopulmonary resuscitation (ACD-CPR) with an ITV or using an ITV with conventional CPR will affect the neurological recovery and survival to hospital discharge following out-of-hospital cardiac arrest is currently under way (ClinicalTrials.gov identifier NCT00189423).

Defibrillation

Ventricular fibrillation and pulseless ventricular tachycardia (VF/VT) are the most common cardiac arrest rhythms in deaths caused by ischaemic heart disease. Defibrillation is the treatment of choice for VF/VT |22|. Monophasic and biphasic are two main types of defibrillation waveform (Fig. 9.4). First-shock defibrillation success rates for long-duration VF/VT are higher for biphasic waveforms |22|. Monophasic defibrillators are no longer manufactured but are still in widespread use. The two commonest variants of biphasic waveform are the truncated exponential and the rectilinear biphasic waveform (Fig. 9.4). Some biphasic waveforms adjust their size and duration with variations in the patient's transthoracic impedance (impedance compensation).

Transthoracic incremental monophasic versus biphasic defibrillation by emergency responders (TIMBER): a randomized comparison of monophasic with biphasic waveform ascending energy defibrillation for the resuscitation of out-of-hospital cardiac arrest due to ventricular fibrillation

Kudenchuk PJ, Cobb LA, Copass MK, *et al. Circulation* 2006; **114**: 2010–18

BACKGROUND. Biphasic shocks seem to give higher first-shock success rates when used to defibrillate VF/VT than do monophasic shock waveforms. Despite this there is no evidence to show they improve overall survival. Consecutive adults

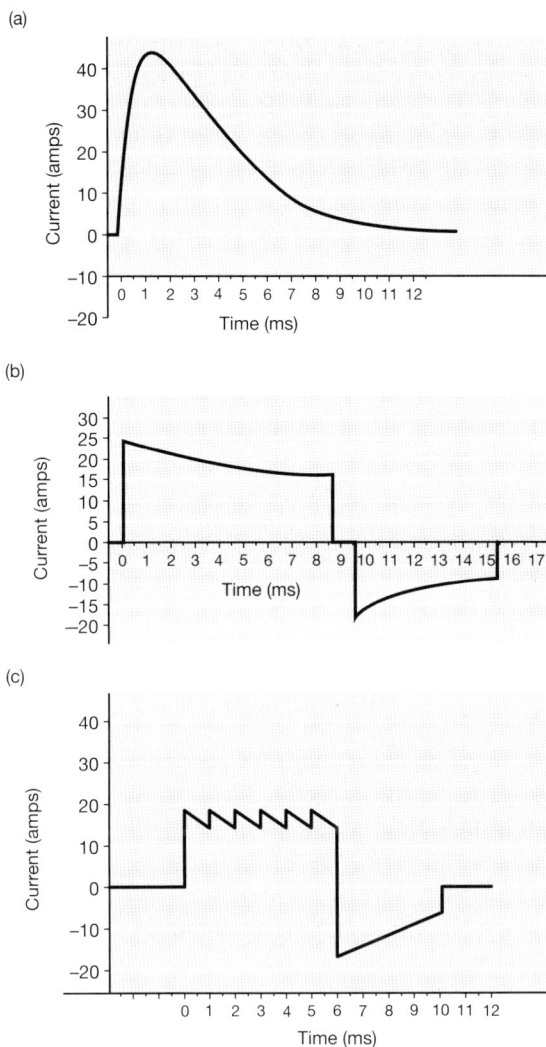

Fig. 9.4 Defibrillation waveforms. (a) Monophasic waveform; (b) biphasic truncated exponential waveform; (c) rectilinear biphasic waveform. Source: Resuscitation Council UK.

with non-traumatic out-of-hospital VF/VT cardiac arrest were randomly allocated to monophasic or biphasic defibrillation from automated external defibrillators administered by pre-hospital medical providers. The primary event of interest was admission alive to the hospital. Secondary events included return of rhythm and circulation, survival and neurological outcome. Providers were blinded to automated defibrillator waveform. Of 168 randomized patients, 80 (48%) and 68 (40%) consistently received only monophasic or biphasic waveform shocks, respectively, throughout resuscitation. The prevalence of ventricular fibrillation,

asystole or organized rhythms at 5, 10 or 20s after each shock did not differ significantly between treatment groups. The proportion of patients admitted alive to the hospital was relatively high: 73% in monophasic and 76% in biphasic treatment groups ($P = 0.58$). Results consistently numerically favoured receipt of biphasic waveform shock, though none reached statistical significance. Notably, 27 of 80 monophasic shock recipients (34%), compared with 28 of 68 biphasic shock recipients (41%), survived ($P = 0.35$). Neurological outcome was similar in both treatment groups ($P = 0.4$). Earlier administration of shock did not significantly alter the performance of one waveform relative to the other, nor did shock waveform predict any clinical outcome after multivariate adjustment.

INTERPRETATION. Although there was a 'trend' towards greater shock success and survival to hospital admission with a biphasic waveform, this was not statistically significant.

Comment

Monophasic defibrillators are no longer manufactured but are still in widespread use. This study provides a small degree of comfort to those who still have the older monophasic defibrillators. Secondary endpoints showed numerical differences suggesting improved outcomes with biphasic defibrillators but these did not reach statistical significance. Other studies have shown that first-shock efficacy for long-duration VF/VT is greater with biphasic than monophasic waveforms, and biphasic waveforms are more effective than monophasic waveforms for cardioversion of atrial fibrillation |22|. This study used defibrillators from a single manufacturer. Depending on the defibrillator manufacturer there are variations of biphasic waveform and different recommendations for shock energy. This makes comparison of defibrillators from differing manufacturers difficult.

Automated external defibrillators (AEDs)

AEDs enable individuals without rhythm recognition skills to safely deliver a shock appropriately to patients in VF/VT. Public access defibrillation (PAD) and first responder AED programmes increase the number of victims who receive bystander CPR and early defibrillation and improve survival from out-of-hospital cardiac arrest. AED programmes with very rapid response times in airports, on aircraft or in casinos, and uncontrolled studies using police officers as first responders report survival rates as high as 49–74% |23|. In the USA members of the public can now buy AEDs for home use.

One AED issue, about which little has been published, has been caused by the recommendation in the 2005 CPR guidelines for use of single shocks in the treatment of VF/VT. The previous guidelines recommended three stacked shocks for the treatment of VF/VT and as a consequence many AEDs currently still in use may be programmed to deliver three stacked shocks in these circumstances. There are several reasons for this. First, very old AEDs are difficult to upgrade and are no longer supported by the manufacturers. Second, the 2005 guidelines process excluded manufacturers, who were therefore not aware of the single shock guideline until their worldwide release in late 2005. Software upgrades for many AEDs were not available until mid-2006. Individuals receiving AED training must therefore be told to switch on the defibrillator and follow the prompts.

Post-resuscitation care

Post-resuscitation care to improve quality of life is the final link in the chain of survival. Recent evidence suggests that unconscious adults with spontaneous circulation after out-of-hospital cardiac arrest should be cooled to 32–34°C for 12–24h when the initial rhythm is VF/VT. Mild hypothermia should also be considered for unconscious adult patients with spontaneous circulation after out-of-hospital cardiac arrest from any other rhythm or after in-hospital cardiac arrest |24|. The initial studies used surface cooling methods such as icepacks, fans and cold air to initiate and maintain hypothermia |25,26|. These can be unreliable and cause both under- and overcooling |27|. Endovascular cooling devices may give better control |28|.

Efficacy and tolerance of mild induced hypothermia after out-of-hospital cardiac arrest using an endovascular cooling system

Pichon N, Amiel JB, François B, et al. Crit Care 2007; **11**: R71 (electronic publication ahead of print)

BACKGROUND. To assess the efficacy, the tolerance and the ability of mild therapeutic hypothermia using an endovascular cooling system to reach and to maintain a target temperature of 33°C after cardiac arrest. This case series comes from the medical–surgical intensive care unit (ICU) of an urban university hospital. Forty patients admitted to the ICU after an out-of-hospital cardiac arrest underwent mild induced hypothermia (MIH). The endovascular system (CoolGard™) works by passing cooled normal saline through a catheter that is placed in the inferior vena cava via the femoral vein. The saline in the catheter cools the blood flowing through the inferior vena cava. The patient's core temperature was monitored continuously for 5 days using a urinary catheter equipped with a temperature sensor. The cooling system monitors the patient's core temperature from the urinary catheter and adjusts the temperature of the saline in the intravascular device to maintain the target patient temperature. The operator can also adjust the rate of temperature change from 0.1 to 0.7°C/h. Neurological status was evaluated daily using Pittsburgh cerebral performance category (CPC). The mechanism of cardiac arrest, the Simplified Acute Physiologic Score (SAPS) II on admission, standard biological variables, and time lags characterizing the duration of cerebral hypoperfusion were recorded. Nosocomial infection rates were collected during and after MIH until day 28. Six patients (15%) died during hypothermia. Among the 34 patients who completed the period of MIH, hypothermia was maintained stable in 31 patients (91%). The mean time to initiate MIH was 98 ± 54 min (range 45–300 min) after resuscitation. It took a mean time of 187 ± 119 min (range 30 to 600 min) to reach 33 °C after initiation of MIH. A temperature of 33 °C was maintained for 37 ± 6 h (range 20–48 h). Rewarming was set at 0.3 °C/h to achieve normothermia. The catheter was removed within 24 h of stopping MIH. Post-rewarming 'rebound hyperthermia', determined as temperature greater than 38.5°C, was observed in 25 patients (74%) during the first 24 h which followed the cessation of MIH. Infectious complications were observed in 18 patients (45%), but no patient developed severe sepsis or septic shock. Biological changes during MIH principally resulted in hypokalaemia <3.5 mol/l (75%).

INTERPRETATION. The intravascular cooling system is effective, safe and allows reaching a target temperature fairly rapidly and steadily over a period of 36 h.

Comment

An intravascular cooling device seems to be more reliable than surface cooling methods to maintain mild hypothermia |27|. These authors used the endovascular device to initiate cooling and maintain hypothermia. Hypothermia was maintained for a longer period than recommended |24|. About three-quarters (74%) of the patients got rebound hyperthermia (>38.5°C) on stopping cooling. This rebound hyperthermia is in itself likely to be harmful |29|. One of the supposed benefits of an endovascular device is controlled rewarming. It may be beneficial to keep the endovascular device in place to maintain normothermia to prevent this rebound hyperthermia. Ideally, cooling should start as soon as possible after ROSC. Unfortunately, endovascular devices for cooling are not easily portable, require the insertion of a large bore venous catheter and are relatively expensive. A simple and effective method to induce mild hypothermia that can start at the scene of the cardiac arrest is the rapid infusion of 30 ml/kg of cold (4°C) fluid |30|.

Conclusion

Devices have been developed that attempt to improve patient care during all four links of the chain of survival. Developments in monitoring may help identify patients at risk of cardiac arrest earlier and enable interventions that can prevent cardiac arrest. Modern CPR devices attempt to replace variation in human performance during CPR. Many are based around the defibrillator. As well as delivering shocks for the treatment of VF/VT, modern defibrillators can advise those without rhythm recognition skills to deliver a shock appropriately, monitor chest compression quality in terms of depth and rate and provide feedback to the rescuer. In the future defibrillators may also be able to monitor the patient's cardiac arrest rhythm and cardiac output during chest compressions. It is feasible that the defibrillator will then advise when the rhythm is favourable to stop chest compressions and deliver a shock with the highest likelihood of success. New 'smarter' defibrillators that are simple to use should enable a wider range of individuals to deliver CPR.

Although most CPR devices (e.g. mechanical chest compression devices) perform the task they were designed for, few have been shown to confer any actual patient benefit in terms of survival to hospital discharge and other useful outcome measures such as good neurological and functional outcomes. Despite this, some of these devices (e.g. LUCAS™, AutoPulse®) are in widespread use. This could be due to good marketing, as well as perceived benefits by those who use them. Some devices, such as mechanical chest compression devices are potentially labour saving. Research in CPR is difficult in terms of setting up trials and recruiting patients. It is likely that many more CPR devices will be marketed and used in the clinical setting, with little evidence of real benefit. Much of the research on CPR devices involves the commercial companies who developed the device. At the very least most companies will supply the device being investigated free of charge to the investigator. It is not easy to say whether this influences what is published.

One problem that users of all these devices face is whether the devices are actually available to use when cardiac arrest occurs. Delay in use negates many of the potential benefits of CPR devices as they often arrive too late.

It is likely that CPR devices will only add benefit to systems where the early steps of the chain of survival are in place. All CPR devices still rely on these basic human interventions: calling for help and starting CPR.

The author has no conflict of interest regarding the content of this article.

References

1. Nolan J, Soar J, Eikeland H. The chain of survival. *Resuscitation* 2006; **71**: 270–1.

2. Nolan JP, Deakin CD, Soar J, Bottiger BW, Smith G. European Resuscitation Council guidelines for resuscitation 2005. Section 4. Adult advanced life support. *Resuscitation* 2005; **67** (Suppl. 1): S39–86.

3. Peberdy MA, Kaye W, Ornato JP, Larkin GL, Nadkarni V, Mancini ME, Berg RA, Nichol G, Lane-Trultt T. Cardiopulmonary resuscitation of adults in the hospital: a report of 14720 cardiac arrests from the National Registry of Cardiopulmonary Resuscitation. *Resuscitation* 2003; **58**: 297–308.

4. Abella BS, Alvarado JP, Myklebust H, Edelson DP, Barry A, O'Hearn N, Vanden Hoek TL, Becker LB. Quality of cardiopulmonary resuscitation during in-hospital cardiac arrest. *JAMA* 2005; **293**: 305–10.

5. Wik L, Kramer-Johansen J, Myklebust H, Sorebo H, Svensson L, Fellows B, Steen PA. Quality of cardiopulmonary resuscitation during out-of-hospital cardiac arrest. *JAMA* 2005; **293**: 299–304.

6. Kause J, Smith G, Prytherch D, Parr M, Flabouris A, Hillman K. A comparison of antecedents to cardiac arrests, deaths and emergency intensive care admissions in Australia and New Zealand, and the United Kingdom – the ACADEMIA study. *Resuscitation* 2004; **62**: 275–82.

7. Edelson DP, Abella BS, Kramer-Johansen J, Wik L, Myklebust H, Barry AM, *et al.* Effects of compression depth and pre-shock pauses predict defibrillation failure during cardiac arrest. *Resuscitation* 2006; **71**: 137–45.

8. Boyle AJ, Wilson AM, Connelly K, McGuigan L, Wilson J, Whitbourn R. Improvement in timing and effectiveness of external cardiac compressions with a new non-invasive device: the CPR-Ezy. *Resuscitation* 2002; **54**: 63–7.

9. Williams KN, Nunn JF. The oesophageal detector device: a prospective trial on 100 patients. *Anaesthesia* 1989; **44**: 412–24.

10. Ashton A, McCluskey A, Gwinnutt CL, Keenan AM. Effect of rescuer fatigue on performance of continuous external chest compressions over 3 min. *Resuscitation* 2002; **55**: 151–5.

11. Ochoa FJ, Ramalle-Gomara E, Lisa V, Saralegui I. The effect of rescuer fatigue on the quality of chest compressions. *Resuscitation* 1998; **37**: 149–52.

12. Harrison-Paul R. A history of mechanical devices for providing external chest compressions. *Resuscitation* 2007; **73**: 330–6.

13. Steen S, Liao Q, Pierre L, Paskevicius A, Sjoberg T. Evaluation of LUCAS™, a new device for automatic mechanical compression and active decompression resuscitation. *Resuscitation* 2002; **55**: 285–99.

14. Timerman S, Cardoso LF, Ramires JA, Halperin H. Improved hemodynamic performance with a novel chest compression device during treatment of in-hospital cardiac arrest. *Resuscitation* 2004; **61**: 273–80.

15. Englund E, Kongstad PC. Active compression-decompression CPR necessitates follow-up post mortem. *Resuscitation* 2006; **68**: 161–2.

16. Deakin CD, Paul V, Fall E, Petley GW, Thompson F. Ambient oxygen concentrations resulting from use of the Lund University Cardiopulmonary Assist System (LUCAS™) device during simulated cardiopulmonary resuscitation. *Resuscitation* 2007; **74**: 303–9.

17. Lewis RJ, Niemann JT. Manual versus device-assisted CPR: reconciling apparently contradictory results. *JAMA* 2006; **295**: 2661–4.

18. Lurie KG, Barnes TA, Zielinski TM, McKnite SH. Evaluation of a prototypic inspiratory impedance threshold valve designed to enhance the efficiency of cardiopulmonary resuscitation. *Respir Care* 2003; **48**: 52–7.

19. Thayne RC, Thomas DC, Neville JD, Van Dellen A. Use of an impedance threshold device improves short-term outcomes following out-of-hospital cardiac arrest. *Resuscitation* 2005; **67**: 103–8.

20. Aufderheide T, Pirrallo R, Provo T, Lurie K. Clinical evaluation of an inspiratory impedance threshold device during standard cardiopulmonary resuscitation in patients with out-of-hospital cardiac arrest. *Crit Care Med* 2005; **33**: 734–40.

21. Pirrallo RG, Aufderheide TP, Provo TA, Lurie KG. Effect of an inspiratory impedance threshold device on hemodynamics during conventional manual cardiopulmonary resuscitation. *Resuscitation* 2005; **66**: 13–20.

22. Deakin CD, Nolan JP. European Resuscitation Council guidelines for resuscitation 2005. Section 3. Electrical therapies: automated external defibrillators, defibrillation, cardioversion and pacing. *Resuscitation* 2005; **67**(Suppl. 1): S25–37.

23. Handley AJ, Koster R, Monsieurs K, Perkins GD, Davies S, Bossaert L. European Resuscitation Council guidelines for resuscitation 2005. Section 2. Adult basic life support and use of automated external defibrillators. *Resuscitation* 2005; **67**(Suppl. 1): S7–23.

24. Nolan JP, Morley PT, Vanden Hoek TL, Hickey RW. Therapeutic hypothermia after cardiac arrest. An advisory statement by the Advancement Life support Task Force of the International Liaison committee on Resuscitation. *Resuscitation* 2003; **57**: 231–5.

25. Hypothermia After Cardiac Arrest Study Group. Mild therapeutic hypothermia to improve the neurologic outcome after cardiac arrest. *N Engl J Med* 2002; **346**(8): 549–56.

26. Bernard SA, Gray TW, Buist MD, Jones BM, Silvester W, Gutteridge G, Smith K. Treatment of comatose survivors of out-of-hospital cardiac arrest with induced hypothermia. *N Engl J Med* 2002; **346**(8): 557–63.

27. Merchant RM, Abella BS, Peberdy MA, Soar J, Ong ME, Schmidt GA, Becker LB, Vanden Hoek TL. Therapeutic hypothermia after cardiac arrest: unintentional overcooling is common using ice packs and conventional cooling blankets. *Crit Care Med* 2006; **34**(12 Suppl.): S490–S494.

28. Pichon N, Amiel JB, Francois B, Dugard A, Etchecopar C, Vignon P. Efficacy and tolerance of mild induced hypothermia after out-of-hospital cardiac arrest using an endovascular cooling system. *Crit Care* 2007; **11**: R71.

29. Zeiner A, Holzer M, Sterz F, Schorkhuber W, Eisenburger P, Havel C, Kliegel A, Laggner AN. Hyperthermia after cardiac arrest is associated with an unfavorable neurologic outcome. *Arch Intern Med* 2001; **161**: 2007–12.

30. Kim F, Olsufka M, Longstreth WT Jr, Maynard C, Carlbom D, Deem S, Kudenchuk P, Copass MK, Cobb LA. Pilot randomized clinical trial of prehospital induction of mild hypothermia in out-of-hospital cardiac arrest patients with a rapid infusion of 4 degrees C normal saline. *Circulation* 2007; **115**: 3064–70.

10

Computers in anaesthesia and ICUs

RANJIT VERMA

Introduction

Technological advances continue to influence the way many aspects of healthcare are delivered. Improvements in the information technology infrastructure mean that newer technology can be brought to bear to enhance clinical practice and ultimately improve the quality of patient care. Often technology that has been tried and tested elsewhere in other disciplines is imported for use in healthcare. Not all technology and information technology developments may be appropriate to use in healthcare delivery. Risks that may be acceptable elsewhere may be inappropriately high in the healthcare sector.

Wireless communication

The ability to use electronic devices wirelessly offers significant advantages. It allows people to work remotely and yet be part of a larger integrated data collection or communication system. Although this is commonplace in industry, healthcare seems to lag behind. Most new technological advances in healthcare now give due consideration to the use of such technology. Wireless technology can be used relatively locally, for example within an operating theatre, within a department or a hospital, or more extensively in global transmission of data over large distances. It is important to remember that such technologies also have their hazards and pitfalls.

Wireless technologies and patient safety in hospitals

Boyle J. *Telemedicine and e-Health* 2006; **12**: 373–82

BACKGROUND. There has been considerable concern that communication devices that use wireless technology can have an adverse effect on electronic apparatus and might potentially harm patients. Electromagnetic interference is frequently blamed with little recourse to actual evidence. This technical review addresses this issue.

INTERPRETATION. Wireless technology is used at the bedside to access patient records, laboratory and other investigative results, literature resources and for patient monitoring. These measures can increase efficiency and productivity, decrease costs and improve the quality of healthcare delivered. This paper reviews current evidence and states as its objective to act as a guide for policy-makers regarding introduction of wireless technologies into hospitals.

Comment

There are pressures within healthcare to minimize error rates, conduct diagnoses on the basis of real-time patient data, improve efficiency and reduce costs. Wireless technology can be used to facilitate this. Several areas can benefit from real-time wireless access, including admissions, laboratories, medical records, radiology, nursing, and so on. There are concerns that this technology might adversely influence existing electronic equipment.

Wireless technology conveys information via electromagnetic waves whose frequencies vary in their position within the electromagnetic spectrum (Fig. 10.1).

Most wireless communications use radio frequency. Infrared has been used for wireless local area networks (LANs) but is limited because it can only be used where there is clear line of sight. Experiments have shown that there is no evidence of electromagnetic interference with infrared when tested against several devices such as infusion pumps, syringe pumps and cardiac pacemakers [1]. Ultra-wideband is a wireless technology that uses very narrow, short pulses in existing radio services without causing interference. Radio frequencies are managed by an international authority that allocates specific spectral bands to devices. These are regulated by local authorities.

Electromagnetic interference with medical devices has resulted in death or serious injury in the past. Examples of interference include a flat line display when a paging company transmitted digital control information to remote sites and a case when a pulse oximeter showed 100% saturation and a heart rate of 60 bpm when the patient was in fact dead [2]. Factors implicated in electromagnetic interference include power level, distance between the source and the device, coupling of wireless devices, the frequency used and modulation imposed on the fields by the sources [3]. Sources of electromagnetic interference in hospitals include mains-powered electrical equipment, magnetic card readers, surgical diathermy, continuous shortwave physiotherapy diathermy, radio pagers, paramedic and other radios, mobile phones, microwave equipment and automatic doors. Of all the sources, mains electricity is most likely to cause problems [4]. Inadequate transformers that

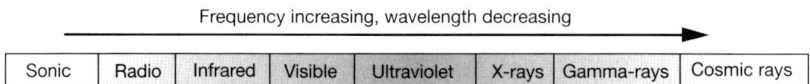

Frequency increasing, wavelength decreasing

| Sonic | Radio | Infrared | Visible | Ultraviolet | X-rays | Gamma-rays | Cosmic rays |

Fig. 10.1 The electromagnetic spectrum.

form part of the equipment and inappropriate location of electrophysiological measurement rooms near medium voltage cables are the most common sources of problems.

Electromagnetic interference can occur from mobile phones |5|. Such interference is more likely when the phones operate at a lower frequency (900 MHz) than when they operate at a higher frequency (1800 MHz). The frequency used by mobile phones varies from country to country and multiband phones use both high and low frequencies. It is has been recommended that a distance of 2 m be observed |6| when in proximity to life support medical devices, until mobile phones using low frequency are gradually phased out |7|. In reality only a small minority of electrical medical equipment is affected by mobile phones even over short distances, with external transcutaneous pacemakers being one important high-risk exception.

Radio LANs such as WiFi and Bluetooth vary in their ability to cause significant electromagnetic interference and have been extensively studied |7–9|. Evidence supports the precautionary view that a 1-m separation should be observed between mobile devices such as laptops and personal digital assistants (PDAs) and critical medical equipment as that used in intensive care or high dependency units.

Apart from interference with equipment, electromagnetic radiation from electronic devices may also harm the human body. Those at risk include healthcare personnel and patients. Consideration needs to be given to such radiation exposure. The main factors include the frequency of the signal and the power output of the transmitter. There is no evidence from laboratory or epidemiology studies that exposure to radio frequencies at levels below the recommended limits |10| has any health significance for humans.

Communication devices in the operating room

Ruskin KJ. *Curr Opin Anaesthesiol* 2006; **19**: 655–9

BACKGROUND. Communication between healthcare personnel working in a theatre environment is a vital part of any healthcare delivery system. Efficient communication in an emergency situation can be critical – not only communication between members of staff but also the ability to access medical records, laboratory results, X-ray reports, etc. Modern technology can facilitate this simply and cost-effectively and help improve quality of patient care and enhance patient safety.

INTERPRETATION. This review outlines the traditional and newer methods of communication that are available or are becoming available in modern hospitals. These include radio pagers, personal digital assistants (PDAs) or small hand-held devices, laptop, notebook and tablet computers, mobile telephones (cell phones) and the use of voice over Internet protocol (VOIP). Use of such technology to communicate efficiently can improve the quality of patient care and improve patient safety.

Comment

This review embraces modern technology and argues that efficient communication can increase patient safety |11|. It offers useful background on new and evolving technologies that are likely to alter how data used in patient care are transferred but may also present new challenges relating to electromagnetic safety, patient confidentiality and security. Communication may entail voice communication, transfer of digital laboratory data or graphical trends or images such as electrocardiogram (ECG) recordings, X-rays, magnetic resonance imaging (MRI) scans and, lately, transmission of video images or video clips.

In hospitals, pagers are the most established and commonest mode of communication |12|. They are inexpensive but limited in their use. However, they offer the best method for simultaneously sending alerts to multiple recipients, which accounts for their long track record. Alpha-numeric pagers are an improvement on traditional pagers because they also allow brief text to be transmitted. Some systems can be set up to receive abnormal (or normal) laboratory results automatically |13|.

Mobile telephones can be used for voice communication, text messaging and transmission of images. They are convenient and cheap but rely on national networks to function efficiently. They use global system for mobile communications (GSM) technology and can work anywhere in the world. However, occasionally their efficiency is compromised inside large buildings because of electromagnetic interference and poor signal reception.

Wireless ethernet (WiFi) technology uses radio frequency energy and requires a local network to function. It has the advantage that it can handle multiple data streams at once. It can be used by a host of peripheral devices such as PDAs, laptops, notebooks and other computers. VOIP is the latest technology that enables communication using local or extended networks. It routes the signal via the Internet and is an alternative to ordinary telephones. Appropriate Internet connections are required at either end. One specialized version, Vocera (Vocera Communications Inc., Cupertino, CA, USA), uses a small badge that can be worn around the neck or clipped to the pocket. Calls can be routed to the public telephone network using a dedicated server and interface |14|.

Congestion within the operating room

Increasing use of technological devices within the operating room leads to increased congestion and can be a source of distraction for people working in the operating room environment. Newer modes of displaying data need to address the requirements of everyone working in the operating suite. No single method can cater for everyone's needs. A combination of display systems may offer the best compromise. The operating room of the future needs to be a tidier place with unobtrusive yet efficient display systems that do not distract from the prime objective of maintaining attention firmly focused on the patient.

Technologies and solutions for data display in the operating room

Bitterman N. *J Clin Monitoring Comput* 2006; **20**: 165–73

BACKGROUND. The operating room is a busy environment that, with ever-increasing items of equipment, can easily become crowded. Added to this, the various platforms that are in use to display information make matters worse. This review examines the display platforms available for use in operating rooms and emerging technologies that may be used in the operating rooms of the future.

INTERPRETATION. No simple display configuration provides an ultimate solution for presenting data in the operating room. It is suggested that a multisensory data display including visual, acoustic and haptic (i.e. using the sense of touch – tactile) manipulation may provide a promising configuration for data display in the operating room. Consideration needs to be given to the operating rooms of the future.

Comment

Increasing numbers of display units in operating rooms lead to increased distraction. This is not conducive to good medical practice, in which observation of patient variables during an operation is critical. As technology increases, this problem may worsen. Applications that increasingly crowd the operating rooms leading to increased congestion are divided into four main groups:

1 surgical machine-controlled applications (robotics, minimally invasive surgery, video endoscopy, master–slave systems) |**15,16**|;

2 designated diagnostic and real-time devices (MRI, computer tomography, 3-D ultrasound) |**15,17**|;

3 information technology applications (electronic patient records [EPRs], picture archiving and communication systems [PACSs], hospital information systems [HISs], laboratory data, etc.) |**17**|; and

4 telecommunication and conferencing systems connecting the operating room to people outside the operating room in real time |**17–19**|.

Computer monitors display multiple outputs in a combination of digital and graphical images. The data displayed are a combination of absolute and relative data |**20**|.

Integrated displays present several outputs simultaneously including graphical displays that indicate deviation from the baseline condition. When used for anaesthesia monitoring they can show multiple physiological variables and deviations from norm can be detected at a glance. Sophisticated versions of integrated displays have been shown to shorten the time taken for anaesthesia personnel to detect deviation |**21,22**|.

Suspended image displays are new, and project the image onto a flat surface, wherever deemed necessary. This could be adjacent to the operating table, for example for the surgeon, or on a partition, for the anaesthetist, or even on the wall for the benefit of everyone present |23,24|. There are several advantages over traditional displays. They improve the level of sterility, reduce clutter and multiple images of the display can be shown simultaneously if necessary. However, they are not without their limitations, which include the need for flat surfaces on which to project and problems due to ambient light in the operating room |23|. Projection of 3-D holographic images is the next logical step, eliminating the need for flat surfaces with the images floating in space |25|. However, ambient operating room lighting remains a problem.

Wearable computers are defined as fully functional, self-contained computers that can be carried and accessed anywhere and at any time while leaving the hands free |26|. Head-up displays or helmet-monitored displays are examples used in aviation |27|, but their use in clinical situations is still unproven. Integration of wearable computers as part of clothing (computerized clothing, smart operating room costume) |28| or units attached to the users body (e.g. to wrists, hands, fingers) offer other possibilities |29|. Although developing fast, the technology is still not adequate to be of any practical value in operating rooms. At present, these units are clumsy, demanding of time, with limited capability and poor display quality. They remain expensive |29,30|.

Auditory data displays are used to sound alarms when measured values deviate from the norm. They are also used to monitor individual variables continuously, for example during pulse oximetry |31|. Other physiological haemodynamic parameters can also be conveyed by tone, pitch, location and volume. Continuous acoustic display is known as *sonification*. Often it is the change in acoustics that is readily perceived by the observer instead of an absolute or individual reading level |32|.

Haptic or tactile displays are perceived on the skin as force, texture, electrical stimulation, vibration or thermal sensation. These were originally developed for people with visual or auditory disability but are being developed in the field of minimally invasive surgery, simulators and the fast developing area of virtual reality |15,16|.

Multimodal/multisensory displays include visual, acoustic and haptic manipulation |24|. A combination of several modalities helps offset limitations associated with individual modalities.

The authors conclude that the choice of appropriate data platforms depends upon the specific surgical team and the operating room characteristics and should not be determined by passing trends or innovations in technology without thorough and objective testing in a simulated operating room comprising as exact a working environment as possible.

Teleanaesthesia, telemonitoring and telemedicine

Traditionally, the use of satellite communication has been prohibitively expensive for clinicians to consider its use in everyday anaesthesia. Advancements in technological devices such as digital cameras and mobile computers, combined with affordable communication systems such as the Internet (the infrastructure of millions of networked computers) and the World Wide Web (the information, data and resources made available on the Internet) make such goals achievable. Indeed, all are likely to play an increasing role in global care of patients in the future, especially for patients in remote locations. Advances in this field are a prerequisite to virtual reality and robotic surgery that is yet to become commonplace.

Remote anaesthetic monitoring using satellite telecommunication and the Internet

Cone SW, Gehr L, Hummel R, *et al*. *Anesth Analg* 2006; **102**: 1463–7

BACKGROUND. Use of telemedicine is not new in other specialties |33–35|. Telemedicine has also been used to monitor vital signs between two geographically isolated places in the past |36|. Technologies used have included various video conferencing techniques |37,38|. Collaboration between two sites and monitoring of vital signs could lead to improved patient safety and quality of care. The purpose of this study was to evaluate the feasibility of the use of telemedicine to prepare an anaesthetic plan, administer anaesthesia and monitor patients during surgery between two geographically separated locations, in real time. The remote site (manned by trained anaesthesia physicians, for the purpose of this study) was in Ecuador ,with the other site being in Richmond, VA, in the USA. Data transmitted from Ecuador and monitored in the USA included preoperative patient evaluations, real-time live video of tracheal intubation and confirmation of tube position, electrocardiograph waveforms, pulse oximetry measurements, arterial blood pressure readings, capnography readings and auscultation breath sounds. The concept of telementoring is introduced where an expert in one location shares information and guides a colleague in a remote location. The importance of this type of collaboration lies not only in enhancing medical care internationally (e.g. in the developing world), but also in improving quality of care in remote inaccessible locations around the earth (e.g. in mountaineering, terrestrial exploration and beyond, as in space travel).

INTERPRETATION. Transmission of a host of physiological data along with simultaneous voice and video transmission, with minimal lag time, is possible with modern satellite and related technology. Teleanaesthesia, defined as telementoring and telemonitoring of preoperative planning, postoperative care and real-time vital signs monitoring during anaesthesia for surgical procedures has the potential to enhance patient safety.

Comment

Seven operations (five under general anaesthesia and two under spinal anaesthesia, involving cholecystectomies, herniorrhaphies and lipoma resection) were successfully operated upon in Equador with mentoring, guidance and real-time monitoring in the USA.

The technology used in this project consisted of equipment for collecting data, equipment for transmitting it over a long distance and equipment for receiving and assimilating data at the receiving end. Patient monitoring and data transmission were conducted by using a rapidly deployable telemedicine unit (RDTU) operated by a technician. A QRS Diagnostics (Plymouth, MN, USA) ECG monitoring system was used for collecting a 12-lead ECG via a serial port of an IBM compatible laptop computer. Oxygen saturation was monitored via a QRS Medical SpirOxCard, which plugs into a laptop computer and emulates a pulse oximeter. Heart and breath sounds were evaluated via a Cardionics Inc. (Webster, TX, USA) electronic stethoscope model 718-7120. Automated non-invasive blood pressure readings were obtained by plugging an ordinary BP cuff into the RDTU and a RS232 interface. End tidal carbon dioxide readings were made using a Datex-Ohmeda (Louiseville, CO, USA) hand-held $EtCO_2$ monitor connected via a serial output to the RDTU. The transmitted signal was digital and reconstituted as a waveform at the other end. Streaming video was obtained by a fixed video-conferencing camera or a hand-held camcorder and transmitted using Microsoft's Net Meeting software, which also supported Chatbox text messaging. The video stream could be changed from camcorder or other camera to the fibreoptic laryngoscope intubation system.

Transmission of the streaming audio/text, video and real-time vital signs was done via InMarSat B satellite phone, providing a 64 kb/s data rate to an Internet service provider in the United States. The physiological data was encrypted and decrypted, archived and made available at the other end by a secure password-protected Internet connection.

The use of such a system in real-time management of anaesthesia is unique and has considerable potential to enhance patient safety and quality of anaesthetic care delivered in various testing locations.

Electronic anaesthetic records and user compliance

No matter how good an electronic record-keeping system might be, user compliance plays a vital part in its success. Motivating individuals to actually use a system, irrespective of cost, time and effort put into establishing it, can be a challenge. Requirement for data input may be mandatory or voluntary. It may be automated or require commitment from the user. In any voluntary system a fine balance is required between effort and reward. If it is too complicated, difficult or onerous it is likely to fail. Systems that are easy to use and reward users, for example by feedback, are more likely to succeed.

Changing medical group behaviours: increasing the rate of documentation of quality assurance events using an anaesthesia information system

Vigoda MM, Gencorelli F, Lubarsky DA. *Anesth Analg* 2006; **103**: 390–5

BACKGROUND. Quality assurance variable recording into electronic medical records can be voluntary or mandatory. In electronic systems it can be self-reported or automated. Accurate anaesthesia documentation is accepted as the norm in modern anaesthesia practice. However, documentation of quality assurance events (e.g. hypotension, arrhythmias) during the course of an anaesthetic can vary and depends on user compliance. This is equally true if an electronic anaesthetic record system is used. This study looked at implementing a series of interventions to change the behaviour of those administering anaesthesia, with consequent increase in incidence of documenting quality assurance events in anaesthetic electronic medical records.

INTERPRETATION. Education, feedback and continual monitoring improved the quality and rate of documentation of quality assurance events amongst anaesthesia personnel in this large anaesthesia department. With a positive approach that includes regular feedback, encouragement and better communication, the improvement was sustained.

Comment

In the authors' institution an anaesthesia record-keeping system (Pics, Wakefield, MA, USA) is used routinely in all operating rooms. The electronic system automatically records vital signs and allows the anaesthesia personnel to document events, medications and quality assurance entries. The electronic quality assurance form in use is based on a previously used paper version and is available throughout the time anaesthesia care is being provided. The quality assurance data are divided into several headings – for example cardiac, respiratory, etc. – and there is a facility by which events that are not included in the predefined headings can be entered.

This project consisted of several distinct stages. During stage 1 (2 months) data was recorded prior to any interventions to establish a baseline level. During stage 2 (1 month) an intensive effort was made to inform all anaesthesia personnel that there was a policy in place that required documenting of quality assurance variables in the anaesthesia records. During stage 3 (1 month) the workflow pattern was changed in that when the users re-accessed the electronic patient record in the post-anaesthetic care unit or intensive care unit (ICU) where the anaesthetic chart would be closed and printed off, the first window with which they were confronted was the quality assurance form. Here, the quality assurance variables could be entered if not done so already or the 'no complications' option could be selected. Although this form was accessible throughout the anaesthetic in the operating rooms, the 'no complication' option was disabled and only made available in the post-anaesthetic care unit or ICU prior to printing of the record. Stage 4 (one-off) consisted of individualized feedback. A report summarizing the previous month's cases along with their quality assurance completion rates was communicated to each individual. Finally, during stage 5 (3 months) individual feedback along with departmental statistics was continued to be provided to individuals via emails.

The above measures resulted in progressive and sustained improvement in quality assurance data reporting, which was sustained after the completion of the study.

Although major events (e.g. death) are reported well, lesser events are usually less well reported |**39,40**|. Paper-based reporting systems are prone to poor response rate, observer bias and variable threshold at which individuals complete the forms |**41**|. Voluntary reporting underestimates the incidence of adverse incidents that occur |**39**|. This study motivated individuals to increase their incidence of reporting quality assurance events. Factors that enabled this to happen included education, improved workflow pattern and targeted individual feedback. To ensure that the improvement in reporting is sustained it was necessary to repeat the above processes at regular intervals.

Electronic anaesthesia record

Real-time data capture of physiological data gives the most accurate evaluation of patient status during anaesthesia. This, along with user input of events during an anaesthetic, completes the anaesthesia record. Use of such electronic anaesthesia records is routine in many hospitals. Although these systems are usually very reliable, they may occasionally fail and cause untoward consequences. Software for such systems needs to be robust and reliable. Failsafe warnings are critical in recognizing failures in communications between devices, be they from human error or device malfunction.

Failure to recognize loss of incoming data in an anaesthesia record-keeping system may have increased medical liability

Vigoda MM, Lubarsky DA. *Anesth Analg* 2006; **102**: 1798–802

BACKGROUND. There is a perception that automated anaesthesia record-keeping systems may limit medical liability because they sample data continuously and give a true picture of what is happening at any given time |42|. This may very well be true but over reliance on such displays can lead to a false sense of security and consequent human error. In this paper the authors describe an unfortunate incident with an untoward outcome following failure of anaesthesia personnel to appreciate the true nature of the data displayed on the screen. Further, failure to document vital signs when the error was realized made a robust defence untenable.

INTERPRETATION. Automated anaesthesia record-keeping systems are useful but increasing number and complexity of data measured or derived from the sampled physiological variables can lead to a cluttered screen on which vital information may be hidden behind superimposing windows. Clinical vigilance is necessary at all times if critical data are not to be missed.

Comment

This is a case report of an untoward outcome where poor documentation of the anaesthesia record was deemed to be indefensible. The automated anaesthetic record-keeping system in use in this institution measured several vital signs during anaesthesia. In addition, the system allowed for input of data by the anesthesiologist throughout anaesthesia as required. During a 7-h craniotomy in a patient with a brain tumour, undertaken in the sitting posture, 93 min of physiological data were not captured by the automated anaesthetic record-keeping system. When the absence of this real-time incoming data was eventually noticed, manoeuvres were initiated to correct this. Following a slow recovery from anaesthesia, the patient was found to have become quadriplegic. The cause of the loss of data was probably a loose connection between the physiological monitor and the automated anaesthesia record-keeping system. Several factors made this case indefensible: namely the failure to recognize that the system was not receiving any data from the monitor for a prolonged period of time and the failure of staff to manually enter the missing data, which at the end of the case was still retained in the trend memory of the physiological monitor. This left the anaesthetic record essentially blank for over an hour and a half of the anaesthetic. Other factors were present, most of which were duly corrected. These included poor ergonomic siting of the monitors in the operating room, in that the monitors were placed behind the anaesthetist. These are now placed in a line of sight. An early alert system has also been incorporated so that a message on the screen alerts the user if there is a failure of communication between the physiological monitors and the automated anaesthesia record-keeping system.

Anaesthesia and information management systems

Electronic anaesthetic records are part of anaesthesia information management systems and have been around for many years. Although good at gathering information, which can later be used by clinicians and managers alike, their cost, reliability, ease of use and integration into the mainline hospital databases can vary. Transferring data gathered from different sources using differing devices running different operating systems and data structures can be difficult and requires considerable user and technological support.

Integration of a handheld based anaesthesia rounding system into an anaesthesia information management system

Fuchs C, Quinzio L, Benson M, *et al. Int J Med Inform* 2006; **75**: 553–63

BACKGROUND. Anaesthetic information management systems (AIMSs) are a fact of life in many hospitals, replacing traditional paper records, and can improve the quality of documentation |43,44|. The depth and breadth of information held in these systems, as well as the mode of data entry, vary. The system used at the University Hospital in Giessen, Germany, records perioperative anaesthesia care. The perioperative record is generated from data gathered from a combination of systems. These include online data gathered from the hospital information system containing patient demographics, the laboratory system, anaesthetic data from previous anaesthetic episodes, and data gathered from the current episode via direct monitor interfaces combined with anesthesiologist input during the anaesthetic. Although preoperative assessment information is collected, it is not integrated and has been traditionally recorded on paper and then transferred into the system. This paper describes how this element of the data-gathering process may be integrated into the electronic patient record by using portable personal digital assistants (PDAs). Data are collected on PDAs and then hot-synchronized into the main record database, which is held on an Oracle 7 database (Oracle 7, Oracle Corp., Redwood Stores, CA, USA).

INTERPRETATION. It is possible to use portable electronic devices, such as PDAs, to gather patient information remote from the main computer terminals and later upload the information into the main database to complete the perioperative record of the anaesthesia episode. However, a two-way communication is necessary if this is to be done efficiently without duplication of data capture.

Comment

The AIMS (NarkoData, IMESO GmbH, Huettenburg, Germany) records relevant aspects of anaesthetic care from patient admission to discharge from the recovery unit. Relevant data are imported from the hospital information system. Data from ventilators and vital signs monitoring are gathered automatically at regular intervals. Further data from quality assurance projects previously undertaken at this institution are optionally imported if thought to be relevant to the patient. These data subsets are steered by strict logical algorithms and alert the anaesthesiologists to risk factors relevant to specific diagnoses. This enhanced data set is imported into the main database once the patient is discharged and the anaesthesia record closed.

Preoperative assessment information was previously routinely recorded on paper and then manually transferred into the main database via one of the desktop computers. This method of data entry is known to be prone to errors originating from several sources, including errors of omission, errors of accuracy and errors of transcription. The system developed uses a Palm (Palm Inc., Milpitas, CA, USA) hand-held PDA as the data input device and automatically uploads the information to the main database. The reason for choosing these models was that they are in common use, easy to use, versatile and relatively inexpensive. Marrying the PalmOS-based data set on the PDA with the data fields held on the main Oracle 7 database required the development of a 'C' program (a programming language: C programs are written in 'C'), in which the relevant fields in the Oracle 7 database were imbedded into the Palm data set. Data are entered into the Palm using drop-down menus and a stylus. Uploading data to the main database is carried out by using a standard docking station connected to a desktop computer via a serial interface. Data integration has several elements to it. The software on the desktop computer coordinates data from several different sources, including anaesthesia records, electronic patient files from the ICU, laboratory, microbiology and patient administration systems as well as the data set on the Palm. The integration and transfer of data is controlled by Java desktop software: requiring not just a simple one-sided communication but a two-way movement of data between the desktop computer and the Palm.

Patients scheduled for surgery are identified on the desktop system and tagged. The relevant part of the information on these patients held on the various sources that can be incorporated onto the subset data set contained on the PDA is transferred onto the PDA. The user is then able to take the PDA to the patient's bedside to fill in the pre-anaesthetic assessment information. After this has been done the PDA is connected to the desktop system again, where the updated fields are uploaded to the main database. This information then becomes readily available in various locations, for example the operating rooms, and is accessed during the anaesthetic episode by the personnel administering the anaesthetic. As a security measure, once synchronization has occurred and the data have been uploaded from the PDA to the main database, the data on the PDA are automatically deleted.

The choice of PDAs rested between the devices that use the two rival operating systems prevalent at the moment, Palm OS and Pocket Windows (previously Windows CE). Palm was chosen by the authors because these units are lighter and contained all the system features that were needed. Inevitably, with advances in technology more options will be required and become available.

PDAs have primarily been used as standalone devices, for example for referencing databases, keeping personal records or for performing calculations, thus underutilising their potential. They have been used in this study as a device that can efficiently and reliably capture data at the bedside and integrate it into an AIMS.

The hospital intranet

The hospital intranet is a facility that can be used to make educational and other resources readily available electronically. It has a reliable infrastructure which can usually be accessed from anywhere in the hospital and can be used by groups of healthcare workers to promote education and improve quality of patient care, for example by making available clinical protocols and policies. Due consideration needs to be given to ensure that the resources put on the intranet are relevant, appropriate and up to date. They should be easy to access, be identified quickly and presented to the user in a simple and user-friendly manner.

Anaesthetic care of the trauma patient: development of a web-based resource

Anderson NK, Jones AD, Martin EE, *et al*. *AANA J* 2007; **75**: 49–56

BACKGROUND. Early mortality (death within 3 h of the trauma event) represents 35% of all trauma deaths and is usually attributable to preventable causes, such as bleeding and hypoxia secondary to airway obstruction |45|. The objective of this project was to develop a web-based resource on the hospital intranet to help anaesthesia providers improve the quality of clinical care given to trauma patients by providing a mechanism of accessing relevant information in a timely and efficient manner.

INTERPRETATION. Extensively researched information to aid management of trauma patients was put on the hospital intranet. Developing such a resource is more complicated than is generally appreciated and has to be done systematically, with due attention being paid to each element.

Comment

The authors divided setting up the intranet website into several distinct parts along the lines described by Campbell |46|. Research to gather all the information to be put on the system was initially carried out. Existing resources (for example, policies and protocols already on the intranet) were used and new material was developed using expert authors. Assessments of learning needs were performed. The learning needs of those with a broad pre-existing knowledge base are different from the learning needs of those who do not have such knowledge. In adults learning is enhanced when information is relevant and likely to be put to immediate use, for example with the imminent arrival of a trauma patient |47|. Use of the hospital intranet was chosen because of its ready availability and because it already contained a considerable amount of material. Content included pictures, embedded Powerpoint presentations, and text in outline and paragraph format. Page layout recognized people's different learning techniques |48| and made extensive use of cross-referencing and hyperlinks enabling users to access relevant information efficiently and quickly.

During development the website was trialled by individuals unrelated to the department and their feedback, along with internal feedback, led to several revisions. In this way, the website evolved even after its introduction. The authors concluded that the website is a useful resource and an invaluable educational tool and thus improves the quality of care offered to trauma patients admitted into their institution.

Patient monitoring in intensive care

Constant monitoring of the patient's state is crucial in intensive care. The high nurse–patient ratio is a significant contributory factor. Periodic observations by nurses helps identify problems and ensure that timely action is taken when necessary. Continuous electronic computerized monitoring of physiological variables may be superior to periodic observations by nurses and may help improve the quality of care offered to these seriously ill patients.

Intracranial pressure monitoring in intensive care: clinical advantages of a computerized system over manual recording

Zanier ER, Ortolano F, Ghisoni L, *et al*. *Crit Care (Lond)* 2007; **11**(1): R7

BACKGROUND. Raised intracranial pressure in patients with traumatic brain injury can have an adverse outcome |49,50|. Accurate and continual monitoring of intracranial pressure using various intracranial pressure sensors has been extensively studied |51,52,53,54|. The objective of this study in patients with severe traumatic brain injury was to determine whether hourly recording of intracranial pressure by nursing staff correlated with continuous electronic monitoring of intracranial pressure.

INTERPRETATION. Manually recorded end-hour intracranial pressure correlated well with end-hour and mean-hour values of intracranial pressure recorded automatically using a computerized monitoring system. However, manual recording missed a number of episodes of high intracranial pressure, some of which were of long duration, which might compromise optimal management of these patients.

Comment

Records of 293 patients admitted over a 5-year period were examined. Sixty-two records fulfilled the inclusion criteria, and from these 30 records were randomly examined in detail. The inclusion criteria included age > 14 years, severe traumatic brain injury (Glasgow coma scale < 8), intracranial or cerebral perfusion pressure monitoring for at least 2 days, and intracranial pressure higher than 20 mmHg for at least 25% of the time. Manual measurements were made by nurses at the end of every hour while the computer recorded measurements 10 times per minute. The end-hour manual recordings correlated well with the computer recordings. A total of 351 episodes of raised intracranial pressure of greater than 20 mmHg lasting at least 5 min were identified during continuous recordings but only 204 episodes were recorded by the manual method: missing 42% of these episodes.

The technology used to monitor and record the intracranial pressure was a Macintosh computer (Apple Computers, Inc., Cupertino, CA, USA) through an analogue to digital converter (MacLab; ADInstruments Pty Ltd, Castle Hill, Australia).

Monitoring intracranial pressure using a continuous computerized monitoring system may benefit clinical management of these patients by identifying potentially harmful episodes of raised intracranial pressure that may otherwise be missed when using manual recording methods.

References

1. Hagihira S, Takashina M, Mori T, Taenaka N, Mashino T, Yoshiya I. Infrared transmission of electronic information via LAN in operating room. *J Clin Monit Comput* 2000; **16**: 171–5.

2. White DR. *EMC, Wireless, Computer and Electronics Desk Reference Encyclopedia.* EMF-EMI Control Inc. (EEC), 1998.

3. IEEE Committee on Man and Radiation (COMAR) Technical Information Statement: Radiofrequency interference with medical devices. *IEEE Eng Med Biol Mag* 1998; **17**: 111–14.

4. Grant L. Surveying a hospital for electromagnetic interference. In: *Practical Methods of Mitigation of EMI and EMF Hazards within Hospitals.* York: Institute of Physics and Engineering in Medicine; 2003, pp. 10–11.

5. Lawrentschuk N, Bolton DM. Mobile phone interference with medical equipment and its clinical relevance: a systematic review. *Med J Aust* 2004; **181**: 145–9.

6. NSW Biomedical Engineering Advisory Group (BEAG), Use of mobile telephones and other wireless communication devices – interference with electronic medical equipment , Guidance document prepared for NSW Health Circular 2003/65. (Issued on 18 September 2003). Available at: http://www.bme.asn.au/doc/guidance/Mobile_Phone_Interference_Guidance_Document.pdf (accessed August 2007).

7. Hanada E, Hoshino Y, Oyama H, Watanabe Y, Nose Y. Negligible electromagnetic interaction between medical electronic equipment and 2.4 GHz band wireless LAN. *J Med Syst* 2002; **26**: 301–8.

8. Hanada E, Hoshino Y. Kudou T. Safe introduction of in-hospital wireless LAN. In: Fieschi M, Coiera E, Li Y-Cj, eds. *Proc 11th World Congress Med Informatics, MEDINFO 2004, San Francisco;* 2004, pp.1426–9.

9. Tan KS. Effects of a wireless local area network (LAN) system, a telemetry system, and electrosurgical devices on medical devices in a hospital environment. *Bimed Instrum Technol* 2000; **34**: 115–18.

10. IEEE Committee on Man and Radiation (COMAR) Technical Information Statement: Human exposure to radio frequency and microwave radiation from portable and mobile telephones and other wireless communication devices. September 2000. Available at: www.ewh.ieee.org/soc/embs/comar/phone.htm (accessed August 2007).

11. Soto RG, Chu LF, Goldman JM, Rampil IJ, Ruskin KJ. Communication in critical care environments: mobile telephones improve patient care. *Anesth Analg* 2006; **102**: 535–41.

12. Heslop L, Howard A, Fernando J, Rothfield A, Wallace L. Wireless communications in acute health-care. *J Telemed Telecare* 2003; **9**: 187–93.

13. Poon EG, Kuperman GJ, Fiskio J, Bates DW. Real-time notification of laboratory data requested by users through alphanumeric pagers. *J Am Med Inform Assoc* 2002; **9**: 217–22.

14. Jacques PS, France DJ, Pilla J, Lai E, Higgins MS. Evaluation of a hands-free wireless communication device in the perioperative environment. *Telemed J E Health* 2006; **12**: 42–9.

15. Rattner DW, Park A. Advanced devices for the operating room. *Sem Laparosc Surg* 2003; **10**: 85–9.

16. Satava RM. Future trends in the design and application of surgical robots. *Sem Laparosc Surg* 2004; **11**: 129–35.

17. Feussner H. The operating room of the future: a view from Europe. *Sem Laparosc Surg* 2003; **10**: 149–56.

18. Merrell RC, Jarrell BE, Schenkman NS, Schoener B, McCullough K. Telemedicine for the operating room of the future. *Sem Laparosc Surg* 2003; **10**: 91–4.

19. Doarn CR, Telemedicine in tomorrow's operating room: A natural fit. *Sem Laparosc Surg* 2003; **10**: 121–6.

20. Cook RI, Woods DD. Implications of automation surprises in aviation for the future of total intravenous anesthesia (TIVA). *J Clin Anesthesia* 1996; **8**: 29S–37S.

21. Westhorpe RN. Ergonomics and monitoring. *Anesth & Intensive Care* 1988; **16**: 71–5.

22. Gurushanthaiah K, Weinger MB, England CE. Visual display format affects the ability of anaesthesiologist to detect acute physiologic changes. *Anesthesiology* 1995; **83**: 1184–93.

23. Brown SI, Frank TG, Cuschieri A, Sharpe R, Cartwright C. Optimization of the projection screen in a display system for minimal access surgery. *Surg Endosc* 2003; **17**: 1251–55.

24. Seales WB, Caban J. Visualization trends: applications in the operating room. *Sem Laparosc Surg* 2003; **10**: 107–14.

25. The Laser Cube. Available at: http://www.laser-magic.com/lasercube.html (accessed August 2007).

26. Barfield W, Caudell T. *Fundamentals of Wearable Computers and Augmented Reality.* London: Lawrence Erlbaum Associates; 2001.

27. Wickens CD, Hollands JC. Attention in perception and display space. In: Wickens CD, Hollans JG, eds. *Engineering Psychology and Human Performance.* New Jersey: Prentice Hall; 2000, pp. 69–118.

28. Wilhelm FH, Handke EA, Roth WT. Measurement of respiratory and cardiac function by LifeShirt™: initial assessment of usability and reliability during ambulatory sleep monitoring. *Biol Psychol* 2002; **59**: 250–1.

29. Block FE, Yablok DO, McDonald JS. Clinical evaluation of the 'head-up' display of anesthesia data. *Int J Clin Monit Comput* 1995; **12**: 21–3.

30. Van Koesveld JJM, Tetteroo GWM, de Graaf EJR. Use of head mounted display in transanal endoscopic microsurgery. *Surg Endosc* 2003; **17**: 943–6.

31. Craven RM, McIndoe AK. Continuous auditory monitoring – how much information do we register? *Brit J Anaesth* 1999; **83**: 747–9.

32. Loeb RG, Fitch WT. A laboratory evaluation of an auditory display designed to enhance intraoperative monitoring. *Anesth Analg* 2002; **94**: 362–8.

33. Broderick TJ, Harnett BM, Doarn CR, *et al.* Real-time Internet connections: implications for surgical decision making in laparoscopy. *Ann Surg* 2001; **234**: 165–71.

34. Cone SW, Gehr L, Hummel R, *et al.* Case report of remote anesthetic monitoring using telemedicine. *Anesth Analg* 2004; **98**: 386–8.

35. Russell KM, Broderick TJ, Demaria EJ, *et al.* Laparoscopic telescope with alpha port and aesop to view open surgical procedures. *J Laproendosc Adv Surg Tech A* 2001; **11**: 213–18.

36. Harnett BM, Satava R, Angood P, *et al.* The benefits of integrating Internet technology with standard communications for telemedicine in extreme environments. *Avit Space Environ Med* 2001; **72**: 1132–7.

37. Ballantyne GH. Robotic surgery, telerobotic surgery, telepresence, and telementoring. Review of early clinical results. *Surg Endosc* 2002; **16**: 1389–402.

38. Orlav OI, Drozdov DV, Doarn CR, Merrell RC. Wireless ECG monitoring by telephone. *Telemed J E Health* 2001; **7**: 33–8.

39. Sanborn KV, Castro J, Kuroda M, Thys DM. Detection of intraoperative incidents by electronic scanning of computerized anesthesia records: comparison with voluntary reporting. *Anesthesiology* 1996; **85**: 977–87.

40. Benson M, Junger A, Fuchs C, *et al.* Using an anesthesia information management system to prove a deficit in voluntary reporting of adverse events in a quality assurance program. *J Clin Monit Comput* 2000; **16**: 211–17.

41. Katz RI, Lagasse RS. Factors influencing the reporting of adverse perioperative outcomes to a quality management program. *Anesth Analg* 2000; **90**: 344–50.

42. Feldman J. Do anesthesia information systems increase malpractice exposure: results of a survey. *Anesth Analg* 2004; **99**: 840–3.

43. Abenstein JP, DeVos CB, Tarhan A, Tarhan S. Eight years' experience with automated record keeping: lessons learned-new directions taken. *Int J Clin Monit Comput* 1992; **9**: 117–29.

44. Edsall DW, Deshane P, Giles C, Dick D, Sloan B, Farrow J. Computerized patient anesthesia records: less time and better quality than manually produced anesthesia records. *J Clin Anesth* 1993; **5**: 275–83.

45. Trunkey DD, Blaisdell FW. Epidemiology of trauma. *Sci Am* 1988; **4**: 1–10.

46. Campbell KN. Helping adults begin the process of learning. *AAOHN J* 1999; **47**: 31–40.

47. Lewis DJ, Saydak SJ, Mierzwa IP, Robinson JA. Gaming: a teaching strategy for adult learners. *J Cont Educ Nurs* 1989; **20**: 80–4.

48. Fidisun D. Andragogy and technology; integrating adult learning theory as we teach with technology. Available at: http://www.mtsu.edu/~itconf/proceed00/fidishun.htm (accessed August 2007).

49. Marmarou A, Anderson RL, Ward J, Choi DW. Impact of ICP instability and hypotension on outcome in patients with severe head trauma. *J Neurosurg* 1991; **75**: S59-S66.

50. Juul N, Morris GF, Marshall SB, Marshall LF. Intracranial hypertension and cerebral perfusion pressure: influence of neurological deterioration and outcome in severe head injury. The executive committee of the International Selfotel Trial. *J Neurosurg* 2000; **92**: 1–6.

51. McGraw CP. Continuous intracranial pressure monitoring: review of techniques and presentation of method. *Surg Neurol* 1976; **3**: 149–55.

52. Szewczykowski J, Korsak-Sliwka J, Kunicki A, Sliwka S, Dytko P. A computerized neurosurgical intensive care system. *Eur J Intensive Care Med* 1975; **1**: 189–92.

53. Tindall GT, Patton JM, Dunion JJ, O'Brien MS. Monitoring of patients with head injuries. *Clin Neurosurg* 1975; **22**: 332–63.

54. The Brain Trauma Foundation. The American Association of Neurological Surgeons. The Joint Section on Neurotrauma and Critical Care. Indications for intracranial monitoring. *J Neurotrauma* 2000; **17**: 479–491.

11

Simulation in anaesthesia and intensive care

RONNIE GLAVIN

Introduction

What does simulation have to offer the practising clinical anaesthetist? Many anaesthetists will have already encountered simulation as participants on simulation-based teaching courses. Some may have roles as teachers or members of faculty on such courses. The use of simulation-based teaching is likely to increase for the following reasons:

1   Simulators are becoming less expensive and so more affordable by individual anaesthetic departments.
2   The increasing adoption of anaesthetic curricula that focus on the educational outcomes of teaching (competency-based training courses) is expanding the content of the curricula. Theoretical knowledge and practical skills are no longer sufficient. Areas of the newer curricula include such domains as communication skills, decision-making and teamworking |1|.

Teaching is a long-established role of simulation, and in 2005 the Best Evidence Medical Education Collaborative |2| published the findings of the Topic Research Group on simulation |3|. This group addressed the question, 'What are the features and uses of high-fidelity medical simulations that lead to most effective learning?' This paper is playing a crucial role in laying down guidelines for educational studies involving simulators across the full range of fidelities.

Another effect of the educational outcomes-based approach is that it not only moves teaching into a wider sphere but it is also driving assessment into these areas. The role of simulation as an assessment tool is developing as educational supervisors and course administrators look for stronger evidence that learners can actually demonstrate satisfactory performance in the competencies under review. Whether in the context of formal summative examinations or as part of ongoing continuing professional development, more and more anaesthetists are likely to encounter simulation in this area. Simulated patients, part-task trainers in resuscitation skills and now medium-fidelity simulators in Objective Structured Clinical Examination (OSCE) components of exams reflect a prevailing trend.

Simulation is also taking on an increasing role as a research tool and is being used to explore aspects of anaesthetic practice with the aim of helping anaesthetists become safer and more effective when managing the different aspects of anaesthetic practice.

Simulation has much to offer anaesthetists and even if its influences are only indirectly felt by the majority of currently practising anaesthetists it seems likely that its role within anaesthesia is set to expand.

Medical simulation – some general perspectives

As medical education advances, so does medical simulation. The first set of articles begins with a historical view, which provides a platform for subsequent discussion. The next article considers a theoretical framework that helps those directly involved with simulation review current practice and consider how to advance their practice in this field. The third article reviews the current role of a national centre and evaluates some of the impact that the centre has had on medical education in that country.

A history of simulation in medical education and possible future directions

Bradley P. *Med Ed* 2006; **40**: 254–62

BACKGROUND. The author provides an overview of medical simulation by reviewing the background to simulation, the different modalities of simulation and their uses and some of the educational theory supporting the role of medical simulation-based training. The author concludes with a brief account of some future directions.

INTERPRETATION. After a prolonged gestation period, recent advances have made available affordable technologies that permit the reproduction of clinical events with sufficient fidelity to permit the engagement of learners in a realistic and meaningful way. At the same time, reforms in undergraduate and postgraduate education, combined with political and societal pressures, have promoted a safety-conscious culture where simulation provides a means of risk-free learning in complex, critical or rare situations. The importance of team-based and interprofessional approaches to learning and healthcare can be promoted.

Comments

Bradley lists the different types of simulator (Table 11.1), having given a brief account of the factors behind their development, which he describes in terms of the resuscitation movement, anaesthetic simulation and medical education reform.

Table 11.1 Classification of simulators

Part-task trainers
Computer-based systems
Virtual reality
  Precision placement and haptic system
  Simple manipulation
Complex manipulation
Simulated patients
Simulated environments
Integrated simulators
  Instructor-driven simulators
  Model-driven simulators

Source: Bradley (2006).

He then looks at the trends that are driving the increased use of simulation-based education in medicine today. These he describes in Fig. 11.1: societal expectation, political accountability and professional regulation.

A further review of the main features of each of the different types of simulator in Table 11.1 is followed by an account of the potential uses of simulation (Table 11.2), making reference to the educational theories underlying the use of simulation and exploring some future directions.

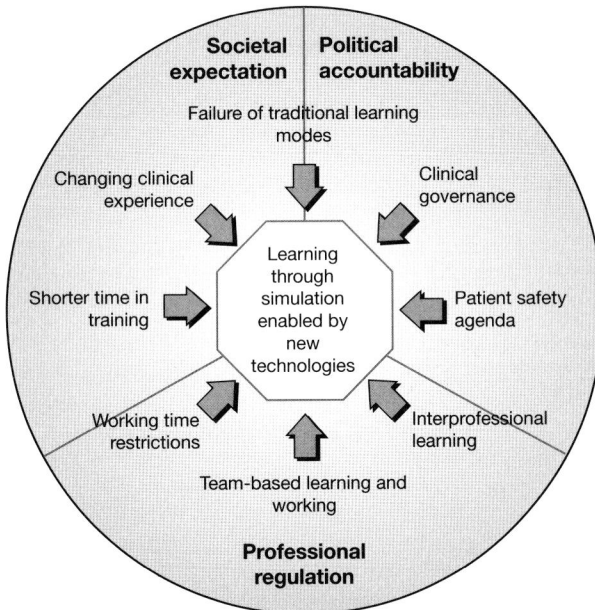

Fig. 11.1 Drives and background to learning through clinical stimulation. Source: Bradley (2006).

Table 11.2 Potential application of simulation

Routine learning and rehearsal of clinical and communication skills at all levels
Routine basic training of individuals and teams
Practice of complex clinical situations
Training of teams in crisis resource management
Rehearsal of planned, novel or infrequent interventions
Induction into new clinical environments and use of equipment
Design and testing of new clinical equipment
Performance assessment of staff at all levels
Refresher training of staff at all levels

Source: Bradley (2006).

Bradley has produced a neat, concise summary of where we are with simulation in medicine at the current time and how we have got there. Anyone who is becoming involved with simulation, especially delivery of simulator-based courses, but is not familiar with the literature on medical simulation would do well to begin with this article. Very few of the individual ideas will be new to anyone who reads a smattering of journal articles every year but Bradley has brought the relevant ideas together in an effective yet economic fashion and has provided a context for the expansion in medical simulation-based education.

Crossing the line: simulation and boundary areas

Kneebone R. *Simulation in Healthcare* 2006; **1**: 160–3

BACKGROUND. Changes in models of healthcare delivery are being driven by changing patterns of care. If simulation is to respond to these changes then it should recreate as closely as possible the conditions of actual practice. Simulation must parallel its real world counterpart in a functional sense. Simulation is less of a physical reality than a conceptual space within which many activities can occur. Many domains will intersect in relation to these various activities.

INTERPRETATION. Kneebone describes three levels of complexity. The most basic is a technical procedure, such as suturing a skin wound. The second level is the clinical context. The learner must take into account the patient's ideas, concerns and expectations. The third level takes into account the wider influences which bear on clinical practice – policy pressures, workforce design, etc. Recreating the levels of complexity requires that the course designer work with others whose realm of expertise comes into contact with the designer through some aspect of simulation – these are the boundaries referred to in the title of the article. Developing some understanding of these areas can in turn help the course designer reflect in a more meaningful way on how well the complexities of the course are matching the requirements for the learners.

Comment

Kneebone is exploring a theory of medical simulation. A theory of simulation would allow practitioners to formulate and test hypotheses and engage with a structured evidence base. In the article Kneebone explores how the demands of recreating the appropriate levels of complexity in simulation are encouraging those who have approached simulation from a clinical background to explore other areas that pertain to simulation. These areas or boundaries are where the clinicians come into contact with other disciplines that have something to offer. Examples of these areas include contributions from psychology, acting, mathematics, engineering, and so on. Kneebone is not saying that practitioners in simulation must gain expertise in all of these fields, but where we interact with practitioners in these fields who are also involved in simulation then we not only learn from them but modify our own understanding of medical simulation. This in turn offers a way to frame problems and so allow practitioners in medical simulation to explore solutions. In summary, if I think only in clinical terms I shall be much less effective at recreating the complexity I require than if I am able to see my problem in terms of features and concepts of these other disciplines.

The importance of this article is that it sets down a vision of what a theory of medical simulation may require to help the healthcare professions make the most effective educational use of this modality.

The Israel Centre for Medical Simulation: a paradigm for cultural change in medical education

Ziv A, Erez D, Munz Y, *et al*. *Acad Med* 2006; **81**: 1091–7

BACKGROUND. Ziv and colleagues describe the impact of simulation-based medical education on the Israeli medical community and explore the impact on patient safety of their 'error-driven' educational approach.

INTERPRETATION. The Medical Simulation Centre in Israel is centrally located, multidisciplinary and multimodality. This contrasts with other centres in the world, which are often confined to one location or one discipline. This has implications for both individual and team performance. The authors list the range of courses and the numbers of different healthcare professionals who have attended these courses. The authors also list some ways in which the national training centre has had an impact on training at a national level in Israel. For example, the development of the simulation-based anaesthesiology board exam brought about a critical appraisal of current training and assessment in anaesthesiology and helped to provide a focus on the key learning outcomes of anaesthesiology training. The education of pre-hospital military teams in trauma management also provided opportunities to learn the limitations of conventional advanced life support training, leading to a change in the training of these teams.

Comment

In this article Ziv and his colleagues have shown how a national centre that delivers a training programme to a substantial number of trainees can identify trends in the behaviour of the learners. If one observes a particular behaviour in only one participant in a simulation-based medical education course then there is a limit to how much one can infer from that. However, if the same behaviours are seen repeatedly then one can, with increasing confidence, begin to make inferences about the strengths and limitations of the training programme. During a single course the faculty at the centre can help learners reflect upon their own strengths and limitations but when all of the courses for a particular group, which consists of all of the learners in that specialty at a particular stage of training in the country, are reviewed then the effectiveness of the training programme is put under scrutiny. The authors refer to the way in which training programmes have been subsequently influenced by this information, especially in the field of multidisciplinary trauma teams. They do not report, however, on whether the impact of these changes in training has had an effect on the subsequent clinical performance of teams. In other words, they do not say whether the educational audit cycle has gone round a second loop or not. The authors argue that this is easier to carry out when the centre is operating at a national level and those with responsibility for the delivery of training have worked together during the development of courses, especially multidisciplinary/ multiprofessional team courses. This involvement with the simulation centre at an early stage has helped key figures in national training programmes become more sympathetic to information coming from the centre. The authors comment on this as a benefit from a national centre but one suspects that it may also arise because Israel is a small country and so it is easier for the different postgraduate medical training programme directors to meet, although their point about early involvement during the development of courses is an important one.

The authors also refer to the importance of the faculty acting as ambassadors for some of the key principles used in the simulation-based medical education when they return to work in their clinical institutions. In this way the medical culture of a country of the size and population of Israel can be influenced by a group of enthusiastic clinicians becoming local champions. Once more it is important to include such people during the development of the courses. The authors claim that the attitudes to medical error are changing from a culture of denial or blame to one of using medical errors as a source of improvement of clinical care.

This paper is important because it demonstrates how a simulation centre can influence not only individual learners but also the content of national training schemes and even the prevailing healthcare culture.

Simulation as a method of teaching

There are many questions that arise in connection with medical simulation as a teaching tool. The next group of papers explore the following themes: the realism of current simulation devices; integration of simulation-based teaching into a multinational teaching programme; the role of debriefing in medical simulation-based teaching; and, finally, the impact of medical simulation-based teaching on clinical outcomes.

Evaluation of four airway training manikins as simulators for inserting the LMA Classic™

Silsby J, Jordan G, Bayley G, et al. Anaesthesia 2006; **61**: 576–9

BACKGROUND. Instructors teaching mask ventilation and tracheal intubation have traditionally used airway manikins. Now that other airway procedures such as laryngeal mask airway (LMA) insertion are being taught, how well can the existing airway manikins facilitate this procedure?

INTERREPRETATION. Twenty volunteer anaesthetists inserted a size-4 LMA five times into each of four airway manikins in random order. Each insertion was assessed using objective and subjective tests. Overall assessment ranked the devices for insertion of the LMA.

Comment

This is a simple study in which anaesthetists with a minimum of 2 years' experience in anaesthesia inserted an LMA using their normal technique and scored the insertion using seven different criteria. A score ranging from 0 to 10 was recorded for each attempt and the anaesthetists inserting the device were asked to rank the four devices.

This paper merits inclusion for two reasons: it is a recent paper, yet it identifies some of the shortcomings of simulation. The authors refer to the need for a device that will not only help instructors teach key skills but which can also undergo some some degree of preclinical testing.

Although the authors do not use the term in the article, this paper is about fidelity. In simulation there are two main types of fidelity – engineering and psychological |4|. In this study we could think of the engineering fidelity as relating to anatomical accuracy, replicating the tone of the tissues and replicating the response of the tissues to the insertion of the mask and the inflation of the cuff. The psychological fidelity relates to how well the device allows the skill under question to be performed. As a simple analogy, consider the 'feel' of loss of resistance when performing a lumber epidural. If all we want to recreate is the actual sensation, then a low engineering fidelity model such as a banana may have high psychological fidelity – the trainee will be able to identify that moment when loss of resistance occurs.

This paper is, therefore, a good example of a study that has exposed some of the limitations of the current generation of part-task trainers in their role for instruction and study of specific airway skills or devices. I have selected it less for the specific content – the ranking of the four devices – than for the general point it makes. As we extend the role of simulation in the teaching, assessment and study of specific areas of the anaesthetic curriculum then we shall continue to encounter limitations. The solution lies with an ongoing dialogue with the manufacturers and as we continue to define our needs in terms of both engineering and psychological fidelity, then that dialogue should prove fruitful. This echoes some of the themes that Kneebone explored in the second paper in this chapter.

Effective management of anaesthetic crises: development and evaluation of a college-accredited simulation-based course for anaesthesia education in Australia and New Zealand

Weller J, Morris R, Watterson L, *et al*. *Simulation in Healthcare* 2006; **1**: 209–14

BACKGROUND. The Effective Management of Anaesthetic Crises (EMAC) course is a two-and-a-half day course that has become an integral component of training for the Fellowship of the Australia and New Zealand College of Anesthetists (ANZCA). The article describes the content of the course, the development of the course and the response of participants to the course.

INTERPRETATION. The EMAC course is divided into five modules: human performance issues, airway emergencies, anaesthetic emergencies, cardiovascular emergencies and trauma management. The ANZCA accredits simulation centres to run the EMAC course. Centres must, therefore, comply with the published standards. The course became a component of training for the Fellowship of ANZCA in 2002. However, participation is not confined to trainees. Career grade anaesthetists can attend the course as part of their Maintenance of Professional Standards (MOPS) programme and the course was also accredited for this in 2002. Over 600 anaesthetists had attended EMAC courses at the time of writing the article, with approximately equal numbers of trainees and specialists.

Comment

The first part of the paper reviews some of the challenges involved in integrating a teaching course integrated into a multinational training programme and the initial impact that this course has had on its participants. The major challenge was to satisfy the body responsible for training and standards (ANZCA) by meeting those standards, while at the same time ensuring the necessary degree of collaboration and cooperation required between different simulation centres to establish and maintain a course that will be delivered to a consistent standard. The paper shows the necessity of setting up a suitable framework before a course can be taught in a consistent manner to a standard approved by a national body.

The second part of the paper reviews participants' opinions about the course. Participants were asked to complete a postal questionnaire. Data from 499 participants were available for analysis (Tables 11.3 and 11.4). Kirkpatrick described

Table 11.3 Best and worst aspects of EMAC (n = number of responses in that category)

Best aspects	Worst aspects
Learning from simulation and debriefs (169)	Simulations (16): lack or realism, lack of familiarity, debriefing process
Non-judgemental collegial approach (50)	Unpleasant stress of scenarios, feeling incompetent (24)
Teaching methods (68): variety of methods, practical, hands on, small group format	Teaching methods (24): too many didactic presentations, more time on simulations
Learn from each other, working with other anaesthetists (48)	Too much material in the time (21)
High standard of instruction (27)	Very long, tiring (16)
Gained insight, motivating (19)	Administrative aspects: facility (12), catering (5), course cost(3), course timing (9)
Specific session or module (63)	Specific session or module (41)
General praise (32)	Nothing they disliked about the course (53)

Source: Weller *et al.* (2006).

a hierarchy, subsequently modified |6|, that categorizes the impact of an educational intervention. The levels are:

- *Level 1*: learner's reactions
- *Level 2a*: modifications of attitudes and perceptions
- *Level 2b*: acquisition of knowledge and skills
- *Level 3*: change in behaviour
- *Level 4a*: change in organizational practice
- *Level 4b*: benefits to patients or clients.

Questionnaire responses are confined to levels 1 and 2a of this hierarchy.

Table 11.4 Responses to open questions asking for a description of any changes participants made to their clinical practice as a result of attending the course (n = 78 respondents)

	n (%)
New problem-solving strategies	47 (60)
Communication with colleagues	16 (21)
Working with a team	21 (27)
Planning for adverse events	17 (22)
Training colleagues in crisis management	10 (13)

Source: Weller *et al.* (2006).

In this paper the impact of the course is measured at the lowest two levels of the hierarchy, since it is confined to responses to a questionnaire. This is not to dismiss collection of such data – it is a necessary starting point and can often provide useful feedback to the course organizers and influence subsequent changes. The other useful purpose of the data is to show the wider community that the course appears to be delivering what it promises. It is interesting that the responses listed in Tables 11.3 and 11.4 show that the impact of the course on those participants who responded was mainly in the area of non-technical skills, even though the course dealt with some very specific practical skills, for example surgical airways.

As the move towards competency-based training becomes ever-more global it will be interesting to see whether ANZCA puts pressure on the course organizers to evaluate the impact of the course at the higher levels of Kirkpatrick's hierarchy.

Value of debriefing during simulated crisis management: oral versus video-assisted oral feedback

Savoldelli GL, Naik VN, Park J, *et al. Anesthesiology* 2006; **105**: 279–85

BACKGROUND. The debriefing process during medical simulation-based education is thought to be of high educational importance but has been poorly studied. Many simulation centres use video feedback as an adjunct that may enhance the impact of the debriefing and in turn maximize learning. This study investigated the value of the debriefing process during simulation and compared the educational efficacy of two types of feedback – oral feedback and video-assisted oral feedback – against a control group (no debriefing). After completing a pre-test scenario participants were randomly assigned to one of the three groups above. Debriefing focused on non-technical skills performance. Participants were then required to manage a post-test scenario.

INTERPRETATION. Participants' non-technical skills did not improve in the control group, whereas the provision of oral feedback, either assisted or not assisted with video review, resulted in significant improvement ($P<0.005$). There was no difference between the groups receiving oral or combined video-assisted and oral feedback.

Comment

Forty-two anaesthesia trainees were enrolled in the study. Before the simulation sessions a group orientation session was held for all participants. The principles of crisis evolution, patient simulation and anaesthesia crisis resource management (ACRM) were discussed. Participants were then familiarized with the simulator manikin, the monitors, anaesthetic machine and operating room environment. Each session consisted of two different scenarios, in which the participant played the role of the primary anaesthetist.

Two evaluators with expertise in simulation and ACRM were recruited and trained. These evaluators analysed the video and scored the performances using a reliable and previously validated system. Interrater reliability was acceptable – intraclass correlation coefficient (single rater) = 0.64. The authors tested for the effect of the level of training. Fourth-year trainees' pre-test scores were higher than first-year trainees' pre-test scores. However, the results of the two-factor ANOVA on total anaesthesia non-technical skills (ANTS) change scores showed no significant effect of the level of training factor ($F_{2,33} = 0.1$, P = not significant). This suggests that, although experienced trainees scored higher at baseline testing, subsequent learning depended on the provision of feedback but was not influenced by the level of training.

The authors note several limitations. The participants were tested immediately after debriefing so long-term retention was not assessed. It is also probable that the video-assisted oral feedback group received less actual instruction because of the time spent reviewing the video. Finally, the authors recognize that debriefing is more of an art than a science and so the generalizability of the findings to other centres, other types of scenario and other learning outcomes beyond non-technical skills in the context of the scenarios of the study is not proven/established.

The key lesson from the study is that participating in a simulated clinical scenario without structured debriefing appears to be of little educational value. The lack of any additional educational value from the use of video-assisted playback has implications for centres that are querying whether to spend money on audiovisual systems for educational purposes. Centres that want to conduct research will, of course, require facilities to record performances.

Does training in obstetric emergencies improve neonatal outcome?

Draycott T, Sibanda T, Owen L, *et al. Br J Obst Gynaecol* 2006; **113**: 177–82

BACKGROUND. In 2000 a new training course was introduced for midwifery and obstetric staff at Southmead Hospital, Bristol, UK. The authors sought to determine whether this course had any impact on perinatal asphyxia and neonatal hypoxic–ischaemic encephalopathy (HIE). Term, cephalic presenting, singleton infants born in the hospital between 1998 and 2003 were identified. Five-minute Apgar scores were reviewed. Infants that developed HIE were prospectively identified throughout this period. The study was a retrospective cohort observational study, comparing the period 'pre-training' (1998–99), with the period 'post training' (2001–03).

INTERPRETATION. Over 99% of targeted staff attended the 1-day training course. The authors showed that infants with 5-min Apgar scores of 6 or less decreased from 86.6 to 44.6 per 10 000 births ($P<0.001$) and those with HIE decreased from 27.3 to 13.6 per 10 000 births ($P = 0.032$). The authors suggest that specific multiprofessional training in obstetric emergencies are practical and may improve neonatal outcome.

Comment

This is an important paper for two reasons. Firstly, the authors sought evidence of clinical outcome (Kirkpatrick hierarchy level 4b) and, secondly, they looked at large numbers. The 1-day course was locally developed but in response to some national guidelines. The course consisted of a morning session for cardiotocograph (CTG) interpretation and an afternoon session in which participants attend six obstetric emergency drill stations, which involve training in the management of shoulder dystocia, postpartum haemorrhage, eclampsia, twin labour, breech presentation, adult resuscitation (including cardiopulmonary resuscitation) and neonatal resuscitation. The course is held bimonthly to accommodate all midwifery and obstetric staff – career grades and trainees. Annual attendance is mandatory. New members of staff are required to attend the next available course. The authors looked at the relevant data prior to the intervention (the new training programme) and compared that with the data collected after the intervention. The authors explore other reasons for the data changes, such as other interventions, continuation of prevailing trends, etc., and conclude that there are no other obvious factors that are likely to have brought about this change.

So, even although the design of the study is a retrospective one rather than a random controlled trial, the clinical and statistical significance of the changes suggest a strong association between the intervention and the outcomes.

This is a very significant paper because it provides further information for the cost–benefit debate related to training. The cost side has been easier to calculate – capital costs for equipment such as part-task trainers, ongoing costs to replace disposables and the costs of taking staff from frontline clinical duties to attend courses or act as faculty. Now we have some of the strongest evidence to date that clinical outcomes can be influenced by such training. The authors did not include any data on financial savings from neonatal bed occupancy or from costs associated with litigation, although they do refer to the impact of negligent intrapartum care on the annual litigation bill of the National Health Service in the UK.

Simulation as a method of assessment

The papers by Weller and by Savoldelli have shown how simulation can play an important role in formative assessment, in which the learner finds out more about his/her strengths or limitations. This is a key role of simulation, as referred to by Bradley. Simulation as an assessment tool in formal, summative high-stakes examinations is not such a well-developed role. Ziv refers to the role of simulation in the Anesthesiology Board examinations in Israel and the Royal College of Anaesthetists have been using simulations in various forms in the OSCE component of the primary component of the Fellowship examinations for several years. Another paper by Savoldelli explores a role that simulation may have to offer in anaesthesiology exams in Canada.

Evaluation of patient simulator performance as an adjunct to the oral examination for senior anaesthesia residents

Savoldelli GL, Naik VN, Hwan SJ, *et al. Anesthesiology* 2006; **104**: 475–81

BACKGROUND. Patient simulators possess features for performance assessment. However, the concurrent validity and the 'added value' of simulator-based examinations over traditional examinations have not been adequately addressed. In this study 20 senior anaesthesia residents were assessed sequentially in resuscitation and trauma scenarios using two assessment modalities: an oral examination, followed by a simulator-based examination. Two independent examiners scored the performances using a previously validated global rating scale. Different examiners were used to rate the oral and simulation performances.

INTERPRETATION. The inter-rater reliability was good to excellent across scenarios and modalities, with intraclass correlation coefficients ranging from 0.77 to 0.87. The within-scenario between modality score correlations were moderate: $r = 0.52$ (resuscitation) and $r = 0.53$ (trauma) ($P < 0.05$). Forty per cent of the average score variance was accounted for by the participants, and 30 per cent was accounted for by the participant-by-modality interaction. These data suggest that trainees who 'know how' in an oral exam may not necessarily be able to 'show how' in a simulation-based assessment.

Comment

Simulation in the form of part-task trainers, especially resuscitation equipment, and standardized patients have been used as assessment tools in OSCE components of examinations in medicine at both undergraduate and postgraduate level. The use of medium- to high-fidelity simulation in formal, summative, high-stakes examinations continues to be controversial and is still under scrutiny. The increased adoption of competency- or outcome-based training in anaesthesia is placing the focus on assessment on the ability of trainees not only to 'know how' but also to 'show how'. As the authors of this study state, simulation-based assessment should not replace oral examinations but should be complementary to them because they assess different aspects of the anaesthetic curriculum. The authors, therefore, set out to investigate the potential of simulation for assessing the performances of senior anesthesia trainees and to correlate and compare simulator performance with a mock oral examination modelled on a genuine formal, summative examination. The biggest limitation of the study is the small number of scenarios, which precluded the use of generalizability theory. Nevertheless, the authors conclude that the trainee scores on the oral examination were not a good predictor of how a particular trainee performed in a simulator assessment. This suggests that the simulator-based assessment is measuring something else. While the oral examination assesses the knowledge of the trainee, the simulator-based examination assesses other areas such as the clinical judgement and management skills of trainees in the context of the study scenarios.

Although the same rating scale was used for both modalities in the study, differences between them emerged. The oral scorings rewarded logical sequencing of reasoning, verbalizing of management plans and the ability to convey opinions in a precise and concise way. The simulator scorings mostly rewarded logical sequencing of management steps, demonstration of proper technical abilities and ability to communicate and lead a medical team. The authors conclude by recommending that larger studies are required before wholesale acceptance of simulation-based assessment in high-stakes examinations.

Simulation and the study of human factors

This role for medical simulation is not new. David Gaba saw this as a key component in his early work in medical simulation |7|. As healthcare in the developed world becomes more complex then this area will continue to gain in importance. The final two papers in this chapter are related in their subject matter of supporting the key knowledge of the anaesthetist during clinical challenges.

A novel point-of-care information system reduces anaesthesiologists' errors while managing case scenarios

Berkenstadt H, Yusim Y, Katznelson R, *et al. Eur J Anaesthesiol* 2006; **23**: 239–50

BACKGROUND. Humans have a limited ability to incorporate information during decision-making. A new electronic system – the On-Line Electronic Help (OLEH) – is a point-of care information system for anaesthesia providers, prepared by the European Society of Anaesthesiologists. In this study, to evaluate the OLEH 48 anaesthetists were presented in random order with six computer screen-based scenarios with the option of using the OLEH and six without that option. Two trained reviewers evaluated the performance of the anaesthetists looking for knowledge-based errors.

INTERPRETATION. The availability of OLEH was associated with higher scores in 11 of the 12 scenarios, and with a decrease in the incidence of critical errors in 10 scenarios.

Comment

The authors developed 24 anaesthesia-related case scenarios, which were in turn reviewed by five senior anaesthetists who were unfamiliar with the OLEH system. The 12 scenarios that achieved the highest scores for relevance and medium scores for complexity were selected. Participants were given a 30-min individual introduction and acquaintance with the OLEH system. They were then given a training scenario before embarking on the study proper. The 48 participants consisted of 12 senior anaesthetists, 12 senior trainee anaesthetists and 24 junior trainee anaesthetists. After the presentation of each case the participant was presented with four to six sequential questions relating to that case. The time needed to perform the task and the extent of use of the OLEH system were recorded.

Although it is well recognized that most overt mishaps in anaesthesia do have a multifactorial cause in which human error plays a significant part, the contribution of insufficient personal knowledge to errors performed during anaesthesia management had not previously been explored. The authors demonstrated in this study that use of this system reduced the incidence of knowledge-based errors without significant prolongation of the time needed for task completion. Although the participants were not allowed access to other sources of information, the authors describe how previous studies have measured the amount of time taken to acquire information. Clearly, a system that allows practitioners to find the relevant information easily and in a timely manner becomes important during clinical events with time constraints.

The main limitation of the study was that the OLEH system was tested in an environment outside the operating theatre, without a patient, anaesthesia monitors, anaesthesia machine and operating room team. The authors acknowledge that using the system in the real environment may also have some deleterious effects on patient care due to distraction. At the time of writing the article the OLEH system was under evaluation using full-scale simulation in an operating theatre.

This study has, however, identified that anaesthetists do have gaps in their knowledge that could lead to adverse events. The OLEH system appears to be easy to use and effective in providing the relevant knowledge. This was a necessary first stage to perform before moving on the second stage of evaluation in full-scale simulation.

Use of cognitive aids in a simulated anaesthetic crisis

Harrison KT, Manser T, Howard SK, *et al*. *Anesth Analg* 2006; **103**: 551–6

BACKGROUND. This study looked at the extent to which the use of a cognitive aid facilitated the correct and prompt treatment of malignant hyperthermia (MH) during a high-fidelity simulation of MH. The authors reviewed the performance of 48 simulated adult MH scenarios: 24 involving trainees in their first year of clinical anaesthesia (CA1) and 24 in their second year of clinical anaesthesia (CA2). The CA2 trainees received a different scenario from the CA1 trainees. Trainees in both years were instructed to bring to the simulated operating room any materials that they routinely took into a regular day of work. No specific training in the management of MH, the use of cognitive aids or the contents of the available MH treatment box was given.

INTERPRETATION. In the CA1 group 19 out of 24 used a cognitive aid, although only 8 of the 19 made extensive or frequent use of the aid. In the CA2 group 18 of 23 used a cognitive aid but only 6 of the 18 used it frequently or extensively. The frequency of cognitive aid use correlated with the MH treatment score for the CA1 group (Spearman $r = 0.59$, $P < 0.01$) and CA2 group (Spearman $r = 0.68$, $P < 0.001$). The teams that performed the best in treating MH used a cognitive aid extensively throughout the simulation. The authors claim that they have demonstrated a strong correlation between the use of a cognitive aid and the correct treatment of MH.

Comment

The authors state that 'a simulated MH event is an excellent model to test how anaesthesia providers respond to a rare but potentially lethal condition'. MH also has the advantage of a widely accepted and defined treatment protocol. Some components of that protocol had a strong association with the use of cognitive aids, in particular determining the correct dose of dantrolene. Others seemed to be less affected by their use, in particular treating hyperkalaemia. The authors also mention some limitations in the study. First, it is not possible to predict what impact on a real patient the omission or late completion of some of the steps would have. Secondly, the scenarios were designed for teaching rather than being set up for the primary purpose of investigation. Thirdly, scenarios were time-compressed. Fourthly, the baseline level of knowledge of the participants was not measured. All had been exposed to some formal teaching and the CA2 participants would have been exposed to at least debriefing of a simulated MH scenario during their CA1 year.

However, even taking the limitations into account, the study has yielded some interesting results. The authors were not only able to look at the impact on performance of the use of cognitive aids but were able to look at the effectiveness of the aids themselves, with some suggestions for future developments. Studies such as this may allow us to develop more effective educational strategies, including how to best make use of cognitive aids during times of unfamiliar or life-critical situations.

Conclusion

Table 11.2, taken from the paper on the history of simulation and future developments by Bradley, lists potential applications of simulation. It is noteworthy how many of these areas were addressed in the papers in this chapter. The papers likely to have the biggest impact are the paper by Draycott *et al.* on the impact of training on clinical outcome and the paper by Savoldelli *et al.* on debriefing.

Training matters; it makes a difference to clinical outcomes. The method of training also matters. Simulation as an educational resource is much more than mere technology. Sound educational principles are required to have an impact on participants.

Many of the other papers echoed these two principles, and have added to our understanding of what simulation can and cannot do effectively. The request from Kneebone for better understanding to help develop a theory of simulation is being answered by many diverse voices.

References

1. Royal College of Anaesthetists. The CCT in Anaesthesia I, II, III and IV. Available at: www.rcoa.ac.uk/index (accessed 27 May 2007).

2. Harden RM, Grant J, Buckley G, Hart IR. BEME Guide No **1**: best evidence medical education. *Medical Teacher* 1999; **21**: 553–62.

3. Issenberg SB, McGaghie WC, Petrusa ER, Gordon DL, Scalese RJ. Features and uses of high-fidelity medical simulations that lead to effective learning: a BEME systematic review. *Medical Teacher* 2005; **27**: 10–28.

4. Maran NJ, Glavin RJ. Low to high fidelity simulation – a continuum of medical education? *Medical Education* 2003; 37(S1): S22–S28.

5. Kneebone R. Simulation in surgical training: educational issues and practical implications. *Medical Education* 2003; **37**: 267–77.

6. Barr H, Freeth D, Hammick M, Koppel I, Reeves S. *Evaluations of Interprofessional Education: a United Kingdom Review of Health and Social Care*. London: CAIPE/BERA; 2000, pp. 25–38.

7. Gaba DM, Fish KJ, Howard SK. *Crisis Management in Anesthesiology*. New York: Churchill Livingstone; 1994, pp. vii–ix.

12

Novel intubation equipment

NICHOLAS LAM, CARIN HAGBERG

Introduction

For many years, the flexible fibreoptic laryngoscope has been an important tool in the management of the difficult airway. Nonetheless, this technique has several shortcomings, including (i) high cost; (ii) the need for additional training beyond standard laryngoscopy; (iii) its inability to physically displace soft tissues such as a large, floppy epiglottis; and (iv) an inability to provide adequate ventilation when used solely for this purpose. There are a multitude of airway devices, including rigid fibreoptic intubation aids that have recently appeared on the market in an attempt to overcome some or all of these issues.

The new intubation tools are largely but not entirely fibreoptic and can be divided into three main categories: laryngoscopes, stylets and conduits. The fibreoptic *laryngoscopes* are designed for use with minimal training beyond that required to perform traditional direct laryngoscopy. They are designed to enable the airway provider to attain improved laryngoscopic views by attaching fibreoptic technology to modified laryngoscopes without much further training in the new equipment. The main advantage of these devices is that they are 'quick and easy' as the learning curve is short and equipment preparation is minimal. When intubation is performed with these devices, the tracheal tube should be styletted in order to facilitate its passage into the glottis. Additionally, there are specially designed tubes, such as the Parker flex-tip tube (Parker Medical, Englewood, CO, USA), which facilitate glottic entry with any of the fibreoptic intubation adjuncts.

Fibreoptic *stylets* are rigid in design and more intuitive to use than the flexible fibreoptic laryngoscope. They allow novice airway providers to easily navigate through the airway and have the advantage of being able to manoeuvre around soft tissues and physically lift an epiglottis, if necessary. Additionally, they require minimal mouth opening compared with the laryngoscopic and conduit type of intubation adjuncts.

Conduit-type fibreoptic adjuncts have the advantage of providing a pathway for ventilation and intubation. However, they are limited by the requirement that a certain amount of mouth opening is required to be present and assume that the conduit will lead the airway provider to the glottic opening. Difficulties may occur as they work best with midline and central positioning in the airway. Lastly, there are usually more steps involved in their use, thus more training may be necessary as compared with other fibreoptic intubation techniques.

This chapter will cover four different laryngoscopic (Videolaryngoscope, Glidescope, Airtraq and AirWay Scope), four stylet (SensaScope, Bonfils, Shikani and Levitan fibreoptic laryngoscopes) and one conduit type (CTrach) of rigid intubation adjuncts.

Video Macintosh Laryngoscope

Comparison of direct and video-assisted views of the larynx during routine intubation

Kaplan MB, Hagberg CA, Ward DS, et al. J Clin Anes 2006; **18**: 357–62

BACKGROUND. The Video Macintosh Laryngoscope (VML; Karl Storz Endoscopy, Tuttlingen, Germany) consists of a 3-mm image light bundle near the tip of a standard laryngoscope blade (Fig. 12.1). Although various blade types and blade sizes are now available, including Macintosh 3, 4, Dorges and all Miller blade sizes, this study was performed with the Macintosh 3 or 4 blade. A camera with a monitor and light cable is inserted into the handle. This prospective, randomized study compared 867 ASA I–IV adults in 11 internationally affiliated hospitals. All patients were placed in the sniffing position and after standardized induction and

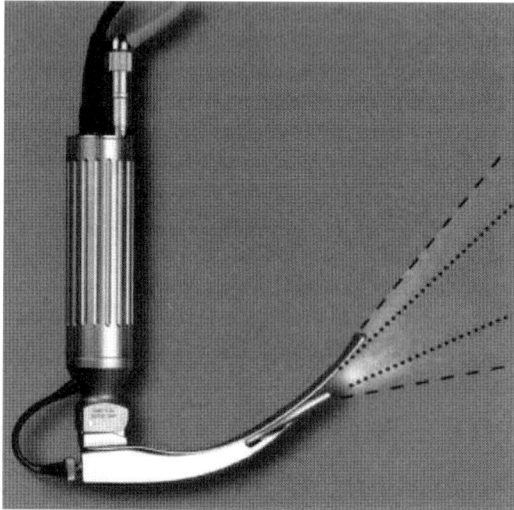

Fig 12.1 The Video Macintosh Laryngoscope showing the field of view from the image fibre bundle. Note that the monitor view (dashed line) extends more anteriorly compared with the direct line-of-sight view (dotted line). Source: Kaplan et al. (2006).

muscle relaxation, laryngoscopy was performed. First, the best laryngoscopic view was obtained with the VML during direct vision using optimal external laryngeal manipulation, if necessary. The view was graded by the laryngoscopist without looking at the video monitor. The view on the monitor was subsequently graded by the same laryngoscopist using the same laryngoscopic position. Subjective assessments regarding the two views (direct view vs. monitor view) were made (better, same or worse). Glottic views were rated according to the Cormack–Lehane (C–L) scoring system, as modified by Yentis and Lee |1|, with difficult laryngoscopy being defined as C–L grade 3 and 4 views. Tracheal intubation was then performed using the monitor view.

INTERPRETATION. Of the 865 patients suitable for analysis, visualization was considered *easy* (C–L grade 1 and 2) in 737 patients and *difficult* (C–L grade 3 and 4) in 21 for both direct and video-assisted views. In seven patients, the view was graded as *easy* by direct visualization and *difficult* on the video monitor view, whereas in 100 patients the view was considered *difficult* by direct visualization and *easy* on the video monitor view ($P<0.001$). Intubation was unsuccessful in three cases using either method. In these patients, C–L grade 2a, 3 and 4 views were obtained, with only the C–L grade 3 view improving to a 2b by video laryngoscopy. These airways were subsequently secured with flexible fibreoptic laryngoscopy. This study did demonstrate that video laryngoscopy provides an improved view of the larynx, as compared with direct visualization. However, in a small percentage of cases, video laryngoscopy provided a worse view. Additionally, it did not decrease the overall incidence of failed intubation.

Comment

The fibreoptic laryngoscope demonstrated a superior view, compared with direct laryngoscopy, in a significant percentage of patients. This is due to the positioning of the image fibre bundle tip close to the blade tip changing the viewpoint from a straight line of sight to a 45° angle in the Macintosh blade type (Fig. 12.1). Also, due to the panoramic lens, a wider viewing angle is transmitted to the video monitor.

Despite the improved view, the rate of unsuccessful intubation may not change using this technique. Even when improving the laryngoscopic view from a C–L grade 3 to 2b, the airway providers were not able to intubate a patient without the use of a flexible fibreoptic laryngoscope. Flexible fibreoptic laryngoscopy was used in two additional patients as a rescue technique.

However, there are many advantages of the VML. Unlike other video laryngoscopes (e.g. GlideScope, Airtraq, Truview EVO2, McGrath and AirWay Scope), the blade design and its use are very similar to standard laryngoscopy. Manipulation of the endotracheal tube using the monitor requires more dexterity than direct visualization but it is easily learned. The VML is extremely useful for teaching direct or indirect laryngoscopy as the image is projected on the monitor for all to see |2|. It is also useful in demonstrating the effect of optimal laryngeal manipulation and cricoid pressure on laryngeal view. Lastly, it is extremely useful in determining the appropriate position of a variety of devices, including gastric tubes, temperature probes, and so on, and can also be used for nasotracheal intubation.

GlideScope®

The use of the GlideScope® for tracheal intubation in patients with ankylosing spondylitis

Lai HY, Chen IH, Chen A, et al. Br J Anaesth 2006; **97**: 419–22

BACKGROUND. The GlideScope® (Verathon Medical, Bothell, WA, USA) is a plastic, non-disposable fibreoptic laryngoscope with an angled laryngeal blade (60°) that is connected to a portable colour LCD monitor. The monitor can be attached to a stand (Fig. 12.2) or be fully integrated into a small portable system. Three sizes of blades are available: adult, paediatric and neonate. The latest version of the GlideScope, the Cobalt GVL® Stat, is designed with a reusable video baton and a disposable blade (available in two sizes: small and large), which is ideal for fast-paced intubation settings. Twenty ankylosing spondylitis patients were selected to undergo tracheal intubation using the GlideScope. The first anaesthesiologist performed direct laryngoscopy with a Macintosh 3 blade and determined the modified Cormack and Lehane (MCLS) |1| grade and percentage of glottic opening (POGO) |3| score. The MCLS divides grade 2 into 2a and 2b, according to whether a portion of the vocal cords are visible (grade 2a) or not (grade 2b)|1|. A second anaesthesiologist then used the GlideScope and provided a separate MCLS and POGO score. A third anesthesiologist, experienced in the use of the GlideScope (> 200 intubations), provided an independent MCLS and POGO before intubating each patient.

INTERPRETATION. Eleven of the 12 patients were judged as difficult to intubate with MCLS grades 3 or 4 by direct laryngoscopy. The GlideScope improved the MCLS grade and POGO score in all but one (two out of the three) MCLS grade 4 and POGO score 0 patients ($P<0.01$). The GlideScope improved all MCLS grade 3 patients to grade 2b or 2a. Nasotracheal intubation using the GlideScope was successful in all patients except

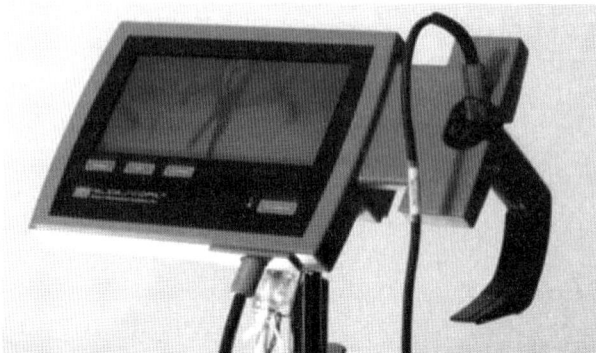

Fig 12.2 GlideScope. A high-resolution camera is integrated into an angled laryngeal blade, allowing a better view of the full glottis and requiring less force. Source: Lai et al. (2006).

the three patients who were predicted to be difficult and had MCLS grade 4 scores by direct laryngoscopy. Even though the glottic view of one of three patients improved from an MCLS grade 4 view to a grade 3 with the GlideScope, intubation was unsuccessful.

Comment

Unlike a standard laryngoscope, all versions of the GlideScope are designed with a 60° angled laryngoscope blade. Its use is similar to direct laryngoscopy, yet a direct view of the glottis is not possible because of the blade design. As such, the GlideScope is not as intuitive to use as the VML and requires short, simple training regarding insertion technique, manipulation of the blade for optimal view and preparation of the tube. The GlideRite® stylet (Verathon Medical, Bothell, WA, USA) is designed for use with any of the GlideScope laryngoscopes to facilitate intubation.

Like the VML, the GlideScope improves the view of the glottic opening. Nonetheless, improved glottic views do not always equate with successful tracheal intubation. The GlideScope is highly portable and has a built-in heating mechanism over its lens, thus the application of antifog solution is unnecessary. In trained hands, it is quick to set up and use, and is therefore useful for unexpected difficult airways |4|.

Airtraq

A comparison of tracheal intubation using the Airtraq or the Macintosh laryngoscope in routine airway management: a randomized, controlled clinical trial

Maharaj C, O'Croinin D, Curley G, *et al. J Anaesth* 2006; **61**: 1093–9

BACKGROUND. The Airtraq (Prodol Meditec SA, LLC, Vizcaya, Spain) is a single-use, self-contained portable and disposable intubation device with a channel for insertion of a tracheal tube. A battery-operated light is present at the tip of the blade with the image transmitted to a proximal viewfinder by a combination of lenses and prisms (Fig. 12.3). When used for tracheal intubation, the Airtraq should be preloaded with an appropriately sized tracheal tube (6.0–8.5 mm). Mannikin studies have demonstrated that the Airtraq offers potential advantages in both easy and difficult laryngoscopy scenarios |5|. This prospective, randomized, controlled study compared the Airtraq with standard laryngoscopy in patients considered to be at low risk for difficult intubation, defined as 'easy airways'. Sixty patients were randomized to be intubated with either the Airtraq or a Macintosh laryngoscope. Only one of four anaesthesiologists was experienced in both techniques. All patients received a standardized general anaesthetic and were paralysed. The intubation difficulty score (IDS), number of intubation attempts, number of optimization manoeuvres (readjustment of head, use of

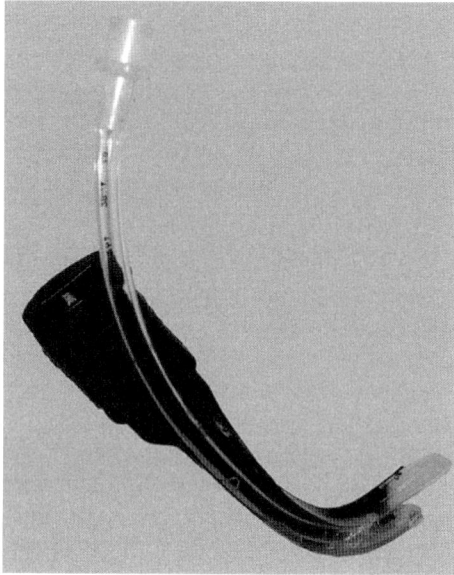

Fig 12.3 The Airtraq laryngoscope with a tracheal tube in place in the side channel. Source: Maharaj *et al.* (2006).

bougies or second assistant) to aid intubation and severity of dental trauma were noted. Cardiovascular changes associated with intubation with each device were noted.

INTERPRETATION. The results showed that the Airtraq is similar to the Macintosh laryngoscope in intubating patients with easy airways. However, the Airtraq reduced intubation difficulty (based on IDS scores) and reduced the number of optimization manoeuvers. Despite reduced dental trauma in manikin studies |6|, this study did not show any difference in dental trauma between the two groups. There was, however, less hypertension and tachycardia in the Airtraq group than in the Macintosh group.

Comment

The Airtraq requires simple training and studies have demonstrated that novice personnel find it easier to use than direct laryngoscopy in manikin studies. Additionally, the sniffing position is not necessary for intubation and patients may be intubated in positions other than supine, which may be very useful in 'out-of-hospital' settings. Being disposable, the Airtraq has the advantage of reducing transmission of infections, but the disadvantage of teaching costs on real patients and environmental wastage. This study showed that the Airtraq is one of the few single-use airway devices that is at least as effective as the standard Macintosh laryngoscope blade. Previous studies comparing standard Macintosh blades with disposable blades have favoured the former. This study demonstrated similar intubation success in patients with easy airways and, despite the reduced intubation difficulties and success in manikin studies, there is still an absence of data regarding patients with difficult airways.

It is recommended that the Airtraq be inserted midline like the GlideScope. Neck flexion or large chests or breasts may hinder this process more than direct laryngoscopy, even with the standard handle. The Airtraq is available in two sizes (small and large), with the smaller size providing more manoeuvrability. The preformed tracheal tube channel limits tube manipulation, which can be problematic for intubation, especially in patients with significant neck flexion and when using the larger-sized Airtraq.

AirWay Scope

Description and first clinical application of Airway Scope for tracheal intubation

Kyoama J, Aoyama T, Kusano Y, et al. J Neurosurg Anesthesiol 2006; **18**: 247–50

BACKGROUND. The AirWay Scope (AWS; Pentax, Tokyo, Japan) aims to bridge the gap of portability and ease of handling of a rigid laryngoscope with the reduced invasiveness of a flexible fibreoptic laryngoscope. The AWS (Fig. 12.4) is an introducer (INTLOCK) connected to a camera unit with an integrated light source and projects an image onto a 2.4-inch liquid crystal display. The INTLOCK should be preloaded with a tracheal tube. This is a case series of 10 consecutive patients, which focuses on the clinical description and application of the AWS. Oropharyngeal classification ranged from Mallampati class I to III, although three patients' airways could not be classified due to their inability to cooperate. After standardized induction and muscle relaxation, the investigator performed airway manipulation and intubation. Intubation time was defined as the time from cessation of bag mask ventilation until resumption of ventilation via the tracheal tube.

INTERPRETATION. All patients were intubated on the first attempt with full glottic exposure obtained (C–L 1). Time for intubation ranged from 24 to 102 s, with 8 out of 10 patients intubated within 60 s. There were no complications noted during intubation procedures.

Comment

The introducer device (INTLOCK) is inserted much like a Miller blade and withdrawn until the glottic view is seen on the attached monitor. The airway provider then manoeuvres the AWS until the sighting device is aligned with the glottic opening. The tracheal tube is advanced through the central channel using the monitor view. Because of the inherent hook shape of the INTLOCK, intubation

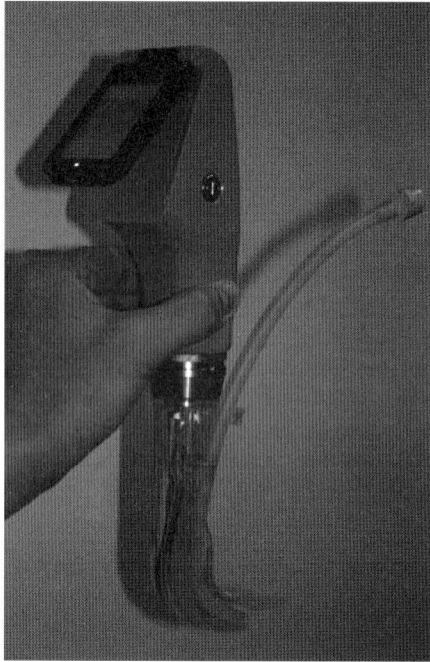

Fig 12.4 The AirWay Scope with a tracheal tube loaded on the Intlock blade. Source: Kyoama *et al*. (2006).

of the patient is relatively independent of neck extension. However, despite the rotating monitor, intubating from the caudal position is difficult due to the lifting axis involved.

This paper does not compare the device to either standard or fibreoptic laryngoscopy, thus interpretation of the data is limited. At present, it is still unknown if the AWS is simlar to or better than the standard laryngoscope in easy or difficult airways.

Similar to the other video fibreoptic laryngoscopes, the AWS affords the benefit of allowing an assistant to visualize his or her performance of external laryngeal manipulation to enhance glottic exposure. This device has a disposable component and is extremely portable, with the capability of running on two AA batteries for 1 h. Another advantage is the presence of a suction channel, which allows passage of a 12-Fr catheter.

Fibreoptic stylets

Using direct rigid laryngoscopy, the incidence of C–L grade 3 or 4 views has been reported to be 5.8% in prospective trials. The most common intubation aide used in these situations is a malleable stylet or gum elastic bougie, placed blindly. However, blind techniques have a higher failure rate than visualized techniques and may cause more trauma. The rationale in the use of fibreoptic stylets is that intubation success is enhanced by visualization of the glottic opening. The stylets require minimal preparation, making them valuable in the unanticipated difficult intubation. They can be less traumatic and time-consuming than multiple attempts at direct laryngoscopy, flexible fibreoptic laryngoscopy or blind endotracheal intubation. Nonetheless, experience is necessary with any device and the airway provider should practice 15–20 times before he or she can be considered competent with any of the fibreoptic stylets |7|.

SensaScope

First clinical experience of tracheal intubation with the SensaScope®, a novel steerable semirigid video stylet

Biro P, Baatig U, Henderson J, et al. Br J Anaesth 2006; **97**: 255–61

BACKGROUND. The SensaScope (Acutronic Medical Systems AG, Hirzel, Switzerland) is a 45-cm-long video stylet with a rigid S-shaped curve (Fig. 12.5). It has a 3-cm-long steerable tip with a 75° range of motion in the sagittal plane, controlled by a lever at the proximal end of the device, very similar to a standard flexible fibreoptic laryngoscope. The proximal end consists of an eyepiece through which the operator can look directly or which can be connected to a video camera and light source. Unlike the flexible fibreoptic laryngoscope, the SensaScope has no working channel and has a 15-mm female connector in the proximal shaft to mount a tracheal tube. This is the first clinical trial of the SensaScope, testing its speed and utility during normal and difficult tracheal intubation of 29 females and three males with normal airways. Eight airway providers were chosen, four of whom were considered skilled with flexible fibreoptic laryngoscopy (> 20 cases performed). No providers had previously used the SensaScope. After a brief demonstration, the airway providers performed tracheal intubation with only verbal advice from the investigator.

INTERPRETATION. Patients were intubated with a mean intubation time (defined as the time of insertion of the laryngoscope until circuit connection to the tracheal tube) of 25 s and all were successfully intubated within 1 min. There was no significant difference in intubation time between the providers who were experienced vs. those who were inexperienced with flexible fibreoptic laryngoscopy. However, in this small study the difference was not statistically significant. The ease of use of the device was reported on a scale of 0 to 10 and determined as 3.8 by the fibreoptic novice and 2.2 by the fibreoptic experts. Of the 32 patients, seven exhibited C–L grade 3 direct laryngoscopic views, which were subsequently converted to C–L grade 1 or 2 views.

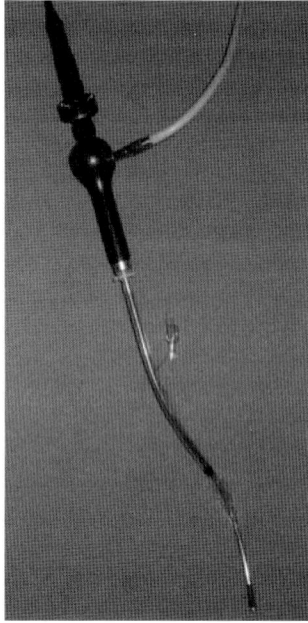

Fig. 12.5 The assembled SensaScope® system with a mounted tracheal tube ready for use. Source: Biro *et al.* (2006).

Comment

The use of the SensaScope requires the application of anti-fog solution but no lubrication. After loading the tracheal tube, direct laryngoscopy is performed with the left hand while holding the SensaScope in the right hand. Once the best laryngeal view is achieved, the SensaScope is introduced as close to the palate as possible and manoeuvred past the vocal cords. The Macintosh blade is then removed, and the SensaScope advanced to the mid-trachea position until the carina is visualized. A preloaded tracheal tube is then advanced into the trachea. In this study, there were no complaints of sore throat or injury related to the intubation process.

Patient selection produced a 22% incidence of a C–L grade 3 view, which is extremely high compared with the figure of 5.8% reported in the literature |8|. The authors felt that this was most likely due to the lower lifting force used by the airway providers and omission of external laryngeal manipulation. Thus, the data related to improving the glottic view with the SensaScope must be viewed with caution.

Limitations of its use in emergency airway management include a preparation time of 3 min (connection, white balance, camera alignment and anti-fog), limitation of the intubation route to the oral approach and lack of data with its use in difficult airways.

The main advantage of this device is its ease of use. This is intuitively true as the rigid portion of the shaft provides greater rotational manoeuverability. Unfortunately, the purpose of this paper was to launch the SensaScope for clinical use, not to demonstrate its ease of use. Future comparative studies involving novice users with flexible fibreoptic laryngoscopy will be helpful to determine its true simplicity of use.

Shikani

A comparison of the Seeing Optical Stylet and the gum elastic bougie in simulated difficult tracheal intubation: a mannikin study

Evans A, Morris S, Petterson J, *et al*. *Anaesthiology* 2006; **61**: 478–81

BACKGROUND. The Shikani or Seeing Optical Stylet (Clarus Medical, Minneapolis, MN, USA) is a semimalleable fibreoptic endoscope. The high-resolution fibreoptic bundle is housed in a stainless-steel stylet. The tracheal tube is loaded onto the stylet and fixed with a locking device so that the tube lies just proximal to the tip of the endoscope (Fig. 12.6). The proximal end is an eyepiece through which the operator can directly look or attach a camera. The proximal end fits onto a handle with the light source powered by a rechargeable battery. A fibreoptic light source may also be utilized. The Shikani has been studied in normal airways of adults, with encouraging results. There have also been studies performed in children with predicted difficult airways. This is a prospective, randomized crossover study comparing the Shikani to the gum elastic bougie (Smiths Medical ASD, Keene, NH/Smiths Medical International, Hythe, Kent, UK) in a manikin adjusted to have a C–L grade 3 laryngoscopic view. Forty-four airway providers of varying experience (2–21 years) were recruited, where the gum elastic bougie is routinely used to aid difficult intubation. All participants were given a brief opportunity to handle the Shikani beforehand. Time to intubation with each method was recorded and any unsuccessful intubation attempts noted.

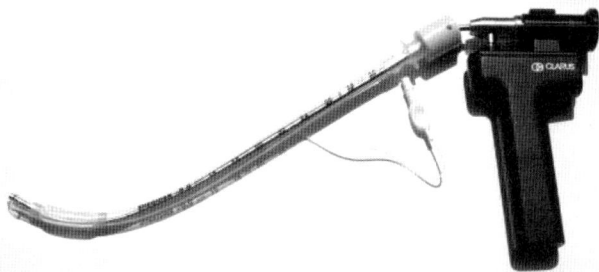

Fig. 12.6 Shikani Seeing Optical Stylet with a mounted tracheal tube ready for use. Source: Evans *et al*. (2006).

INTERPRETATION. The mean time for intubation with the Shikani was 20.8 s (11–62 s) compared with 30 s (13–220 s) ($P = 0.001$) with the gum elastic bougie. Esophageal intubation occurred six times with the bougie. On each occasion in which this occurred, intubation was subsequently successful.

Comment

This study demonstrated that use of the Shikani was faster and more reliable for the performance of tracheal intubation than use of the gum elastic bougie in manikins with difficult airways. However, caution should be exercised when applying these results to patients with abundant airway tissue and secretions. Additionally, the timing was skewed towards the Shikani as it was already preloaded with the tracheal tube. On the other hand, the operators were all new to the use of the Shikani and were much more experienced with the gum elastic bougie. Unfortunately, the study was not designed with enough power to examine the accuracy of intubation. Nonetheless, there were no oesophageal intubations in the Shikani group. Intuitively, a visualized intubation technique should result in a decreased incidence of oesophageal intubation compared with a blind technique such as a bougie. Although it has been suggested that the Shikani be used without a laryngoscope and the operator providing anterior displacement of the lower jaw, the Shikani was used like a bougie in conjunction with a laryngoscope in this study.

The Shikani has the advantage over the flexible fibreoptic laryngoscope in terms of ease of use. Lateral and rotational manoeuvres are much more intuitive than with a flexible laryngoscope. Also, its semirigid nature allows tissues to be manually displaced in cases where oedema or soft tissue has obscured the operator's visualization of the airway anatomy.

The drawbacks of the Shikani are that it is not possible to perform nasal intubation and there is no suction channel. Nonetheless, there is a special adapter that can be attached to the stylet enabling either oxygen insufflation, instillation of local anaesthesia or suction around the stylet and within the tracheal tube. Also, the J-shaped curve does not allow the scope to pass far beyond the cords. Indeed, the SensaScope with the flexible tip and S-curve bypasses this problem. The Flexible Airway Scope Tool (FAST, Clarus Medical, Minneapolis, MN, USA), a member of the Shikani family of devices, is a totally malleable fibreoptic cable but without a guidable tip: it can be used for verification of correct tube placement and to assist nasotracheal or LMA Fastrach/CTrach intubation.

Levitan FPS (First Pass Success) stylet

Design rationale and intended use of a short optical stylet for routine fiberoptic augmentation of emergency laryngoscopy

Levitan R. *Am J Emerg Med* 2006; **24**: 490–5

BACKGROUND. The Levitan FPS (Clarus Medical, Minneapolis, MN, USA) is a 30-cm malleable optical stylet. Like the Shikani, the malleable steel stylet encloses optical and light-transmitting optical fibres that connect to an eyepiece and a removable light source (Fig. 12.7). The proximal end consists of an eyepiece and a light source and accepts the 15-mm connector of a tracheal tube. The light source can be a standard fibreoptic illuminated laryngoscope handle or miniature light-emitting diode. On the right of the tube is a small hole for a removable oxygen connector for insufflation of oxygen through the distal end of the stylet. The Levitan is a shorter, streamlined version of the Shikani with no imaging screen or power connection. This paper is a descriptive study of the Levitan fibreoptic intubation stylet by its inventor. In preparation, the tracheal tube should overhang the stylet tip by approximately 1 cm to keep blood and secretions from obscuring the lens. This is aided by blowing oxygen through the tube. Positioning the tube in this way also minimizes tissue trauma. The stylet is shaped in a 'field hockey stick' style with a 35° bend at the proximal end.

INTERPRETATION. For C–L 1–2 laryngoscopic views, the FPS stylet can be used as a normal stylet and correct tracheal placement can be verified fibreoptically upon final passage of the tube. During difficult laryngoscopy (C–L 3 view), the FPS is placed under direct vision until its distal tip is close to but below and away from the epiglottis. The operator then moves his or her head to bring their dominant eye to the eyepiece and manoeuvres the tip of the FPS through the glottic opening. Moving the handle towards the right corner of the mouth to slide the stylet backward may be helpful to direct the tip upward. Care must be made not to shape the hockey stick beyond 35° as this will

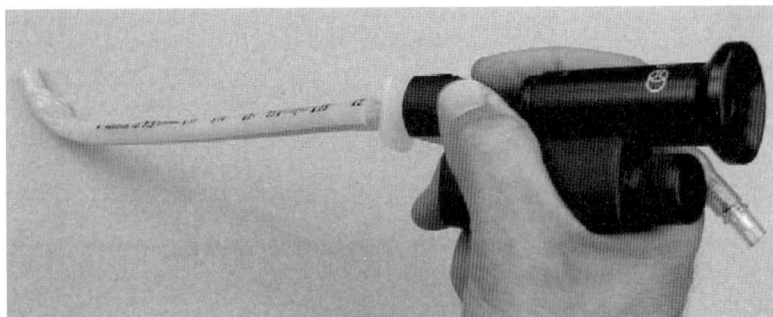

Fig. 12.7 Levitan FPS scope with the miniature LED light source held in a pencil grip manner. Source: Levitan (2006).

impede or prevent tube advancement through the glottis. Once the stylet passes through the glottis, the laryngoscope is removed and the left hand is free to slide the tracheal tube into the trachea. In C–L grade 4 views, the FPS can be used with a 70° bend without a laryngoscope. The left hand lifts the jaw and tongue and the stylet is rotated into the oropharynx following a midline palatal approach.

Comment

The Levitan was developed as a device for routine augmentation of emergency direct laryngoscopy. It is intended to be easy to use and simple to set up. Rescue devices that are used infrequently are useless in emergencies unless they are extremely intuitive. Like the other optical stylets, the Levitan does require practice and training for proficient use.

The Levitan has similar advantages compared with the Shikani; however, it is shorter and easier to manoeuvre. Set-up may take longer due to the prescribed length of the shaft requiring the endotracheal tube to be cut to the appropriate length. Similarly, the FPS cannot be used for nasal intubation.

Bonfils

Prehospital emergency endotracheal intubation using the Bonfils Intubation Fiberscope

Byhahn C, Meininger D, Walcher F, et al. Eur J Emerg Med 2007; **14**: 43–6

BACKGROUND. **The Bonfils Retromolar Intubation Fiberscope (Karl Storz Endoscopy, Tuttlingen, Germany) is a 40-cm-long, reusable, rigid fibreoptic stylet with a 40° curved tip (Fig. 12.8). A flexible eyepiece that can be looked through directly or attached to a camera is located on the proximal end. Like the Shikani, a special 15-mm endotracheal tube connector can be attached for oxygen**

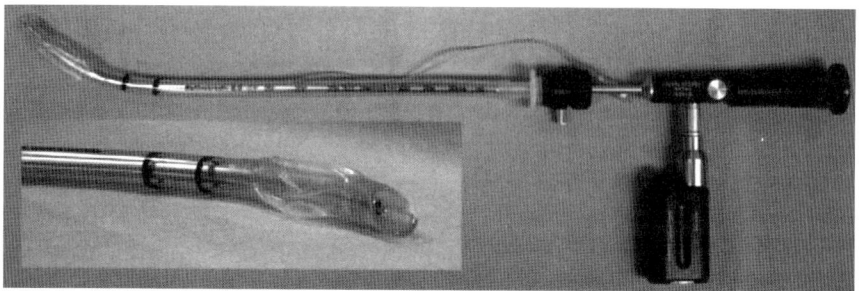

Fig. 12.8 Battery-powered Bonfils Intubation Fiberscope armed with an 8.0-mm inner diameter endotracheal tube. Note that the tip of the fibrescope must be placed inside the endotracheal tube (see inset). Source: Byhahn et al. (2007).

insufflation, suction, or instillation of local anaesthetic. The light source can be battery-powered or fibreoptic. Additionally, the Bonfils comes in a DCI (direct coupler interface) intubation system in which there is no eyepiece but rather a camera unit which snaps into place at the proximal end. The tracheal tube should be loaded in similar fashion to the Shikani intubation stylet. This is a case series of six pre-hospital emergency endotracheal intubations in patients with difficult airways using the Bonfils, including two patients who required cervical spine immobilization and one patient who had sustained a cardiac arrest and failed intubation with direct laryngoscopy.

INTERPRETATION. Up to 64% of patients in rigid collars have a C–L grade 3 or 4 view |9|. In this case series, the use of the Bonfils allowed intubation without removing the front portion of the rigid collar, thus saving time and increasing cervical safety. Despite the fact that all cases occurred in the prehospital setting, patients had 'dry' airways not contaminated with blood or secretions which would have rendered the use of any fibreoptic stylet difficult.

Comment

The Bonfils is one of the most studied fibreoptic stylets. It has a steep learning curve and the authors suggest that 10 supervised intubations be undertaken before the airway provider can be deemed to have achieved sufficient skill to use it in suboptimal conditions.

It has been demonstrated that minimal neck extension is required to use the Bonfils compared with direct laryngoscopy. The Bonfils can be used by itself, like the other fibreoptic stylets, with the left hand lifting the jaw to create a retropharyngeal space. However, with this method, the time to intubation is significantly longer than when used in conjunction with direct laryngoscopy. Although this is not a problem in preoxygenated patients, it may be a problem in those who have not been preoxygenated. The use of a laryngoscope to create the retropharyngeal space significantly reduces the intubation time, and the authors suggest using a laryngoscope in all intubations with this device.

Fibreoptic conduit

CTrach

An evaluation of poor LMA CTrach™ views with a fiberoptic laryngoscope and the effectiveness of corrective measures

Liu EH, Goy RW, Chen FG. *Br J Anaesth* 2006; **97**: 878–82

BACKGROUND. The LMA CTrach (LMA North America, Inc, San Diego, CA, USA) is an intubating laryngeal mask airway (ILMA) with fibreoptic channels incorporated into the laryngeal mask conduit and a detachable LCD viewfinder (Fig. 12.9). It is available in three adult sizes (3–5) and comes with 6.0- to 8-mm silicon-tipped, wire-reinforced tracheal tubes. Despite the high success rate of intubation with the CTrach, it is often difficult to view the glottis (48% of the cases) |10|. This study recruited 69 patients with difficult CTrach views and evaluated the reasons for the poor glottic views. Evaluation was performed with the aid of a fibreoptic laryngoscope passed through the CTrach without lifting the epiglottic elevator bar. This study demonstrated that the reasons for the difficult views included epiglottic downfolding, arytenoid obstruction or secretions. Secondly, manoeuvres to overcome the poor glottic views were assessed. With epiglottic downfolding, the CTrach was advanced more deeply; if this did not resolve the poor view, partial withdrawal by 6 cm followed immediately by reinsertion was attempted while hand ventilating the patient (up–down method). Withdrawal of the CTrach by 1 cm and applying forward lift was used to overcome the poor view associated with arytenoid obstruction. Complete removal and cleaning of fibreoptic ports was used to overcome the problem of secretions.

INTERPRETATION. Epiglottic downfolding was the major cause of a poor view in 82.6% (57/69) of patients of which 89.5% (51/57) were corrected by the up–down manoeuvre. In six patients the up–down manoeuvre failed to achieve a full glottic view even after removal and reinsertion of the CTrach. Of these, three were successfully intubated blindly and three were subsequently intubated with a standard Macintosh laryngoscope. During direct laryngoscopy, these three patients had C–L grade 1–3 laryngoscopic views. Obstruction was caused by the arytenoids in 10.2% (7/69) of patients and by secretions in 7.2% (5/69), all of which were corrected by the rescue manoeuvres.

Comment

Poor view with the CTrach is common due to device technical failures, despite correct positioning. Nonetheless, in this paper, epiglottic downfolding was the most

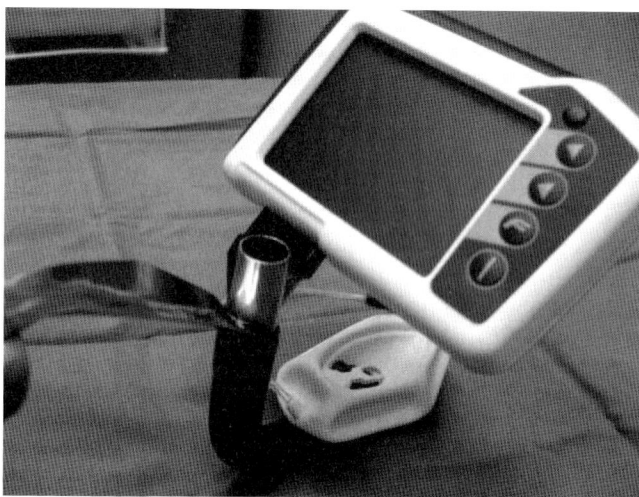

Fig. 12.9 CTrach laryngeal mask airway. Source: Timmermann *et al. Br J Anaesth* 2006; **96**: 516–21.

common reason for poor glottic views. Despite this finding, ventilation was not an issue. When full view of the glottis was obtained, the first attempt success rate was high. Although the manoeuvres described help to achieve a full view of the glottis, they are not universally successful. These manoeuvres may also be applicable to the Fastrach. In clinical practice, it would be difficult to determine which manoeuvre to use without performing fibreoptic laryngoscopy to diagnose the cause of the poor CTrach view. Additionally, the up–down manoeuvre may have to be performed more than once to retract the epiglottis back up with the cuff of the CTrach.

Direct laryngoscopic views had no bearing in obtaining a difficult glottic view with the CTrach. This may be because laryngoscopy was performed in the sniffing position and the CTrach was placed in the neutral position. The patient population in this study had modest body mass indexes (BMIs); only 16 patients exhibited a C-L grade 3 view and none exhibited a grade 4 view. It is worth noting that in obese patients redundant airway tissue often collapses in front of the glottic opening and ventilation through the tube during the procedure can help in visualizing the glottis.

Other manoeuvres that may help include changing the patient position from neutral to sniffing position, changing the size of the CTrach and using the tracheal tube to raise the epiglottic elevator in an attempt to flip the downfolded epiglottis. Although this manoeuvre is successful about 50% of the time, the authors discourage this method for fear of causing glottic trauma.

Conclusion

Fibreoptic laryngoscope-type equipment is generally easier to use than other fibreoptic intubation adjuncts. It has been shown to improve glottic views in general, but the improved view may or may not correlate with increased intubation success. Nevertheless, this type of equipment is extremely useful for teaching purposes and enables assistants to see the effects of their external laryngeal manipulation. Disposability, as with the Airtraq and the AWS, is advantageous in terms of preventing disease transmission.

Fibreoptic *stylets* have been shown to be useful for difficult intubations in case series and manikin studies. These devices can be used alone or in conjunction with a laryngoscope. Their rigid design aims to avoid the rotational and lateral steering difficulties associated with the flexible fibreoptic scope. As such, all of the rigid fibreoptic stylets are restricted from nasal intubation but at the same time have the ability to manoeuvre around collapsed or oedematous tissues.

The CTrach is unique in that oxygenation and ventilation are possible during the process of intubation, thus improving the safety profile of this device. Although rescue manoeuvres have been developed to improve visualization of the glottis, poor views continue to occur and lead to an increased chance of intubation failure. One unique feature of the CTrach, compared with any other fibreoptic intubation adjunct, is the ability to perform the intubation blindly when visualization is not possible. Nonetheless, blind intubation is still associated with a higher failure rate.

Despite the advent of fibreoptic intubation adjuncts, flexible fibreoptic laryngoscopy and direct laryngoscopy remain the mainstay of airway management. However, even in the best of hands, both have failed when used alone or in conjunction with alternative techniques or devices. The fibreoptic adjuncts described in this chapter attempt to bridge the gap between the standard rigid laryngoscope and the flexible fibreoptic laryngoscope and will most likely multiply and continue to be modified in the future. Rigid indirect laryngoscopes, optical stylets and intubating laryngeal masks can facilitate rapid tracheal intubation in both normal and difficult airways. All anaesthesiologists should develop and maintain skills in one or more of these alternative techniques. Video techniques, in general, have improved enormously in the last decade, with smaller cameras producing higher-quality images. Suitable devices should be available wherever anaesthesia is administered and all anaesthesiologists should develop skill in their use.

References

1. Yentis SM, Lee DJ. Evaluation of an improved scoring system for the grading of direct laryngoscopy. *Anaesthesia* 1998; **53**: 1041–4.

2. Kaplan MB, Ward D, Hagberg CA, Berci G, Hagiike M. Seeing is believing: the importance of video laryngoscopy in teaching and in managing the difficult airway. *Surg Endosc* 2006; **20** (Suppl 2): S479–S483.

3. Levitan RM, Ochroch EA, Kush S, Shofer FS, Hollander JE. Assessment of airway visualization: validation of the percentage of glotttic opening (POGO) scale. *Acad Emerg Med* 1998; **5**: 919–23.

4. Hung O, Murphy M. Unanticipated difficult intubation. *Curr Opin Anaesthesiol* 2004; **17**: 479–81.

5. Maharaj CH, Costello JF, Higgins BD, Harte BH, Laffey JG. Learning and performance of tracheal intubation by novice personnel: a comparison of the Airtraq® and Macintosh laryngoscope. *Anaesthesia* 2006; **61**: 671–7.

6. Maharaj CH, Higgins BD, Harte BH, Laffey JG. Evaluation of intubation using the Airtraq or Macintosh laryngoscope by anaesthetists in easy and simulated difficult laryngoscopy – a mannikin study. *Anaesthesia* 2006; **61**: 469–77.

7. Halligan M, Charters P. A clinical evaluation of the Bonfils Intubation Fibrescope. *Anaesthesia* 2003; **58**: 1087–91.

8. Rose DK, Cohen MM. The incidence of airway problems depends on the definition used. *Can J Anaesth* 1996; **43**: 30–4.

9. Heath KJ. The effect on laryngscopy of different cervical spine immobilization techniques. *Anaesthesia* 1994; **49**: 843–5.

10. Maurtua MA, Maurtua DB, Zura A, Doyle JD. Improving intubation success using the CTrach Laryngeal Mask Airway™. *Anesthesiology* 2007; **106**: 640–1.

Part IV

Critical care

Vasopressin and its analogues in critical care – do they live up to expectations?

SARAH MITCHELL, JENNIFER HUNTER

Why use vasopressin?

In acute medical practice, anaesthetists are familiar with the use of vasopressin analogues such as desmopressin to treat diabetes insipidus and bleeding disorders such as von Willebrand disease, or to prevent further haemorrhage from oesophageal varices (with terlipressin). Organ donation teams use vasopressin as a supplementary vasopressor to reduce inotrope requirements in potential donors |1|. Does vasopressin have any advantages as a vasopressor? The normal plasma concentration is 4 pg/ml, which is sufficient to produce its osmotic effect, but to exert a vasopressor effect levels of 10–200 pg/ml are required |2|. Relative vasopressin insufficiency has been found after 36 h in patients with septic shock |3|. In vasodilatory septic shock, plasma vasopressin levels averaged only 3.1 ± 1.0 pg/ml compared with 22.7 ± 2.2 pg/ml in patients with cardiogenic shock |4|. During treatment for septic and other vasodilatory shock states, catecholamine hyposensitivity can occur. Vasopressin is used as an adjunct to ongoing catecholamine therapy to improve vital organ blood flow, especially to the kidney, and to limit the doses of catecholamines. It also stimulates cortisol production |5|. For these reasons, it can be used as a second-line vasopressor in vasodilatory shock |6|; however, evidence relating to improved survival is scarce. The treatment of haemorrhagic shock unresponsive to intravenous fluids is another potential area for the use of vasopressin.

Renal effects

One of the most significant beneficial effects of vasopressin is on the renal circulation, with animal studies showing a preservation of renal function compared with noradrenaline |7| and an improvement in creatinine clearance |8,9|. It is speculated that the improvement is secondary to selective afferent arteriolar vasodilatation mediated by nitric oxide, and selective efferent vasoconstriction |10|.

Terlipressin

Tricyl-lysine-vasopressin is a synthetic analogue of vasopressin. It is thought to divert blood away from the splanchnic circulation to improve renal blood flow |11|. In one review from the Cochrane database on its use in hepatorenal syndrome (HRS), mortality at 14 days was reduced by 34% |12|. A meta-analysis of terlipressin therapy in HRS showed it to be efficacious and safe, but a significant number of patients who initially responded, relapsed after stopping the drug |13|. Terlipressin has also been used to treat intractable hypotension secondary to sepsis |14,15|.

Physiology

Vasopressin, also known as antidiuretic hormone, is a nonapeptide synthesized in the hypothalamus as a pro-hormone and secreted from the posterior pituitary gland. Its most important role is in fluid balance. It is released in response to an increased plasma osmolality and hypovolaemia. It increases water reabsorption through the collecting ducts in the nephron.

Vasopressin can also have cardiovascular effects, especially in haemodynamically unstable patients. With normal functioning of the renin–angiotensin and sympathetic nervous systems, endogenous vasopressin is not crucial for blood pressure stability |16|. Vasopressin secretion is stimulated by arterial hypotension and severe hypovolaemia |17|, which are detected by baroreceptors in the aortic arch and carotid sinus. Its release is inhibited by firing of stretch receptors in the left atrium and aortic arch.

Vasopressin is similar in structure to oxytocin, differing in only two out of nine amino acids (Figure 1). At low concentrations, vasopressin has been shown to act at oxytocin receptors activating nitric oxide release to cause vasodilatation in pulmonary arteries, the umbilical vein and the aorta |18|. It has been postulated that this may make vasopressin a useful agent in cardiac arrest associated with pulmonary hypertension |19|.

Vasopressin receptors

Vasopressin acts at three types of receptors in the body – V_{1a}, V_2 and V_3 (previously known as V_{1b}) receptors (Table 1). These receptors are coupled to G-proteins for signal transduction. V_{1a} and V_3 receptors are linked with Gq proteins causing phospholipase C stimulation, which in turn activates inositol triphosphate and the release of intracellular calcium. V_{1a} receptors are found in platelets and in vascular smooth muscle, where stimulation causes vasoconstriction. These are thought to be primarily responsible for the vasopressor effects of vasopressin. Terlipressin is a specific V_{1a} receptor agonist. V_3 receptors are found in the central nervous system, and are involved in the secretion of corticotrophin-releasing hormone from the anterior pituitary gland. V_2 receptors lie within the collecting duct of the kidney

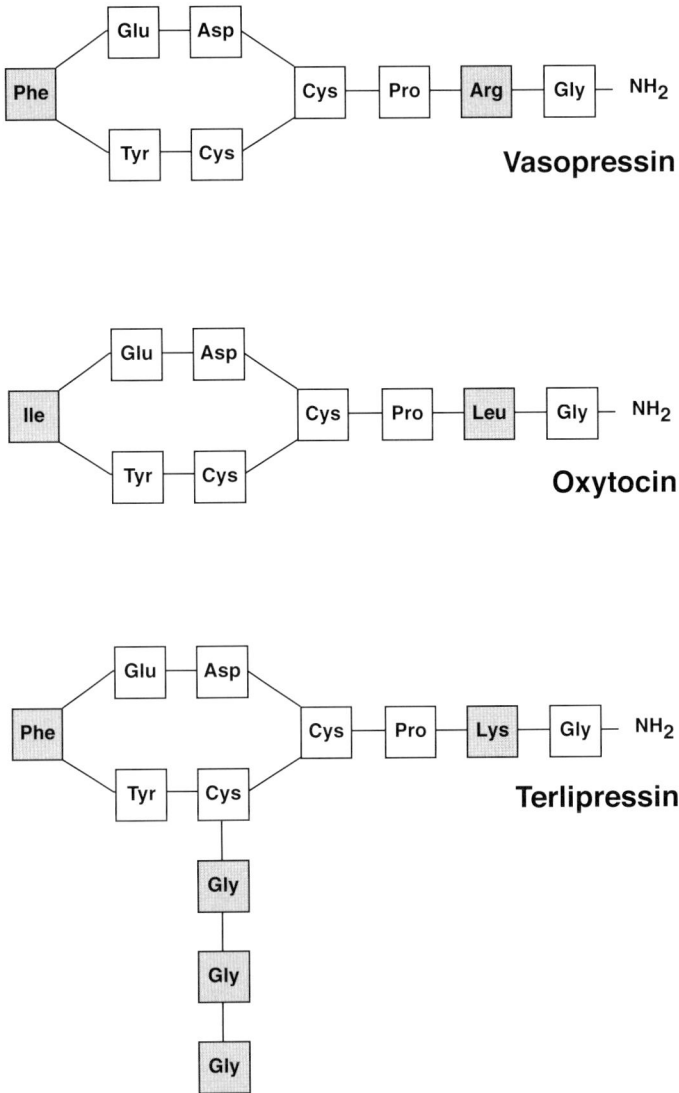

Fig. 1 The structure of vasopressin, oxytocin and terlipressin. The shaded amino acids mark the differing structure of the polypeptides.

and modulate water reabsorption. Stimulation of V_2 receptors is mediated by Gs proteins, which, via adenylate cyclase, results in increased levels of cyclic adenosine monophosphate (cAMP) and increased water absorption |16|.

Table 1 A comparison of the three types of vasopressin receptor

Receptor	V$_{1a}$	V$_2$	V$_3$ (previously V$_{1b}$)
Location	Vascular smooth muscle Platelets Liver Central nervous system	Collecting duct of kidney	Central nervous system
Signal transduction	Gq protein	Gs protein	Gq protein
Effects of stimulation	Vasoconstriction	Increased water absorption	Secretion of corticotrophin-releasing hormone

Adapted with permission from Treschan and Peters. *Anesthesiology* 2006; **105**: 599–612.

Clinical use

Vasopressin must be given parenterally as it is hydrolysed by trypsin if given orally. An intravenous dose exerts its effects within 6 min. It has a short plasma half life of between 10 and 30 min as it is metabolized by peptidases in the liver and kidney |20|. It is usually given as an infusion: a fixed rate of between 0.01 and 0.04 iu/min i.v. is recommended in adult patients. In cardiac arrest and haemorrhagic shock it has also been given as a bolus of 40 iu i.v. (Table 2). A vial of vasopressin 20 iu costs £20. The price of terlipressin is similar.

Terlipressin has a much longer half life of 6 h and is generally given as a bolus (1–2 mg i.v., 4-hourly). In addition to its use in patients with varices or HRS (Table 2), a study is under way looking at a low-dose terlipressin infusion (1.3 µg/kg/h) compared with an infusion of vasopressin in 30 patients with septic shock (www.ClinicalTrials.gov/ct/show/NCT00481572).

Cardiac arrest

During cardiac arrest, levels of many stress hormones (including cortisol) rise. Increased endogenous vasopressin levels during CPR are associated with a better outcome |21|. Vasopressin stimulates the release of corticotrophin-releasing hormone, increasing cortisol levels |22|, which may be one mechanism for its effect. Vasopressor effects may also improve vital organ perfusion |21|.

The 2005 American Heart Association Guidelines for Cardiopulmonary Resuscitation suggest that, as the effects of vasopressin have not been shown to differ from those of epinephrine in cardiac arrest, one dose (40 iu i.v.) can be given instead of the second dose of epinephrine (Table 2) |23|. The European Resuscitation Guidelines, for the same reasons, do not include vasopressin in the 2005 Guidelines on Adult Life Support |24|.

Table 2 The indications for and doses of vasopressin and its analogues. Source: Treschan and Peters. *Anesthesiology* 2006; **105**: 599–612.

Drug	Indication	Dose	Comment
Arginine vasopressin	CPR in adults	40 iu i.v. bolus may replace second dose of adrenaline	2005 AHA Guidelines on CPR, no recommendation for use in children
	Haemorrhagic shock	From 0.04 iu/min to 40 iu bolus i.v.	Few case reports published Trial under way (www.vitris.at)
	Refractory hypotension in septic shock	0.01–0.04 iu/min i.v.	Doses above 0.1 iu/min may increase serious side-effects
	Vasodilatory shock after cardiopulmonary bypass	0.1 iu/min i.v.	
	Anaesthesia for neuroendocrine tumours	10–20 iu bolus i.v. plus 0.1 iu/min	Case reports published
	Anaphylactic shock	Range 2–40 iu bolus	Few case reports published Must be combined with adrenaline
Terlipressin	Bleeding from oesophageal varices in portal hypertension	1–2 mg i.v. every 4–6 h	Evidence for efficacy, 34% relative risk reduction in mortality
	Hepatorenal syndrome	1–2 mg i.v. every 4–6 h	Several small non-randomized studies with consistent results of improved renal function and systemic haemodynamics
	Refractory hypotension in septic shock	1–2 mg i.v. every 4–6 h	One prospective study comparing terlipressin with noradrenaline, effects on outcome not yet evaluated
	Refractory intraoperative hypotension	1 mg i.v.	Three clinical trials with total of 60 patients; one case report on myocardial ischaemia after terlipressin application
Desmopressin	Von Willebrand disease and haemophilia A	0.3 µg/kg i.v.	Clinical use since 1977 and clear evidence for efficacy
	Diabetes insipidus	5–40 µg nasally or 1–4 µg i.v. (in 24 h) or 0.3–0.6 mg p.o. (in 24 h)	Clinical use since 1976 and clear evidence for efficacy

The largest multicentre trial of vasopressin |25| provoked much discussion |26–28|. The double-blinded study recruited 1186 patients with out-of-hospital cardiac arrests. Patients were randomized to receive two doses of either vasopressin 40 iu i.v. or adrenaline 1 mg i.v.. There was an improvement in rate of survival to hospital admission and subsequent discharge in asystolic patients treated with vasopressin compared with those treated with epinephrine (hospital admission rate 29.0% vs. 20.3%; $P=0.02$; hospital discharge rate 4.7% vs. 1.5%, $P=0.04$). It is interesting to note the very low survival rate in either group. In contrast to the asystolic patients, no benefit was seen in patients with ventricular fibrillation or pulseless electrical activity from vasopressin, although previous studies had shown an improvement with it |29|. However, analysis of a subgroup of patients who received vasopressin followed by adrenaline showed a significant improvement in rates of survival to hospital admission and discharge compared with epinephrine alone (25.7% vs. 16.4%; $P=0.002$: 6.2% vs. 1.7%; $P=0.002$, respectively) |25|.

This has led to interest in the combination of vasopressin and epinephrine in treating cardiac arrest. An observational study in 2007 showed that a combination of vasopressin and adrenaline during CPR in patients with asystole improved short-term survival, neurological outcome and hospital discharge rate |30|. A large European trial recruited over 2000 patients comparing the combination of vasopressin and adrenaline with adrenaline alone in out of hospital cardiac arrests (www.ClinicalTrials.gov/ct/show/NCT00127907) and we await the results.

The American College of Emergency Physicians in 2006 concluded that there was insufficient evidence to establish a benefit of vasopressin over adrenaline in increasing survival to discharge or improving neurological outcome in adult patients with non-traumatic cardiac arrest |31|. At present, despite some early promising results, there is conflicting evidence: the consensus on the use of vasopressin during cardiac arrest is that there is little advantage to changing current practice.

Haemorrhagic shock

Current opinion is also divided on the early treatment of haemorrhagic shock with vasopressin. Strategies for limiting blood loss remain controversial and include limited or hypotensive resuscitation, and the use of hypertonic solutions |32,33|. Several animal studies and human case reports have discussed the use of vasopressin in such circumstances: there is a large European trial (VITRIS: a multicentre, randomized, controlled trial assessing arginine vasopressin vs. saline placebo in refractory traumatic haemorrhagic shock) starting to look into this indication |34|.

A study in pigs compared colloid resuscitation with saline resuscitation or vasopressin alone after initiation of haemorrhagic shock. Group 1 received vasopressin 0.4 iu/kg followed by a vasopressin infusion; group 2 Ringer's lactate 25 ml/kg and 25 ml/kg of gelatin solution; and in the control group 3, only an equal volume of saline was given. After 30 min, any haemodynamically stable pigs had the haemorrhage controlled surgically. All the vasopressin pigs survived until bleeding was surgically controlled yet none of the pigs in either fluid group survived to that point. The authors concluded that vasopressin may help by diverting blood away from the injury and improving flow to vital organs |35|.

A randomized controlled trial compared outcome in pigs following traumatic brain injury and haemorrhagic shock treated after 20 min with vasopressin or a saline bolus. All five vasopressin pigs survived but only two out of five pigs in the saline group survived to 300 min |36|. A possible mechanism is that vasopressin prevented hypotension and reduced fluid requirements, helping to preserve blood flow to the brain.

Case reports (level 3 evidence) also highlight the use of vasopressin in haemorrhagic shock which is unresponsive to fluid therapy. Two patients, who bled unexpectedly during abdominal surgery and had long periods of prolonged hypotension unresponsive to fluid therapy and catecholamine infusions, were managed successfully with the addition of an infusion of vasopressin 0.04 iu/min |37|.

Septic shock

There is a high frequency of sepsis in the critically ill. In Europe, the intensive care mortality from septic shock is 54% |38|. An Austrian study found a relative vasopressin deficiency (< 10 pg/ml) in 22% of septic shock patients |39|. Primarily, the elevation in blood pressure with vasopressin is due to vasoconstriction in vascular smooth muscle increasing systemic vascular resistance. Vasopressin may also interfere with nitric oxide signalling, and inactivate K-ATP channels: both mechanisms are involved in the vasodilatation of septic shock |2|. Very low concentrations of vasopressin (10^{-9} mol/l) in laboratory studies have been shown to work synergistically with catecholamines, causing vasoconstriction |40|. A reduction in vasopressin responsiveness has been demonstrated in rats with septic shock and the authors suggest that progressive stimulation of the nitric oxide relaxation pathway may contribute to this hyporesponsiveness |40|.

The Surviving Sepsis Guidelines published in 2004 (currently under review) provide structured plans for the initial and ongoing treatment of patients with septic shock. This advice is given: 'Vasopressin use may be considered in patients with refractory shock despite adequate fluid resuscitation and high-dose conventional vasopressors. It is not recommended as a first line agent. If used in adults it should be infused at a rate of 0.01–0.04 U/min. It may decrease stroke volume' |6|.

The vasopressin dilemma

Vasopressin is increasingly acknowledged as an adjunct vasopressor in catecholamine-resistant shock states |41|, but there is a dilemma about when to start administration. A retrospective study in Austria suggested that mortality rapidly increases if noradrenaline dosages exceed 0.6 μg/kg/min before vasopressin is commenced |**42**|.

The Vasopressin and Septic Shock Trial (VASST Study), which was completed in 2006 from intensive care units across Canada and Australia, studied 779 patients with septic shock already receiving an infusion of noradrenaline. This study blindly randomized patients to a supplementary infusion of either vasopressin (at a rate of 0.03 iu/min i.v.) or a second noradrenaline infusion. Initial results suggest vasopressin reduced 28-day and 90-day mortality in those patients with less severe (noradrenaline infusion at < 15 μg/kg/min on enrolment) septic shock (26.5% vs. 35.7%, $P = 0.05$, and 35.8% vs. 46.1%, $P = 0.04$, respectively) |**43**|.

Side-effects of vasopressin

There have been concerns over the side-effects of vasopressin. Doses higher than 0.04 iu/min have been associated with myocardial ischaemia, a reduction in cardiac output and cardiac arrest |**6**|. But it is interesting that in one prospective trial patients on high-dose noradrenaline infusions developed significantly more tachyarrhythmias than those on a supplementary vasopressin infusion |**44**|.

Several studies have found that, although fluid resuscitation with vasopressin slowed cardiovascular collapse, it led to lactic acidaemia and a reduction in cardiac index when compared with fluid resuscitation alone |**36,45**|. In a retrospective study of an infusion of vasopressin 4 iu/h (equivalent to 0.067 iu/min), cardiac index decreased in patients with a hyperdynamic circulation (from 5.4 l/min/m² before vasopressin therapy to 4.9 l/min/m² after 72 h of treatment), but it remained unchanged in patients with a normal cardiac index (from 3.1 l/min/m² to 3.0 l/min/m²) |**42**|. The authors noted a decrease in central venous pressure and increase in stroke volume index despite significant reductions in inotropic support, suggesting that low-dose vasopressin improves cardiac performance. Mechanisms of improved myocardial performance include an increase in myocardial calcium concentration and increased myocardial blood flow |**42,44**|.

With the hypothesized diversion of blood away from the splanchnic circulation, it is not surprising that increased bilirubin levels and raised liver enzymes have been reported in patients treated with vasopressin |**46**|. In one retrospective study of 316 intensive care patients, those with a raised serum bilirubin were more likely to die, but an increase in liver enzymes made no difference to mortality |**42**|.

Treatment with vasopressin can lead to ischaemic lesions peripherally – in 30% of patients in one study |**47**|. Although such lesions often develop more rapidly with vasopressin, the incidence was not found to be significantly different between patients with septic shock treated with noradrenaline alone or treated with both vasopressin and noradrenaline |**44**|.

Animal studies have suggested that vasopressin alone causes significant gut hypoperfusion |**8,48**|. In contrast, a retrospective study in intensive therapy unit

(ITU) patients comparing supplemental vasopressin infusion with noradrenaline infusion alone in vasodilatory shock found evidence of mesenteric occlusion in only 4.3% of patients treated with vasopressin at post mortem |**42**|, confirming reports that gastrointestinal perfusion was improved in patients with vasodilatory shock treated with vasopressin and noradrenaline compared with noradrenaline alone |**44**|.

There is concern that the use of vasopressin may exacerbate gut hypoperfusion in haemorrhagic shock. A small observational study in pigs treated with vasopressin during uncontrolled haemorrhage produced diarrhoea 3 h after treatment in all eight pigs, which resolved by 24 h. One week after the experiment, samples of gut, liver and kidney demonstrated no histopathological changes |**49**|. This study used vasopressin alone in high doses for a period of 30 min in healthy pigs – it remains to be seen whether further studies can demonstrate a similar lack of side-effects.

Conclusion

Vasopressin has recently been studied extensively in the critically ill. Evidence suggests that we should use it as a second-line vasopressor in vasodilatory shock at low doses. Selective vasodilatation and vasoconstriction in differing vascular beds produce a beneficial effect on the kidney. In contrast, there is insufficient evidence for the use of vasopressin in cardiac arrest, although it is not contraindicated |**50**|. The early results on vasopressin as an adjunct in haemorrhagic shock are promising and we look forward to the results of the Canadian study (http://www.vitris.at).

References

1. Kutsogiannis DJ, Pagliarello G, Doig C, Ross H, Shemie SD. Medical management to optimize donor organ potential: review of the literature. *Can J Anaesth* 2006; **53**: 820–30.

2. Landry DW, Oliver JA. The pathogenesis of vasodilatory shock. *N Engl J Med* 2001; **345**: 588–95.

3. Sharshar T, Blanchard A, Paillard M, Raphael JC, Gajdos P, Annane D. Circulating vasopressin levels in septic shock. *Crit Care Med* 2003; **31**: 1752–8.

4. Landry DW, Levin HR, Gallant EM, Ashton RC Jr, Seo S, D'Alessandro D, Oz MC, Oliver JA. Vasopressin deficiency contributes to the vasodilation of septic shock. *Circulation* 1997; **95**: 1122–5.

5. Antoni FA. Vasopressinergic control of pituitary adrenocorticotropin secretion comes of age. *Front Neuroendocrinol* 1993; **14**: 76–122.

6. Dellinger RP, Carlet JM, Masur H, Gerlach H, Calandra T, Cohen J, *et al.* Surviving Sepsis Campaign guidelines for management of severe sepsis and septic shock. *Intensive Care Med* 2004; **30**: 536–55.

7. Levy B, Vallee C, Lauzier F, Plante GE, Mansart A, Mallie JP, Lesur O. Comparative effects of vasopressin, norepinephrine, and L-canavanine, a selective inhibitor of inducible nitric oxide synthase, in endotoxic shock. *Am J Physiol Heart Circ Physiol* 2004; **287**: H209–15.

8. Di GD, Morimatsu H, Bellomo R, May CN. Effect of low-dose vasopressin infusion on vital organ blood flow in the conscious normal and septic sheep. *Anaesth Intensive Care* 2006; **34**: 427–33.

9. Lauzier F, Levy B, Lamarre P, Lesur O. Vasopressin or norepinephrine in early hyperdynamic septic shock: a randomized clinical trial. *Intensive Care Med* 2006; **32**: 1782–9.

10. Guzman JA, Rosado AE, Kruse JA. Vasopressin versus norepinephrine in endotoxic shock: systemic, renal, and splanchnic hemodynamic and oxygen transport effects. *J Appl Physiol* 2003; **95**: 803–9.

11. Ortega R, Gines P, Uriz J, Cardenas A, Calahorra B, De Las HD, *et al.* Terlipressin therapy with and without albumin for patients with hepatorenal syndrome: results of a prospective, nonrandomized study. *Hepatology* 2002; **36**: 941–8.

12. Gluud LL, Kjaer MS, Christensen E. Terlipressin for hepatorenal syndrome. *Cochrane Database Syst Rev* 2006 (4): CD005162.

13. Fabrizi F, Dixit V, Martin P. Meta-analysis: terlipressin therapy for the hepatorenal syndrome. *Aliment Pharmacol Ther* 2006; **24**: 935–44.

14. O'Brien A, Clapp L, Singer M. Terlipressin for norepinephrine-resistant septic shock. *Lancet* 2002; **359**: 1209–10.

15. Leone M, Albanese J, Delmas A, Chaabane W, Garnier F, Martin C. Terlipressin in catecholamine-resistant septic shock patients. *Shock* 2004; **22**: 314–19.

16. Treschan TA, Peters J. The vasopressin system: physiology and clinical strategies. *Anesthesiology* 2006; **105**: 599–612.

17. Bisset GW, Chowdrey HS. Control of release of vasopressin by neuroendocrine reflexes. *Q J Exp Physiol* 1988; **73**: 811–72.

18. Thibonnier M, Preston JA, Dulin N, Wilkins PL, Berti-Mattera LN, Mattera R. The human V3 pituitary vasopressin receptor: ligand binding profile and density-dependent signaling pathways. *Endocrinology* 1997; **138**: 4109–22.

19. Smith AM, Elliot CM, Kiely DG, Channer KS. The role of vasopressin in cardiorespiratory arrest and pulmonary hypertension. *QJM* 2006; **99**: 127–33.

20. Ferguson JW, Therapondos G, Newby DE, Hayes PC. Therapeutic role of vasopressin receptor antagonism in patients with liver cirrhosis. *Clin Sci (Lond)* 2003; **105**: 1–8.

21. Lindner KH, Haak T, Keller A, Bothner U, Lurie KG. Release of endogenous vasopressors during and after cardiopulmonary resuscitation. *Heart* 1996; **75**: 145–50.

22. Kornberger E, Prengel AW, Krismer A, Schwarz B, Wenzel V, Lindner KH, Mair P. Vasopressin-mediated adrenocorticotropin release increases plasma cortisol concentrations during cardiopulmonary resuscitation. *Crit Care Med* 2000; **28**: 3517–21.

23. 2005 American Heart Association Guidelines for Cardiopulmonary Resuscitation and Emergency Cardiovascular Care. *Circulation* 2005; **112**: IV1–203.

24. Nolan JP, Deakin CD, Soar J, Bottiger BW, Smith G. European Resuscitation Council guidelines for resuscitation 2005. Section 4. Adult advanced life support. *Resuscitation* 2005; **67**: S39–86.

25. Wenzel V, Krismer AC, Arntz HR, Sitter H, Stadlbauer KH, Lindner KH. A comparison of vasopressin and epinephrine for out-of-hospital cardiopulmonary resuscitation. *N Engl J Med* 2004; **350**: 105–13.

26. Aberegg SK. Vasopressin versus epinephrine for cardiopulmonary resuscitation (letter to editor re. Wenzel *et al.* 2004). *N Engl J Med* 2004; **350**: 2207.

27. Ballew KA. Vasopressin versus epinephrine for cardiopulmonary resuscitation (letter to editor re. Wenzel *et al.* 2004). *N Engl J Med* 2004; **350**: 2207.

28. Nolan JP, Nadkarni V, Montgomery WH. Vasopressin versus epinephrine for cardiopulmonary resuscitation (letter to editor re. Wenzel *et al.* 2004). *N Engl J Med* 2004; **350**: 2206.

29. Lindner KH, Dirks B, Strohmenger HU, Prengel AW, Lindner IM, Lurie KG. Randomised comparison of epinephrine and vasopressin in patients with out-of-hospital ventricular fibrillation. *Lancet* 1997; **349**: 535–7.

30. Mally S, Jelatancev A, Grmec S. Effects of epinephrine and vasopressin on end-tidal carbon dioxide tension and mean arterial blood pressure in out-of-hospital cardiopulmonary resuscitation: an observational study. *Crit Care* 2007; **11**: R39.

31. Wyer PC, Perera P, Jin Z, Zhou Q, Cook DJ, Walter SD, *et al.* Vasopressin or epinephrine for out-of-hospital cardiac arrest. *Ann Emerg Med* 2006; **48**: 86–97.

32. Tyagi R, Donaldson K, Loftus CM, Jallo J. Hypertonic saline: a clinical review. *Neurosurg Rev* 2007; **30**: 277–89.

33. Heier HE, Bugge W, Hjelmeland K, Soreide E, Sorlie D, Haheim LL. Transfusion versus. alternative treatment modalities in acute bleeding: a systematic review. *Acta Anaesthesiol Scand* 2006; **50**: 920–31.

34. Lienhart HG, Wenzel V, Braun J, Dorges V, Dunser M, Gries A, *et al.* Vasopressin for therapy of persistent traumatic hemorrhagic shock: The VITRIS.at study. *Anaesthesist* 2007; **56**: 145–50.

35. Stadlbauer KH, Wagner-Berger HG, Raedler C, Voelckel WG, Wenzel V, Krismer AC, *et al.* Vasopressin, but not fluid resuscitation, enhances survival in a liver trauma model with uncontrolled and otherwise lethal hemorrhagic shock in pigs. *Anesthesiology* 2003; **98**: 699–704.

36. Sanui M, King DR, Feinstein AJ, Varon AJ, Cohn SM, Proctor KG. Effects of arginine vasopressin during resuscitation from hemorrhagic hypotension after traumatic brain injury. *Crit Care Med* 2006; **34**: 433–8.

37. Sharma RM, Setlur R. Vasopressin in hemorrhagic shock. *Anesth Analg* 2005; **101**: 833–4.

38. Vincent JL, Sakr Y, Sprung CL, Ranieri VM, Reinhart K, Gerlach H, *et al.* Sepsis in European intensive care units: results of the SOAP study. *Crit Care Med* 2006; **34**: 344–53.

39. Jochberger S, Mayr VD, Luckner G, Wenzel V, Ulmer H, Schmid S, *et al.* Serum vasopressin concentrations in critically ill patients. *Crit Care Med* 2006; **34**: 293–9.

40. Leone M, Boyle WA. Decreased vasopressin responsiveness in vasodilatory septic shock-like conditions. *Crit Care Med* 2006; **34**: 1126–30.

41. Dunser MW, Lindner KH, Wenzel V. A century of arginine vasopressin research leading to new therapeutic strategies. *Anesthesiology* 2006; **105**: 444–5.

42. Luckner G, Dunser MW, Jochberger S, Mayr VD, Wenzel V, Ulmer H, *et al.* Arginine vasopressin in 316 patients with advanced vasodilatory shock. *Crit Care Med* 2005; **33**: 2659–66.

43. Russell JA, Walley KR, Singer J, Gordon AC, Hebert P, Cooper J, *et al.* A randomised controlled trial of low dose vasopressin versus norepinephrine infusion in patients who have septic shock. *Am J Resp Crit Care Med* 2007; **175**: A508.

44. Dunser MW, Mayr AJ, Ulmer H, Knotzer H, Sumann G, Pajk W, *et al.* Arginine vasopressin in advanced vasodilatory shock: a prospective, randomized, controlled study. *Circulation* 2003; **107**: 2313–19.

45. Johnson KB, Pearce FJ, Jeffreys N, McJames SW, Cluff M. Impact of vasopressin on hemodynamic and metabolic function in the decompensatory phase of hemorrhagic shock. *J Cardiothorac Vasc Anesth* 2006; **20**: 167–72.

46. Dunser MW, Mayr AJ, Ulmer H, Ritsch N, Knotzer H, Pajk W, *et al.* The effects of vasopressin on systemic hemodynamics in catecholamine-resistant septic and postcardiotomy shock: a retrospective analysis. *Anesth Analg* 2001; **93**: 7–13.

47. Dunser MW, Mayr AJ, Tur A, Pajk W, Barbara F, Knotzer H, *et al.* Ischemic skin lesions as a complication of continuous vasopressin infusion in catecholamine-resistant vasodilatory shock: incidence and risk factors. *Crit Care Med* 2003; **31**: 1394–8.

48. Hiltebrand LB, Krejci V, Jakob SM, Takala J, Sigurdsson GH. Effects of vasopressin on microcirculatory blood flow in the gastrointestinal tract in anesthetized pigs in septic shock. *Anesthesiology* 2007; **106**: 1156–67.

49. Stadlbauer KH, Wenzel V, Wagner-Berger HG, Krismer AC, Konigsrainer A, Voelckel WG, *et al.* An observational study of vasopressin infusion during uncontrolled haemorrhagic shock in a porcine trauma model: effects on bowel function. *Resuscitation* 2007; **72**: 145–8.

50. Mitchell SLM, Hunter JM. Vasopressin and its antagonists: what are their roles in acute medical care? *Br J Anaesth* 2007; **99**: 154–8.

13

Serious medical errors in intensive care

AMY FAHRENKOPF, CHRISTOPHER LANDRIGAN

Introduction

In its groundbreaking 1999 report, *To Err is Human*, the Institute of Medicine estimated that adverse events due to medical errors cause 44 000–98 000 deaths each year in the United States |1|, making medical error the sixth to ninth leading cause of death in America. Subsequent studies have found adverse events to be common throughout the industrialized world |2,3|, including the UK, where they occur in more than 10% of all hospital admissions |4|.

Adverse events due to medical errors have long been recognized to be particularly common in critical care settings, where patients are most fragile, and where the frequency of intensive interventions is highest. Early chart review studies identified frequent harms due to care |5–7|, but the full magnitude of the problem was not recognized until the advent of direct observational studies. In 1995, Donchin *et al.* conducted a groundbreaking study in an Israeli ICU in which errors were detected by continuous direct observation, supplemented by staff reports |8|. An average of 1.7 errors per patient per day were discovered, 46% of which were attributable to physicians. In Rothschild *et al.*'s 2005 Critical Care Safety Study |9|, direct 24-h-per-day observation of interns in two critical care units was combined with daily chart review, solicitation of reports from clinical staff and computerized detection of adverse events to comprehensively capture serious errors in care; 80.5 adverse events, 36.2 preventable adverse events and 149.7 serious errors were detected per 1000 patient-days. Sixty-one per cent of serious medical errors occurred in the delivery of treatments, including medications; 53% were due to slips and lapses in the execution of routine tasks, rather than knowledge-based mistakes |9|. As the high incidence of error in intensive care has been recognized, a series of intervention studies have been conducted in an effort to identify ways to improve the safety of critical care. Implementation of computerized physician order entry (CPOE), ward-based clinical pharmacists and reduction in provider work hours have each been shown to substantially reduce the incidence of serious medical errors. Bates *et al.* found that implementation of a CPOE system led to an initial 55% reduction, and an eventual 81% reduction, in serious medical errors |10,11|, a finding that has been substantiated repeatedly |**12–15**|. Leape and colleagues found that the involvement of clinical pharmacists in ICU rounds led to a 66% decrease in the incidence of preventable adverse drug events in the ICU |**16**|. In a randomized controlled trial, the Harvard Work Hours, Health, and Safety Group found that implementation of a schedule that eliminated the traditional 24-h work shifts of interns led to a substantial reduction in serious medical errors in the critical care setting. Overall, interns working traditional 24- to 30-h shifts suffered twice as many polysomnographically documented attentional failures at night and made 36% more serious medical errors and 460% more serious diagnostic errors than those whose scheduled work was limited to 16 consecutive hours |**17,18**|.

In this chapter, we will review how the state of the science of ICU patient safety has continued to advance from 2006 through 2007 by discussing 10 key studies. The past year has seen the identification of new safety hazards in the ICU, publication of multicentre studies of critical care safety and the development of novel interventions to improve care. These studies serve to illustrate the breadth and depth of research being conducted regarding critical care safety, and suggest how intensivists and hospital leaders may take concrete steps towards improving the safety and quality of care.

Patient safety in intensive care: results from the multinational Sentinel Events Evaluation (SEE) study

Valentin A, Capuzzo M, Guidet B, *et al. Intensive Care Med* 2006; **32**: 1591–8

BACKGROUND. This observational, cross-sectional study sought to assess the prevalence of sentinel events affecting patient safety in ICUs on a multinational level, and to identify factors associated with these events. Conducted in 205 ICUs worldwide (Table 13.1) over a 24-h period of time, the SEE study asked nurses and physicians on duty during the time of the study to fill out questionnaires at the bedside of all patients, reporting the time and nature of sentinel events. The questionnaires were anonymous and did not ask about the outcome of the unintended events. Study authors also collected data on length of stay and severity of illness for each patient, as well as information regarding the size and staffing of each ICU.

INTERPRETATION. During the 24-h study period, there were a total of 584 reported events affecting 391 of 1913 patients. The most common type of event was unplanned dislodgements of lines, catheters or drains (158 patients) followed by medication errors (136 patients), equipment failures (112 patients), losses, leakages or obstructions of airways (47 patients) and inappropriate shut-offs of alarms (17 patients). Patients were at increased risk of experiencing a sentinel event if they required a higher intensity of care, had a higher severity of illness, or had a longer length of stay in the ICU. Study authors believe this multinational study demonstrates that sentinel events are a systemic problem common to all ICUs, and that further collaboration is needed to address each of the five common types of events.

Table 13.1 Participating countries, with number of ICUs and patients studied, in the multinational sentinel events evaluation study

Country	ICUs (n)	Patients (n)
Australia	1	13
Austria	26	187
Belgium	2	30
Brazil	2	41
Czech Republic	13	124
Denmark	7	64
Estonia	1	1
Finland	2	14
France	6	50
Germany	12	184
Greece	6	65
Hong Kong	3	37
India	7	89
Indonesia	1	6
Italy	34	257
Latvia	1	6
Macedonia	1	15
Netherlands	2	11
Norway	1	7
Poland	1	9
Portugal	18	136
Romania	1	10
Singapore	1	7
Slovakia	1	2
Slovenia	2	10
Spain	18	197
Switzerland	9	93
United Kingdom	25	239
United States	1	9

Source: Valentin et al. (2006).

Comment

This multinational study confirms that adverse events in ICUs are common worldwide, and frequently secondary to systemic problems across nations and healthcare systems. In addition, the results help identify which types of errors are common across ICUs and which types of patients are most at risk for adverse events. Few systemic variables emerged as potential predictors of adverse events, and only patient–nurse ratio remained in the final multivariate model as a non-linear term, though the heterogeneity of ICUs may have attenuated the opportunity to identify specific systemic predictors of harm. Limitations of the study were that: (i) the investigators collected information on errors, but did not collect data on patient harm that may have resulted; (ii) the presence or absence of certain proven interventions (e.g. CPOE, clinical pharmacists) was not assessed as potential predictors of errors; and (iii) detected errors were not validated. Definitions and detection rates may, therefore, have varied widely by site. While these limitations introduce some uncertainty regarding the precise rates of errors and the accuracy of detected predictors, this study does advance the science by effectively confirming the widespread nature of errors in ICU care. It helps to open the door to more collaborative research, and demonstrates the urgent need to improve ICU care worldwide.

Medication errors and adverse drug events in an intensive care unit: direct observation approach for detection

Kopp BJ, Erstad BL, Allen ME, *et al*. *Crit Care Med* 2006; **34**: 415–25

BACKGROUND. This prospective study used an intensive, direct observational methodology to determine the epidemiology of adverse drug events in an ICU. Earlier direct observational studies have evaluated the epidemiology of error as a whole in ICU care |8,9|, but this study sought to delve more deeply into the nature of errors in drug ordering, preparation and delivery, which are among the most common errors in critical care. The study was conducted at a 16-bed medical/surgical ICU in an urban academic medical centre. Two pharmacy residents trained in critical care pharmacy practice collected data during a 24-h pilot period as well as the four observation periods, consisting of sequential 12-h shifts for four consecutive days. An attending physician and senior clinical pharmacist then reviewed and graded adverse drug events (ADEs) collected by the observers.

INTERPRETATION. A total of 185 incidents were identified by the two observers: 132 were deemed preventable and/or of clinical importance by the event evaluators; 22 preventable errors were detected that led to actual patient harm (preventable ADEs); and 110 potential ADEs were identified. One serious preventable error occurred for every five doses of medication administered. The most common type of errors were errors of omission (23%), followed by errors due to wrong dose (20%), wrong drug (16%), improper administration (15%) and drug–drug interaction (10%). Actual preventable ADEs were most commonly due to errors in drug prescribing (77%) or administration (23%). The main types of medications involved were cardiovascular medications, antibiotics and sedation/anaesthesia medications.

Comment

Using a more intensive design, this study identified a higher rate of actual and potential ADEs than earlier studies that have relied upon voluntary reporting or chart review. The authors used a rigorous, well-established classification schema developed by Bates *et al.* to classify and rate incidents |10,11|. As in previous studies, inter-rater agreement on event classification was high; agreement on incident severity and preventability was lower. By demonstrating that potential or actual adverse drug events occur in one of every five medication doses, this study emphasizes the urgent need to improve the organization and culture of safety in ICUs generally, as well as the systems of medication prescribing and delivery in particular.

Patient safety event reporting in critical care: a study of three intensive care units

Harris CB, Krauss MJ, Coopersmith CM, *et al. Crit Care Med* 2007; **35**: 1068–75

BACKGROUND. This prospective interventional study was designed to observe change in error-reporting in three ICUs at a large, urban tertiary care centre when an anonymous, voluntary card-based event-reporting system was introduced. Prior to the introduction of the new system, error reports were collected through a non-anonymous online reporting system. The card was internally developed following interviews with healthcare providers regarding barriers to reporting. The card was piloted in the medical ICU (MICU), revised then introduced and studied in the MICU, the surgical ICU (SICU) and the cardiothoracic ICU (CTICU).

INTERPRETATION. A total of 714 patient safety events were reported using the card-based system during the 14-month study period. There was a significant increase in event reporting from 20.4 reports per 1000 patient-days pre-intervention to 41.7 reports per 1000 patient-days post intervention; rate ratio 2.05 (95% CI, 1.79–2.34). Nurses reported the majority of events (67.1% vs. 23.1% for physicians and 9.5% for other healthcare providers); however, there was a 45-fold increase in the number of events reported by physicians as opposed to a 1.7-fold increase for nurses. Physicians were also more likely to report events that caused harm (33.9% physician reports vs. 27.2% nurses reports and 13.0% from other staff, $P<0.005$).

Comment

While studies such as those by Valentin *et al.* (2006) and Kopp *et al.* (2006) continue to define the epidemiology of errors in critical care, increasing efforts have also been invested in stimulating routine reporting of adverse events by critical care nurses and physicians, so that better data can be routinely generated and acted upon at a local level. Owing to fears of both legal consequences and professional censure, many clinicians have previously expressed reluctance to report errors in care. For the medical system to effectively decrease medical errors and improve patient safety, it is imperative that hospitals develop effective event-reporting systems, both to identify the kinds of errors occurring and to track changes over time.

This study by Harris and colleagues highlights the importance of having a well-designed event-reporting system that obtains the buy-in of clinical staff. By involving physicians and nurses in the design of the new safety cards and allowing anonymous reporting, there was a significant improvement in the number of events reported. This study also highlights differences in the types of errors different members of the healthcare team are likely to report. By improving physician event reporting, researchers were able to capture more errors that actually caused harm.

In the United States, there has been an increased focus on the importance of developing confidential reporting systems since passage of the Patient Safety and Quality Improvement Act of 2005. This act creates Patient Safety Organizations

(PSOs) to 'collect, aggregate, and analyse confidential information reported by health care providers' (further information available at http://www.ahrq.gov/qual/psoact.htm). The potential of this legislation to stimulate increased reporting and providers' awareness of safety concerns, however, will unquestionably be mediated by local efforts such as that described by Harris and colleagues. This study thus serves as an important model of how hospitals can develop effective reporting systems that may be of wide interest in critical care as well as other settings.

Impact of computerized physician order entry on medication prescription errors in the intensive care unit: a controlled cross-sectional trial

Colpaert K, Claus B, Somers A, *et al. Crit Care* 2006; **10**: R21

BACKGROUND. This prospective, controlled cross-sectional trial was designed to study the impact of computerized physician order entry (CPOE) on medication errors in a SICU, a previously under-studied area. The ICU was divided into three units, of which one instituted CPOE with clinical decision support, while the others retained a paper-based ordering system. An independent clinical pharmacist analysed all orders on randomly selected patients over a 5-week period of time. A panel of clinicians and pharmacists then reviewed all identified medication errors and graded their severity. Clinical staff on the units were unaware the study was being conducted.

INTERPRETATION. In total, 2510 orders were reviewed in this Belgian SICU, representing 80 patient-days per unit. A total of 375 medication errors were identified. There were significantly fewer errors on the CPOE unit (3.4%) than on the paper-based units (27.0%; $P<0.001$), including both fewer intercepted errors (12 vs. 46; $P<0.001$) and non-intercepted potential adverse drug events (21 vs. 48; $P<0.001$). There were also fewer ADEs in the CPOE unit (2 vs. 12 events; $P<0.001$).

Comment

Numerous studies have now demonstrated the potential of CPOE systems to improve safety, but adoption remains relatively low worldwide. One reason for slow adoption has been the concern that systems designed or implemented in a suboptimal manner can potentially introduce new types of errors |**19,20**|. Consequently, there remains a need to study diverse CPOE systems, and ensure their safe adoption and implementation.

The current study assessed the effects of a CPOE system in an understudied setting using concurrent controls and a rigorous methodology for assessing events. Concurrent evaluation of intervention and control units eliminated the potential for temporal trends to bias study results, which strengthens the findings reported. The fact that the study was conducted in Europe also increases its value, as most literature on CPOE systems has come from the USA. Evaluation of the utility of CPOE and other safety interventions across healthcare systems is extremely important.

Patient handover from surgery to intensive care: using Formula 1 pit-stop and aviation models to improve safety and quality

Catchpole KR, De Leval M, McEwan A, *et al. Pediatr Anesth* 2007; **17**: 470–8

BACKGROUND. This prospective interventional study sought to improve safety and quality of patient handover from surgery to ICUs utilizing concepts from two other industries: aviation and Formula 1 racing. Researchers met with racing teams to adapt pit-stop techniques to patient handovers. In addition, aviation training captains observed several handovers and identified areas for improvement. A new handover protocol was developed with clearly identified roles, checklists, and specialized training for staff for the transfer of children having undergone cardiac surgery to the cardiac ICU of a major children's hospital. An observer experienced in the observation of human error in surgical settings observed and graded all handovers, both pre and post observation. Handovers were evaluated for technical errors, information omissions and time duration.

INTERPRETATION. Fifty handovers were observed: 23 pre-intervention and 27 post intervention. The mean number of technical errors per handover decreased from 5.42 (95% CI 4.18–6.66) to 3.15 (95% CI 2.44–3.86) and information omissions were reduced from 2.09 (95% CI 0.95–3.23) to 1.07 (0.52–1.62). Thirty-nine per cent (9/23 patients) had more than one error in both technical and information handover as compared with 11.5% (3/27 patients) post intervention. Mean duration of handover time was unchanged: 10.8 min (95%CI, 9.2–12.4) pre-intervention vs. 9.4 min (95% CI 8.09–10.69) post intervention. Study authors emphasized that having a handover protocol can improve information sharing and that medicine should not hesitate to take advantage of expertise from other industries.

Comment

Patient handover is becoming an increasingly important area of concentration for patient safety. Handover technique is particularly important in the care of medically complex patients, such as those admitted to the ICU following surgery. Traditionally, the transfer of information between caregivers follows no set protocol and caregivers are rarely trained in how to effectively communicate information to colleagues. This process, or lack thereof, leaves patients vulnerable to errors due to information omissions or miscommunication. As such, the development of simple, easily trainable handover protocols should be an important goal of the medical community.

A limitation of this study is its small size, which limits the power to fully evaluate the effects of the intervention on different types of errors, or on the time spent by providers handing over care. Likewise, the generalizability of the results remains somewhat unclear. The adoption of handoff techniques from other industries, however, is certainly a promising strategy, as suggested by the results of this interesting pilot study. Further research regarding teamwork functioning and handover strategies will be an important area of future critical care safety research.

An intervention to decrease catheter-related bloodstream infections in the ICU

Pronovost P, Needham D, Berenholtz S, *et al. N Engl J Med* 2006; **355**: 2725–32

BACKGROUND. This collaborative cohort study of 108 ICUs evaluated the effect on the incidence of catheter-related bloodstream infections (CRBIs) of implementing five evidence-based procedures recommended by the Centres for Disease Control and Prevention (CDC). These were: hand washing; using full barrier precautions during catheter insertion; cleaning the skin with chlorhexidine; avoiding the femoral site when possible; and expeditiously removing unnecessary catheters. Each ICU designated a nurse or physician team leader in charge of dissemination of safety information. In addition, checklists were introduced with procedure kits; catheter removal was discussed daily on rounds; and teams received feedback regarding infection rates. Data on the number of CRBIs were collected monthly by a trained, hospital-based infection control practitioner.

INTERPRETATION. The analysis included 1981 ICU-months and over 375 000 catheter-days of data. The median rate of catheter-related bloodstream infections fell from 2.7 (mean, 7.7) per 1000 catheter-days at baseline to 0 (mean, 2.3) at 3 months ($P<0.002$) and the median level of 0 infections per 1000 catheter-days was sustained at 18 months ($P<0.002$) (Table 13.2). A Poisson multilevel regression model showed a continuous decrease in the infection incidence-rate ratio following implementation of the interventions, falling from a baseline rate of 1.00 to 0.76 (95% CI 0.57–1.01) during the intervention to 0.62 (95% CI 0.47–0.81) at 3 months, etc. to an eventual rate of 0.34 (95% CI 0.23–0.50) at 16–18 months as compared with baseline. The authors concluded that broad use of this simple, inexpensive intervention significantly decreased the morbidity, mortality and total costs associated with CRBIs.

Comment

In this landmark study, Pronovost *et al.* found that with an inexpensive series of interventions CRBIs were greatly reduced in over 100 ICUs, and reductions in harm were sustained 18 months after implementation. The preventability of nosocomial infections in general – and CRBIs in particular – has historically been a source of some controversy among medical professionals. Frequently, there is no observed error in care (e.g. the inadvertent introduction of a pathogen into a sterile field) prior to the occurrence of an infection and, as a consequence, it might be presumed that most line infections are inevitable. Pronovost, however, convincingly demonstrates, through a large, rigorous multicentre study, that two-thirds of these infections can

Table 13.2 Rates of CRBIs from baseline to 18 months post implementation*

Study period	No. of ICUs	No. of bloodstream infections per 1000 catheter-days (median and interquartile range)				
		Overall	Teaching	Non-teaching hospital	<200 beds	≥200 beds
Baseline	55	2.7 (0.6–4.8)	2.7 (1.3–4.7)	2.6 (0–4.9)	2.1 (0–3.0)	2.7 (1.3–4.8)
During implementation	96	1.6 (0–4.4)†	1.7 (0–4.5)	0 (0–3.5)	0 (0–5.8)	1.7 (0–4.3)†
After implementation						
0–3 months	96	0 (0–3.0)‡	1.3 (0–3.1)†	0 (0–1.6)†	0 (0–2.7)	1.1 (0–3.1)‡
4–6 months	96	0 (0–2.7)‡	1.1 (0–3.6)†	0 (0–0)‡	0 (0–0)†	0 (0–3.2)‡
7–9 months	95	0 (0–2.1)‡	0.8 (0–2.4)‡	0 (0–0)‡	0 (0–0)†	0 (0–2.2)‡
10–12 months	90	0 (0–1.9)‡	0 (0–2.3)‡	0 (0–1.5)‡	0 (0–0)†	0.2 (0–2.3)‡
13–15 months	85	0 (0–1.6)‡	0 (0–2.2)‡	0 (0–0)‡	0 (0–0)†	0 (0–2.0)‡
16–18 months	70	0 (0–2.4)‡	0 (0–2.7)‡	0 (0–1.2)†	0 (0–0)†	0 (0–2.6)‡

*Because the ICUs implemented the study intervention at different times, the total number of ICUs contributing data for each period varies. Of the 103 participating ICUs, 48 did not contribute baseline data. P-values were calculated by the two-sample Wilcoxon rank-sum test.
†$P \leq 0.05$ for the comparison with the baseline (pre-implementation) period.
‡$P \leq 0.002$ for the comparison with the baseline (pre-implementation) period.
Source: Pronovost et al. (2006).

be eliminated simply by consistent implementation of published best practices. The best possible baseline rate using these best practices is far lower than typical infection rates in many hospitals. CRBIs can no longer be viewed as inevitable; rather, they are sentinel events that demand careful consideration of extant care practices and focused efforts to improve them. CRBIs account for as many as 28 000 ICU deaths per year in the USA, and cost as much as $2.3 billion per year to treat |21|. Dissemination and implementation of the straightforward interventions evaluated in this study could greatly reduce both the human and financial burden of this important patient safety problem.

Decline in ICU adverse events, nosocomial infections and cost through a quality improvement initiative focusing on teamwork and culture change

Jain M, Miller L, Belt D, King D, *et al*. *Qual Saf Health Care* 2006; **15**: 235–9

BACKGROUND. Like the Pronovost *et al.* (2006) study, this interventional study sought to improve patient safety through consistent implementation of published best practices in ICU care, as well as teamwork enhancements. In a single ICU, the incidence of adverse events, nosocomial infections, length of stay (LOS) and costs was evaluated following implementation of a broad multidisciplinary quality improvement initiative. The study was implemented at a 28-bed medical–surgical ICU in October and November 2002 as part of a collaborative effort run by the Institute for Healthcare Improvement. The intervention included four key components: (1) physician-led multidisciplinary rounds; (2) daily 'flow' meetings to assess bed availability; (3) implementation of 'bundle' care sets for ventilators and central lines; and (4) culture change through team decision-making. Adverse event, cost, infection and length of stay data were collected through administrative and nursing records from 2001 through 2004.

INTERPRETATION. There was a significant decrease in the rate of ventilator associated pneumonias (VAPs) (7.5 to 3.2 per 1000 ventilator days, $P = 0.004$) and CRBIs (5.9 to 3.1 per 1000 line days, $P = 0.03$) after implementation of the quality improvement initiative. There was a strong decline over time in the number of adverse events, as seen in Figure 13.1. Cost and length of stay trended downward over time.

Comment

While this single-centre study is far smaller than that of Pronovost and colleagues (2006), it provides another illustrative example of the potential safety benefits of consistently implementing evidence-based care practices. In addition to CRBIs, the investigators found a reduction in ventilator-associated pneumonias and adverse events following implementation of evidence-based practices for preventing CRBIs and VAPs, as well as rounding, teamwork and culture changes. While causal inferences and generalizability are always limited in a single-centre, non-

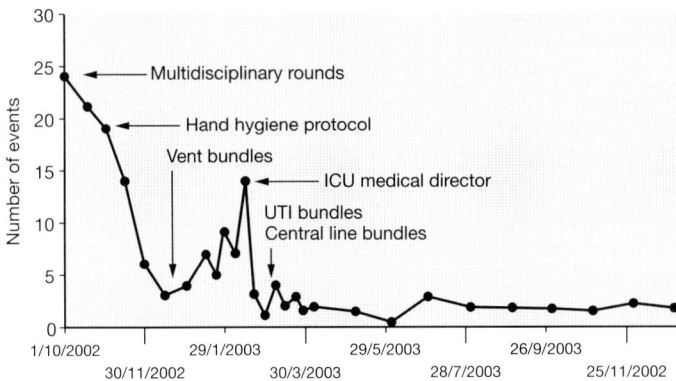

Fig. 13.1 Run chart: improvement in rates of adverse events in the ICU following implementation of a multi-faceted quality improvement initiative. Source: Jain *et al.* (2006).

randomized study, and while it is not possible to confidently determine which elements of this multipronged intervention were most crucial, this investigation provides a promising example of the potential to improve care across multiple domains through a focused, multidisciplinary effort.

Of note, this study also serves as an example of how quality improvement (QI) methodologies may be combined with more traditional epidemiological methods and established heath services research methodologies in patient safety research. A well-established method for identifying adverse events – a 'trigger tool' – was used by nurse data extractors in their chart reviews, but rates over time were assessed using a run chart, an evaluation metric derived from QI research that may be unfamiliar to many clinicians. Concurrently, infection rates were compared using a pre-post design, and traditional chi-square statistics. Each of these methodologies has limitations, but in this case the consistent improvements demonstrated across several methods of analysis are complementary, and reinforce the value of the intervention in this pilot study.

Recovery from medical errors: the critical care nursing safety net

Rothschild JR, Hurley AC, Landrigan CP, *et al. Joint Comm J Qual Pat Safety* 2006; **32**: 63–72

BACKGROUND. In this follow-up to the Critical Care Safety Study, Rothschild *et al.* evaluated the role of critical care nurses in intercepting potential adverse events before they reached the patient, and in ameliorating events that reached the patient, but could have caused more harm were they not recognized and addressed expeditiously. While nurses unquestionably provide most of the

direct, hands-on care that patients receive |8|, their importance in preventing and mitigating harm has not been adequately studied.

INTERPRETATION. Using a direct observational methodology, supplemented with daily chart abstraction and collection of staff reports, Rothschild *et al.* found in a coronary care unit that on average, nurses recover (i.e. prevent or ameliorate) slightly more than two potentially harmful medical errors per 8-h shift, or more than 7300 medical errors per year in a 10-bed ICU. Sixty-nine per cent of the recovered medical errors that were detected were intercepted before reaching the patient; 13% reached the patient but were recovered before causing harm; and 18% reached the patient and caused harm, but were recovered before causing further harm. In 51% of cases the potential for harm was severe or life-threatening. Medication errors represented 73% of all medical errors recovered.

Comment

Rothschild has demonstrated that nurses play a critical role in preventing harm in ICUs, through their routine interception of errors. This is an especially significant finding because most safety interventions – including computerized physician order entry (CPOE), pharmacist review of physician orders, and resident work hour reforms – have focused on physicians rather than nurses. Recent work, however, has begun to suggest that nurses, as doctors, become more error-prone when working under adverse conditions, including excessive hours (as discussed further below), and excessive patient loads |22|. As efforts are made to improve the safety of care delivery, a focus on improving the performance of nurses will be essential, not only to decrease their commission of errors, but also to optimize their crucial capacity to intercept and ameliorate harm.

Effects of critical care nurses' work hours on vigilance and patients' safety

Scott LD, Rogers AE, Hwang WT, *et al*. *Am J Crit Care* 2006; **15**: 30–7

BACKGROUND. A series of studies conducted over the past several years have demonstrated that working extended hours increases the risk of error among physicians in training, particularly among those working in critical care environments |17,18|. Scott *et al.* enrolled a random nationwide sample of 502 critical care nurses in a study of nurses' work, sleep and patient safety. Enrolled nurses completed daily logs of their work hours and sleep for 28 days, and reported any episodes of on-the-job sleepiness and medical errors or 'near-errors' in which they were involved.

INTERPRETATION. Respondents consistently worked longer than their scheduled shifts (86% of shifts), and longer work duration was associated with an increased risk of reporting errors and near errors in care. Sixty-two per cent of all shifts exceeded 12.5h: 65% of nurses reported difficulty staying awake on the job at least once during the data collection period, and 20% fell asleep on the job. Nurses working ≥12.5-h shifts were

Table 13.3 Relationship between nurses' work hours, errors and 'near-errors'

Work duration (h)*	No. of shifts (%)	No. of shifts with at least one error (%)	Odds ratio (P)	No. of shifts with at least one near error (%)	Odds ratio (P)
≤8.5	543 (9)	11 (2)	1.00	27 (5)	1.00
>8.5 to <12.5	1720 (29)	46 (3)	1.42 (0.30)	72 (4)	1.13 (0.59)
≥12.5	3748 (62)	146 (4)	1.94 (0.03)	247 (7)	1.64 (0.05)
Total	6011	203	NA	346	NA

*The duration of six work shifts could not be classified because of missing data.
NA, not applicable.
Source: Scott et al. (2006).

nearly twice as likely to make a medical error (OR = 1.94; P = 0.03) as those working shifts ≤8.5 h (Table 13.3).

Comment

In this investigation, Scott *et al.* demonstrated that critical care nurses working extended shifts report significantly decreased alertness on the job and approximately twice as many medical errors. While medical errors were assessed by self-report in this study, and hence some uncertainty surrounds the precision of reporting, the primary finding that long hours were associated with increased error rates has now been demonstrated among nurse and physician populations in multiple intensive clinical studies, laboratory investigations, and national cohort studies |17,18,23–26|. The current study supports the importance of long work hours as a risk for error among critical care nurses.

In light of the consistent research documenting the relationship between long work hours and errors, the Institute of Medicine recently recommended that nurses be limited to no more than 12 consecutive hours of work in any setting |27|. Scott *et al.*'s study demonstrates that this recommendation is directly germane to the critical care environment. In this setting, strategies to prevent error are likely to be particularly important, given the potential for errors to cause severe harm in fragile, critically ill patients.

Sleep and well-being of ICU housestaff

Parthasarathy S, Hettiger K, Budhiraja R, Sullivan B. *Chest* 2007; **131**: 1685–93

BACKGROUND. This prospective, single-centre study sought to measure the effects of reducing housestaff work hours following implementation of the 2003 ACGME work hours limitations. Subjective and objective measures of sleepiness in housestaff and fellows rotating through an ICU were collected. All study participants (34 internal medicine residents and 10 critical care fellows) filled out questionnaires at the beginning and end of 2 month-long ICU rotations before and after work-hour changes, regarding sleepiness, baseline fatigue and well-being. Participants also filled out sleep and work logs, wore actigraphs to assess periods of quiescence, and underwent multiple sleep latency testing. Intercepted errors in written medication orders were collected on the units through chart review of a random sample of written orders; non-intercepted errors were not collected, nor were adverse events due to errors.

INTERPRETATION. Following the implementation of work hours limitations, residents experienced a small, statistically significant improvement in work hours (82 ± 7 vs. 76 ± 4 h per week), sleep time (6.7 ± 1.0 vs. 7.1 ± 1.2 h per night), subjective sleepiness and quality of life. However, objectively measured sleepiness (mean sleep latency) remained unchanged (P = 0.6), with many subjects scoring in the pathological range both before and after implementation of the ACGME duty hour standards. There was a significant decrease in the number of intercepted medical errors detected before compared with intervention, from 7.5 ± 3.4 to 2.1 ± 0.9 errors per 100 patient-days ($P = 0.01$). There was also a significant decrease in the number of residents reporting drowsy driving, from 62% before to 32% after intervention ($P = 0.02$). Fellows' sleep hours, sleepiness, error rates and drowsy driving rates did not change. Both the pre- and post-intervention groups experienced deterioration of sleep time, subjective sleepiness and quality of life indices over the course of their ICU rotations.

Comment

This investigation by Parthasarathy *et al.* found an improvement in residents' sleep time, subjective sleepiness and intercepted medication errors following implementation of the ACGME duty hour standards. The absolute improvement in sleep and work hours was small, however, and objectively measured sleepiness remained unchanged. Many subjects remained pathologically sleepy even after implementation of the standards. While there was a decrease in intercepted medication errors, no data on non-intercepted or harmful errors was collected, making the reported results difficult to interpret; further, the large decrease in errors seems disproportionate to the modest improvement in sleep and work hours, suggesting that other unmeasured factors may have affected this outcome.

In the USA, implementation of the ACGME standards has resulted in only 5–6% improvements in interns' sleep and work times, and compliance with the standards has been poor; 24- to 30-h shifts remain common |**28**|. Numerous studies have recently demonstrated the risks to patients and residents alike of residents' traditional 24-h shifts |**17,18,23,25,29,30**|. In light of the persistent presence of pathological sleepiness before and after implementation of the standards in their study, Parthasarathy and colleagues suggest that limiting residents' work to < 16 consecutive hours may be called for. Similarly, the Sleep Research Society (http://www.sleepresearchsociety.org/ResidentWork.aspx) and the Committee of Interns and Residents (http://www.cirseiu.org/docUploads/residentworkhours.pdf) have called for limitations in residents' work to a maximum of 16–18 consecutive hours in any setting; optimal work hour limits in critical care settings may well be even lower. While further research is needed into the best means of reducing work hours to safe levels while improving the quality of teamwork and handovers of care, it is clear that the status quo is unsafe.

Conclusion

In this chapter, we have reviewed 10 key studies that serve as representative examples of the diverse patient safety evaluations and interventions currently under way in critical care settings worldwide. There were many additional outstanding studies conducted between 2006 and 2007 that we could not review here due to space constraints. Altogether, there has been tremendous growth over the past few years in the quality and number of critical care safety studies.

While errors in critical care remain extremely common, significant strides have been taken to improve the safety of care in this high-stakes environment. Implementation of computerized order entry, pharmacist involvement in medication ordering and work hours reduction are well-proven means of reducing errors; efforts to implement these interventions effectively are now under way in a variety of settings worldwide. Many additional interventions, including implementation of evidence-based 'care bundles' to reduce catheter-related bloodstream infections and ventilator-associated pneumonias, are also proving to be extremely important. In addition, recent efforts have investigated strategies to improve teamwork functioning, care handovers, reporting of data on errors and the culture of safety in ICUs. Metrics to measure complex outcomes such as 'safety culture' are emerging, and pilot studies have demonstrated that focused efforts to improve teamwork and culture can lead to significant improvements in care.

In the next few years, we anticipate further research that will refine our understanding of hazards in critical care and result in effective interventions to reduce harm. The dissemination of these findings, through professional publications, professional societies, ongoing provider education, and collaborative ICU research and improvement networks, will be of critical importance in bringing best practices to bear in the care of critically ill patients worldwide. Multicentre efforts to study and improve care will be of particular value as the science of critical care safety advances. We are confident that as diverse efforts to improve safety across domains of care are disseminated and broadly implemented, the safety and quality of critical care will continue to improve.

References

1.	Kohn LT, Corrigan JM, Donaldson SM, eds. Institute of Medicine. *To Err is Human: Building a Safer Health System*. The National Academies Press, Washington, DC; 1999. Available at: http://www.nap.edu/openbook.php?isbn=0309068371

2.	Wilson RM, Harrison BT, Gibberd RW, Hamilton JD. An analysis of the causes of adverse events from the quality in Australian health care study. *Med J Aust* 1999; **170**: 411–15.

3.	Blendon RJ, Schoen C, DesRoches C, Osborn R, Zapert K. Common concerns amid diverse systems: health care experiences in five countries. *Health Aff (Millwood)* 2003; **22**: 106–21.

4.	Vincent C, Neale G, Woloshynowych M. Adverse events in British hospitals: preliminary retrospective record review. *BMJ* 2001; **322**: 517–19.

5.	Rubins H, Moskowitz M. Complications of care in a medical intensive care unit. *J Gen Intern Med* 1990; **5**: 104–9.

6. Giraud T, Dhainaut JF, Vaxelaire JF, Joseph T, Journois D, Bleichner G, *et al.* Iatrogenic complications in adult intensive care units: a prospective two-center study. *Crit Care Med* 1993; **21**: 40–51.

7. Ferraris VA, Propp ME. Outcome in critical care patients: a multivariate study. *Crit Care Med* 1992; **20**: 967–76.

8. Donchin Y, Gopher D, Olin M, Badihi Y, Biesky M, Sprung CL, *et al.* A look into the nature and causes of human errors in the intensive care unit. *Crit Care Med* 1995; **23**: 294–300.

9. Rothschild JM, Landrigan CP, Cronin JW, Kaushal R, Lockley SW, Burdick E, *et al.* The Critical Care Safety Study: the incidence and nature of adverse events and serious medical errors in intensive care. *Crit Care Med* 2005; **33**: 1694–700.

10. Bates DW, Teich J, Lee J, *et al.* The impact of computerized physician order entry on medication error prevention. *J Am Med Inform Assoc* 1999; **6**: 313–21.

11. Bates DW, Leape LL, Cullen DJ, *et al.* Effect of computerized physician order entry and a team intervention on prevention of serious medication errors. *JAMA* 1998; **280**: 1311–16.

12. Raschke RA, Gollihare B, Wunderlich TA. A computer alert system to prevent injury from adverse drug events. *JAMA* 1998; **280**: 1317–20.

13. Evans RS, Pestotnik SL, Classen DC, *et al.* A computer-assisted management program for antibiotics and other antiinfective agents. *N Engl J Med* 1998; **338**: 232–8.

14. King WJ, Paice N, Rangrej J, Forestell GJ, Swartz R. The effect of computerized physician order entry on medication errors and adverse drug events in pediatric inpatients. *Pediatrics* 2003; **112**: 506–9.

15. Potts AL, Barr FE, Gregory DF, Wright L, Patel NR. Computerized physician order entry and medication errors in a pediatric critical care unit. *Pediatrics* 2004; **113**: 59–63.

16. Leape LL, Cullen DJ, Clapp MD, *et al.* Pharmacist participation on physician rounds and adverse drug events in the intensive care unit. *JAMA* 1999; **282**: 267–70.

17. Lockley SW, Cronin JW, Evans EE, Cade BE, Lee CJ, Landrigan CP, Rothschild JM, *et al.* Effect of reducing interns' weekly work hours on sleep and attentional failures. *N Engl J Med* 2004; **351**: 1829–37.

18. Landrigan CP, Rothschild JM, Cronin JW, Kaushal R, Burdick E, Katz JT, *et al.* Effect of reducing interns' work hours on serious medical errors in intensive care units. *N Engl J Med* 2004; **351**: 1838–48.

19. Han YY, Carcillo JA, Venkataraman ST, Clark RS, Watson RS, Nguyen TC, *et al.* Unexpected increased mortality after implementation of a commercially sold computerized physician order entry system. *Pediatrics* 2005; **116**: 1506–12.

20. Walsh KE, Adams WG, Bauchner H, Vinci RJ, Chessare JB, Cooper MR, *et al.* Medication errors related to computerized order entry for children. *Pediatrics* 2006; **118**: 1872–9.

21. Burke JP. Infection control – a problem for patient safety. *N Engl J Med* 2003; **348**: 651–6.

22. Weissman JS, Rothschild JM, Bendavid E, Sprivulis P, Cook EF, Evans RS, *et al.* Hospital workload and adverse events. *Med Care* 2007; **45**: 448–5.

23. Barger LK, Ayas NT, Cade BE, Cronin JW, Rosner B, Speizer FE, *et al.* Impact of extended-duration shifts on medical errors, adverse events, and attentional failures. *Public Library of Science Medicine* 2006; **3**(12): e487.

24. Arnedt JT, Owens J, Crouch M, Stahl J, Carskadon MA. Neurobehavioral performance of residents after heavy night call versus after alcohol ingestion. *JAMA* 2005; **294**: 1025–33.

25. Philibert I. Sleep loss and performance in residents and nonphysicians: a meta-analytic examination. *Sleep* 2005; **28**: 1392–402.

26. Rogers AE, Hwang WT, Scott LD, Aiken LH, Dinges DF. The working hours of hospital staff nurses and patient safety. *Health Aff (Millwood)* 2004; **23**: 202–12.

27. Institute of Medicine (2006) *Keeping patients safe: transforming the work environment of nurses.* The National Academies Press, Washington DC 2003. Available at: http://www.nap.edu/openbook.php?isbn=0309090679

28. Landrigan CP, Barger LK, Cade BE, Ayas NT, Czeisler CA. Interns' compliance with accreditation council for graduate medical education work-hour limits. *JAMA* 2006; **296**: 1063–70.

29. Barger LK, Cade BE, Ayas NT, Cronin JW, Rosner B, Speizer FE, *et al.* Extended work shifts and the risk of motor vehicle crashes among interns. *N Engl J Med* 2005; **352**: 125–34.

30. Ayas NT, Barger LK, Cade BE, Hashimoto DM, Rosner B, Cronin JW, *et al.* Extended work duration and the risk of self-reported percutaneous injuries in interns. *JAMA* 2006; **296**: 1055–62.

14

The Surviving Sepsis campaign

PAUL HOLDER, NIGEL WEBSTER

Introduction

Infection resulting in a systemic inflammatory response and organ system failure (when it is known as severe sepsis) represents a significant challenge to all medical practitioners. It is the most common cause of death in non-coronary intensive care units (ICUs). In the UK, the prevalence of severe sepsis in adult ICUs is 27.7%, which amounts to an estimated 23 211 cases per year [1]. Whilst the lack of universal diagnostic criteria before 1992 makes analysis of data prior to this time difficult, the incidence of sepsis appears to have risen steadily over the last three decades and there is little to suggest that this trend will not continue. It has been suggested that the number of septic patients will continue to rise at 1.5% per annum [2]. There is a 44.7% hospital mortality rate associated with severe sepsis, which means that there are an estimated 10 375 deaths per year in the UK [1], and worldwide the condition kills approximately 1400 people per day [3]. Patients who survive sepsis do so at the cost of a decreased quality of life [4]. This burden of morbidity and mortality remains unacceptably high. It exists despite increases in available research grants and clinical monies, and general improvements in the quality of critical care.

In an effort to improve these statistics, a collaboration of the Society of Critical Care Medicine in the USA, the European Intensive Care Society and the International Sepsis Forum launched the surviving sepsis campaign in 2002 with a founding statement that is known as the Barcelona declaration. In this document the significant burden of sepsis is highlighted, as is the necessity of rapid and appropriate therapy if the best outcome is to be achieved. Furthermore, the group presented a statement of intent to perform several activities: develop comprehensive strategies for action against sepsis; embark on a comprehensive programme of education of healthcare workers to diagnose and appropriately treat sepsis earlier; increase funding for the development of diagnostic tests and treatments for sepsis; ensure availability of counselling for patients and their families affected by sepsis; and develop worldwide standards of care. Moreover, the group committed to a goal of a 25% relative reduction in the mortality from sepsis over 5 years [5].

The first action in response to this declaration occurred within 2 years, when representatives from the fields of critical care and infectious diseases gathered to develop guidelines, which represented the distillation of all available evidence which could be utilized by the physician at the bedside to improve outcome.

These guidelines are presented as a list of interventions at various stages of the disease process. Each is given a grading depending on the level of evidence which supports them, based on an established grading system (Table 14.1) |6|. There are a large number of recommendations which are not in fact evidence based (grade D and E), and their introduction into widespread practice should not, therefore, be supported as being part of the practice of evidence-based medicine. There are, however, a minority of guidelines which have a firm evidence base. The majority of the evidence-based recommendations are in fact negative points such as 'low-dose dopamine should not be used for renal protection as part of the treatment of severe sepsis (grade B)'. We suggest that evidence-based recommendations giving positive guidance on how practitioners can improve their treatment of the patient with severe sepsis would be more appropriate.

The guidelines

Initial resuscitation

The resuscitation of a patient with severe sepsis or sepsis-induced tissue hypoperfusion should begin as soon as it is diagnosed and should not be delayed pending ICU admission. During the first 6 h of resuscitation, the following should be part of a treatment protocol: central venous pressure 8–12 mmHg (12–15 mmHg in ventilated patients), mean arterial pressure >65 mmHg, urine output >0.5 ml/kg/h, and a central venous (superior vena cava) or mixed venous oxygen saturation >70%. If the latter is not achieved with fluid then transfuse to a haematocrit of >30% and or give dobutamine (grade B).

The rationale behind this recommendation centres on a single published trial in which this package of care was compared with a 'standard' regimen in which the

Table 14.1 Grading system

Grading of recommendations	Grading of evidence
A Supported by at least two level I investigations	I Large, randomized trials with clear-cut results; low risk of false-positive (alpha) error or false-negative (beta) error
B Supported by one level I investigation	II Small, randomized trials with uncertain results; moderate-to-high risk of false-positive (alpha) and/or false-negative (beta) error
C Supported by level II investigations only	III Non-randomized, contemporaneous controls
D Supported by at least one level III investigation	IV Non-randomized, historical controls and expert opinion
E Supported by level IV or V evidence	V Case series, uncontrolled studies and expert opinion

Source: Dellinger et al. Crit Care Med 2004; **32**: 858–73.

central venous oxygen was not taken into account whilst the other variables were the same |7|. This reference can support the use of only this single aspect of the package of care. The other aspects are not supported by a randomized trial; if these are to be included in the guidance they should be at a lower level of recommendation. Furthermore, the use of a different CVP target in patients who are intubated and receiving ventilatory support is not covered in the quoted reference. The use of central venous oxygenation and mixed venous oxygenation interchangeably is also a matter of some debate. Whilst the two have been demonstrated to be related, the use of a single target of 70% would seem somewhat unsafe. Indeed, the potentially large gap between these two measurements has been repeatedly demonstrated and central venous oxygen saturation has been concluded to be an unsuitable surrogate |8|.

Fluid therapy

Fluid therapy may consist of natural or artificial colloids. There is no evidence-based support for one type of fluid over another (grade C).

Three references are quoted to support this recommendation; they each are pooled, small randomized trials which are not targeted to examine the intervention in the subgroup of sepsis |9–11|. The use of a meta-analysis to extract useful results from several inadequately sized trials has been criticized, although it does fit within the category of grade C evidence in this system.

Vasopressors

Low-dose dopamine should not be used for renal protection as part of the treatment of severe sepsis (grade B).

This recommendation is supported by a well-conducted double-blinded multicentre randomized control trial of 328 patients. There was no difference between the dopamine and placebo groups with respect to the degree of renal impairment, the number requiring renal replacement therapy, length of stay or mortality |12|.

Further support for this recommendation is given in the form of a meta-analysis, which includes 17 randomized clinical trials that demonstrated no significant difference with respect to the prevention of acute renal failure, the need for renal replacement therapy, or mortality |13|.

Inotrope therapy

A strategy of increasing cardiac index to achieve an arbitrarily predefined elevated level is not recommended (grade A).

This recommendation is supported by two randomized controlled trials. In the first, 762 critically ill patients were randomized to receive either standard therapy, therapy in which the cardiac index was increased to a supranormal level, or that which raised the mixed venous oxygen saturation to a normal level. No significant difference in the number of organ systems failing, length of ICU stay or mortality was demonstrated between the groups |14|.

In the second, 109 patients were randomized to control or to attain goals of cardiac index and oxygen delivery with the use of dobutamine. The treatment group had a significantly higher mortality than the control group |15|.

Steroids

Intravenous corticosteroids are recommended in patients with septic shock requiring vasopressors to maintain blood pressure (grade C).

Support for this statement is in the form of a single trial of 300 patients with septic shock who were randomized to control or to receive hydrocortisone and fludrocortisone. There was a significant decrease in mortality in those patients with a relative adrenal insufficiency (as defined by an inadequate response to a synthetic ACTH challenge) who were treated with steroids |16|.

Doses of steroids > 300 mg hydrocortisone should not be used in severe sepsis or septic shock for the purposes of treating septic shock (Grade A).

This recommendation is supported by two trials and a meta-analysis. The first, a prospective randomized double-blind trial of 182 patients with severe sepsis or septic shock, compared the administration of high-dose methylprednisolone (30 mg/kg) with control. The results demonstrated a significant increase in the mortality at 14 days in the treatment group |17|.

Secondly, a multicentre randomized, double-blind placebo controlled trial of 223 patients with sepsis where patients received high-dose methylprednisolone or placebo in addition to standard therapy: no significant difference was noted in mortality between the two groups |18|.

A meta-analysis pooled nine randomized, controlled trials of corticosteroid therapy in sepsis and septic shock among critically ill adults. The authors conclude that the evidence provides no support for the use of corticosteroids in patients with sepsis or septic shock, and suggests that their use may be harmful |19|.

Recombinant activated protein C

Recombinant activated protein C (rhAPC) is recommended in patients with a high risk of death and with no absolute contraindications related to bleeding risk or relative contraindication that outweighs the potential benefit of rhAPC (grade B).

The evidence to support this recommendation is a randomized, double-blind, placebo-controlled, multicentre trial in 1690 patients. Treatment with rhAPC was associated with a reduction in the relative risk of death of 19.4% (95% confidence interval 6.6–30.5) and an absolute reduction in the risk of death of 6.1% ($P = 0.005$). However, the incidence of serious bleeding was significantly higher in the treatment group |20|.

Blood product administration

Once tissue hypoperfusion has resolved and in the absence of extenuating circumstances, red cell transfusion should occur only when the haemoglobin decreases to < 7.0 g/dl to target a haemoglobin of 7.0–9.9 g/dl (grade B).

The evidence for this recommendation is a trial of 838 critically ill patients who were randomized to a restrictive transfusion regime transfusion trigger of 7.0 g/dl and haemoglobin concentrations maintained at 7.0–9.0 g/dl, or to a liberal strategy transfusion trigger of 10.0 g/dl with haemoglobin concentrations maintained at 10.0–12.0 g/dl. The 30-day mortality was similar in the two groups. However, the 30-day mortality rates were significantly lower with the restrictive transfusion strategy among patients who were less acutely ill. The hospital mortality was significantly lower in the restrictive strategy group. The authors concluded that a restrictive strategy of red cell transfusion is at least as effective as and possibly superior to a liberal transfusion strategy in critically ill patients, with the possible exception of patients with acute myocardial infarction and unstable angina |21|. However, this study was performed using non-leucodepleted blood and some have argued that this may account for the adverse outcome in those given more blood products.

Erythropoietin (EPO) is not recommended as a specific treatment of anaemia associated with severe sepsis but may be used when septic patients have other reasons for use (crade B).

The evidence to support this comes from two studies from the same group. In the first, 160 patients were randomized to receive either EPO or placebo for a minimum of 2 weeks or until ICU discharge. The number of units of blood transfused was significantly less in the treatment group than in the placebo group. However, there were no significant differences between the two groups either in mortality or in the frequency of adverse events |22|.

In the second trial, the methodology was repeated in a larger, multicentre trial in which 1302 patients were randomized to receive EPO or placebo. The treatment group was less likely to undergo transfusion but mortality and adverse clinical events were not significantly different |23|.

Antithrombin administration is not recommended for the treatment of severe sepsis or septic shock (grade B).

The evidence base for this statement is in the form of a single multicentre trial of 2314 patients randomized to receive antithrombin III or placebo. No significant difference in mortality at 28, 56 or 90 days was demonstrated |24|.

Mechanical ventilation of sepsis-induced acute lung injury/ARDS

High tidal volumes, coupled with high plateau pressures, should be avoided. Clinicians should reduce tidal volumes to a volume of 6 ml/kg (predicted body weight) in conjunction with maintaining end-inspiratory plateau pressures of <30 cmH$_2$O (grade B). Four small studies are referenced with respect to this recommendation; however, they are somewhat contradictory. In one study, 53 patients with early acute respiratory distress syndrome (ARDS) were randomized to protective ventilation or conventional ventilation. The protective strategy was associated with improved survival at 28 days, a higher rate of weaning from mechanical ventilation, and a lower rate of barotrauma. But protective ventilation was not associated with a higher rate of survival to hospital discharge |25|. The next study, in which 120 patients deemed at high risk of developing ARDS were randomized to protective or standard ventilatory strategies, failed to demonstrate any difference in mortality or the number of episodes of organ dysfunction |26|. The third study enrolled 116 patients with ARDS and no organ failure other than the lung. They were randomized to receive ventilation below or above 10 ml/kg. The protective approach did not reduce mortality at day 60, the duration of mechanical ventilation, the incidence of pneumothorax or the occurrence of multiple organ failure |27|. The last of the small trials quoted examines 52 patients with ARDS who were randomized to receive either 10–12 ml/kg or 5–8 ml/kg (ideal body weight) tidal volume. There were no significant differences in any of the studied outcomes between the two groups |28|.

The evidence that supports this recommendation is in the form of a single-blinded controlled trial of 861 patients randomized to ventilation with a tidal volume of 12 ml/kg or 6 ml/kg, in which the lower tidal volume group had a reduced hospital mortality from 39.8% to 31% when compared with the higher tidal volume group |29|.

Hypercapnia can be tolerated in patients with ALI/ARDS if required to minimize plateau pressures and tidal volumes (grade C).

Whilst two small non-randomized series did demonstrate this to be safe |30,31|, evidence is also accepted from the protective ventilation trials, which use permissive hypercapnia as an integral part of protective ventilation |29|.

Unless contraindicated, mechanically ventilated patients should be maintained semirecumbent, with the head of the bed raised to 45° to prevent the development of ventilator-associated pneumonia (grade C).

A single study of 86 patients (recruitment stopped after interim analysis) in which mechanically ventilated patients were randomized to be semirecumbent or supine has demonstrated that the frequency of nosocomial pneumonia was significantly lower in the semirecumbent group than in the supine group |32|.

A weaning protocol should be in place and mechanically ventilated patients should undergo a spontaneous breathing trial to evaluate the ability to discontinue mechanical ventilation when set criteria are met (grade A). The first reference to support this recommendation compares two lengths of spontaneous ventilation trials and sets out to find the optimum length of such a trial: as such, it does not appear to support this recommendation |33|.

In the second reference study, a randomized trial of 300 patients underwent a 2-h trial of spontaneous breathing, which, if successful, led to the notification of their physician. The control group was monitored as per standard protocols. The intervention group had a significantly lower duration of mechanical ventilation and a significantly lower incidence of complications (self-extubation, re-intubation, tracheostomy, or mechanical ventilation for more than 21 days) |34|.

The third quoted reference is a randomized controlled trial comparing 2-h spontaneous breathing trials with either a T-piece or pressure support ventilation of 7 cmH$_2$O. None of the statistical analysis or any of the conclusions compare spontaneous breathing trials to another method of assessing appropriateness of extubation and, thus, do not appear to support this recommendation |35|.

Of the quoted references only one randomized trial supports the recommendation and, thus, this should be downgraded to a B recommendation.

Sedation, analgesia and neuromuscular blockade in sepsis

Protocols should be used when sedation of critically ill, mechanically ventilated patients is required. The protocol should include the use of a sedation goal, measured by a standardized subjective sedation scale (grade B).

A trial in which 321 patients were randomized to a group of protocol-directed sedation or non-protocol-directed sedation demonstrated a significantly shorter duration of mechanical ventilation, shorter length of ICU and hospital stay, shorter duration of sedation and a lower tracheostomy rate in the protocol group [36].

Either intermittent bolus sedation or continuous sedation to predetermined end points with daily interruption/lightening of continuous sedation with awakening and re-titration are recommended methods for sedation administration (grade B).

In a randomized controlled trial of 128 adults receiving mechanical ventilation and continuous infusions of sedative drugs, patients in the treatment group had their sedative infusions interrupted until they were awake on a daily basis. In the control group, the infusions were interrupted only at the discretion of the clinicians. The treatment group had significant improvements over the control group in duration of mechanical ventilation and length of ICU stay. Rates of complications such as self-extubation were not significantly different between the two groups [37].

Renal replacement therapy

In acute renal failure, and in the absence of haemodynamic instability, continuous venovenous haemofiltration (CVVHF) and intermittent haemodialysis (IHD) are considered equivalent. CVVHF offers easier management of fluid balance in haemodynamically unstable patients (grade B).

The first reference quoted to provide evidence to support this recommendation is a multicentre, randomized, controlled trial in which 166 patients were randomized to CVVHF or IHD. There were no significant differences in mortality, length of ICU stay or recovery of renal function [38].

Further evidence is provided with a meta-analysis of 13 trials comparing CVVHF and IHD. Only three of the studies were randomized and less than half of the studies compared groups which had comparable severities of illness. The authors concluded that there was insufficient evidence to draw strong conclusions regarding the superiority of one modality over another [39].

Bicarbonate therapy

Bicarbonate therapy for the purpose of improving haemodynamics or reducing vasopressor requirements is not recommended for treatment of hypoperfusion-induced lactic acidaemia with pH > 7.15 (grade C).

Two studies are quoted, with a combined number of 24 patients, who were sequentially given saline or bicarbonate one after the other. No difference was noted in any haemodynamic variables in either study [40,41].

Deep venous thrombosis prophylaxis

Severe sepsis patients should receive deep venous thrombosis (DVT) prophylaxis with either low-dose unfractionated heparin or low-molecular-weight heparin. For those with a contraindication, the use of a mechanical prophylactic device is recommended. In very high-risk patients, a combination of these methods is desirable (grade A). Whilst no study has specifically examined the question of DVT prophylaxis in sepsis, evidence is presented from the wider critically ill population. The incidence of DVT was studied in 119 critically ill patients and low-dose heparin prophylaxis was assessed in a randomized, double-blind study. DVT occurred in 29% of control patients and in 13% of patients receiving heparin 5000 U subcutaneously twice daily |42|. A previous study in medical patients with the same methodology recorded a decrease from 26% to 4% with low-dose heparin |43|. A further study randomized 1102 patients to receive low-molecular-weight heparin or placebo and found a significant decrease in the risk of thromboembolism (relative risk 0.37; 97.6% CI 0.22 to 0.63; $P<0.001$) |44|. Whilst the authors state that the references refer to large populations of ICU patients, in fact the majority of patients appear to be in the general hospital population. No references are provided to support the recommendations concerning mechanical prophylaxis.

Stress ulcer prophylaxis

Stress ulcer prophylaxis should be given to all patients with severe sepsis. H_2 receptor inhibitors are more efficacious than sucralfate and are the preferred agents. Proton pump inhibitors have not been assessed in a direct comparison with H_2 receptor antagonists; however, they demonstrate equivalency in ability to increase gastric pH (grade A).

Again, no studies specifically pertaining to ICU patients are quoted. The first two references show that the use of sucralfate is as efficacious as antacid given regularly in the critically ill |45,46|. The third trial compares ranitidine and sucralfate in patients requiring mechanical ventilation: those receiving ranitidine had a significantly lower rate of clinically important gastrointestinal bleeding than those treated with sucralfate. There were no significant differences in the rates of ventilator-associated pneumonia, the duration of the stay in the ICU or mortality |47|. Given the evidence quoted, this recommendation would therefore appear to be no more than a grade B.

Bundles

As a means to introducing these recommendations into practice as a standard of care, some of the recommendations have been collected together as two bundles. The first, the 'sepsis resuscitation bundle', contains the recommendations of initial resuscitation with the goal that all tasks should be completed within the first 6 h of care (Table 14.2) |6|. 'The sepsis management bundle' has a 24-h window in which to achieve the targets covering low-dose steroids, rhAPC, glycaemic control and limitation of inspiratory plateau pressures (Table 14.3) |6|.

Table 14.2 Example bundle from the Surviving Sepsis campaign – sepsis resuscitation bundle

1 Measure serum lactate
2 Obtain blood cultures prior to antibiotic administration
3 Administer broad-spectrum antibiotic, *within 3 h of ED admission and within 1 h of non-ED admission*
4 In the event of hypotension and/or a serum lactate > 4 mmol/l
   a Deliver an initial minimum of 20 ml/kg of crystalloid or an equivalent
   b Apply vasopressors for hypotension not responding to initial fluid resuscitation to maintain mean arterial pressure (MAP) > 65 mmHg
5. In the event of persistent hypotension despite fluid resuscitation (septic shock) and/or lactate > 4 mmol/l
   a Achieve a central venous pressure (CVP) of ≥ 8 mm Hgb.
   b Achieve a central venous oxygen saturation ($ScvO_2$) $\geq 70\%$ or mixed venous oxygen saturation ($S\tilde{v}O_2$) $\geq 65\%$

Table 14.3 Example bundle from the Surviving Sepsis campaign – sepsis management bundle

Efforts to accomplish these goals should begin immediately, but these items ought to be completed within 24 h of presentation for patients with severe sepsis or septic shock

1 Administer low-dose steroids for septic shock in accordance with a standardized ICU policy. *If not administered*, document why the patient did not qualify for low-dose steroids based upon the standardized protocol
2 Administer drotrecogin alfa (activated) in accordance with a standardized ICU policy. *If not administered*, document why the patient did not qualify for drotrecogin alfa (activated)
3 Maintain glucose control ≥ 70, but < 150 mg/dl
4 Maintain a median inspiratory plateau pressure < 30 cmH$_2$O for mechanically ventilated patients

    This chapter now examines new information that has become available since the publication of the guidelines to see whether any of the recommendations need to be rethought.

Sepsis resuscitation bundle

Economic implications of an evidence-based sepsis protocol: can we improve outcomes and lower costs?

Shorr AF, Micek ST, Jackson WL Jr, Kollef MH. *Crit Care Med* 2007; **35**: 1257–61

BACKGROUND. **The use of sepsis management protocols, based on the principles of early goal-directed therapy recommended by the Surviving Sepsis Campaign to guide resuscitation and early management of sepsis has been proposed as a way of improving outcomes in sepsis. In this study, the authors developed a protocol using the surviving sepsis guidelines. The protocol emphasized the initial**

identification of the septic patient, aggressive fluid resuscitation, timely antibiotic administration, and appropriateness of antibiotics, along with other supportive measures. They then compared the outcome of patients managed previous to and after the introduction of this protocol. The study included a total of 120 patients.

INTERPRETATION. There were significant improvements in the survival (70.0% vs. 51.7%, $P = 0.04$), length of hospital stay (approximately 5 days less in the protocol group, $P = 0.23$) and cost of hospital stay (approximately $5000, $P = 0.008$) after implementation of the sepsis management protocol.

Comment

Although a small study, the results would suggest that the introduction of a sepsis protocol can result not only in improved survival but also in considerable savings.

Implementation of a bundle of quality indicators for the early management of severe sepsis and septic shock is associated with decreased mortality

Nguyen HB, Corbett SW, Steele R, et al. Crit Care Med 2007; **35**: 1105–12

BACKGROUND. One method of ensuring the implementation of the Surviving Sepsis Guidelines is to measure quality markers and give feedback to physicians regarding their performance. In this study, five quality indicators were derived to examine compliance with the 6-h sepsis bundle (Fig. 14.1). These quality indicators were: (1) initiate central venous pressure/central venous oxygen saturation monitoring within 2 h; (2) give broad-spectrum antibiotics within 4 h; (3) complete early goal-directed therapy at 6 h; (4) give corticosteroids if the patient is on a vasopressor or if adrenal insufficiency is suspected; and (5) monitor for lactate clearance. Over a 2-year period the investigators examined the level of compliance with the bundle and the outcomes of the 330 patients.

INTERPRETATION. Over the 2-year period, compliance increased from 0 to 51.2% for patients in whom the bundle was completed (Fig. 14.1). In a multivariate regression analysis including the five quality indicators, completion of early goal-directed therapy was associated with decreased mortality (odds ratio 0.36; 95% confidence interval 0.17–0.79; $P = 0.01$). In-hospital mortality was less in patients who had the bundle completed (20.8 vs. 39.5%; $P < 0.01$).

Comment

The utilization of the initial resuscitation bundle as a package of care has been shown to have an impact on patient survival. As such, it is difficult to argue against the use of a protocolized approach covering the early management of patients who present with sepsis, especially when they are detected early outwith the critical care environment. It has been suggested, however, that it may be more to do with identifying the patient as belonging to a group with sepsis rather than the bundle components that is important.

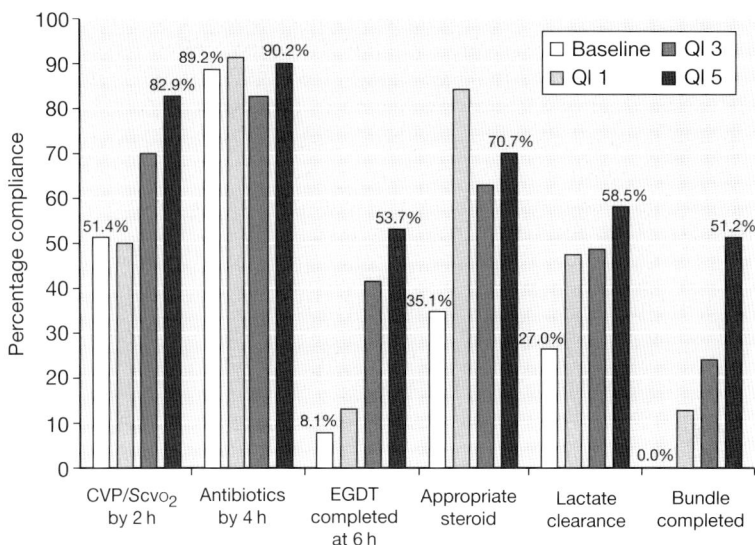

Fig. 14.1 Percentage compliance with the individual aspects of the bundle – baseline compared with the end of 3 months (QI 1), 9 months (QI 3); and 15 months (QI 5). Source: Nguyen et al. (2007).

Mixed venous oxygen saturation cannot be estimated by central venous oxygen saturation in septic shock

Varpula M, Karlsson S, Ruokonen E, et al. Intensive Care Med 2006; **32**: 1336–43

BACKGROUND. Central venous oxygen saturation has been suggested to approximate with the mixed venous oxygen saturation. The authors of this study set out to test this hypothesis in 16 patients with septic shock by taking paired central and true mixed venous samples and measuring the saturation.

INTERPRETATION. The authors demonstrated that the mixed venous saturation was consistently lower than the central venous saturation, and that the difference between these two oxygen saturation parameters varies highly even with similar vasoactive treatment. Therefore, $S\tilde{v}O_2$ should not be estimated on the basis of $ScvO_2$ (Fig. 14.2). However, the authors did show that both $ScvO_2$ and $S\tilde{v}O_2$ are low in early septic shock and conclude that they are useful variables in the detection of shock and during the resuscitation period.

Comment

Whilst the use of central venous oxygen saturation is not interchangeable with true mixed venous oxygen saturation, its use as part of early resuscitation does not appear to be unsound.

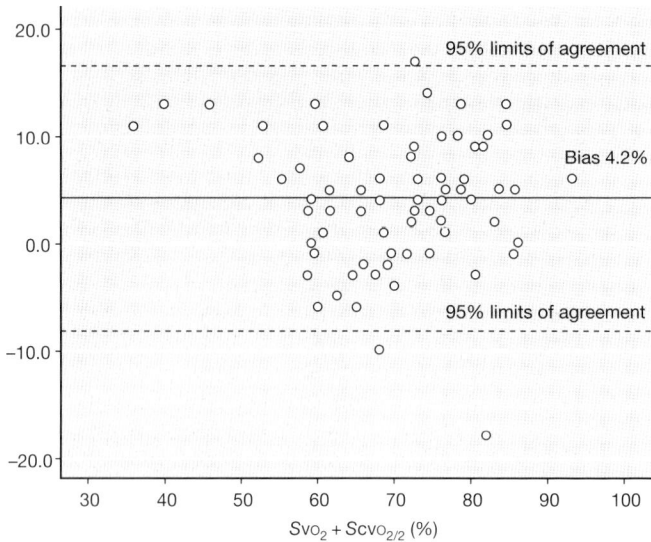

Fig. 14.2 Bland–Altman plot of the differences between $S\bar{v}O_2$ and $ScvO_2$ against their mean values. Source: Varpula *et al.* (2006).

The sepsis management bundle

Steroids in sepsis

Adrenal function in sepsis: the retrospective Corticus cohort study

Lipner-Friedman D, Sprung CL, Laterre PF, *et al. Crit Care Med* 2007; **35**: 1012–18

BACKGROUND. The Surviving Sepsis campaign recommends the use of low-dose corticosteroids in patients with septic shock. Support for this statement is in the form of a single randomized control trial of 300 patients with septic shock who were randomized to control or to receive hydrocortisone and fludrocortisone. The trial demonstrated a significant decrease in mortality in those patients with a relative adrenal insufficiency (as defined by an inadequate response to a synthetic ACTH challenge) who were treated with steroids |16|. The CORTICUS study attempts to clarify the utility of low-dose steroids in severe sepsis (http://clinicaltrials.gov/ct/show/NCT00147004). This was a multicentre, international, double-blind randomized, controlled trial. The primary endpoint was 28-day all-cause mortality in ACTH test non-responders. Secondary endpoints dealt with mortality in the entire population, organ failure resolution and safety.

The study was designed to enrol 800 patients so that it would have sufficient power to detect a 10% difference in mortality. However, because of difficulty with recruitment, the trial was halted after 500 persons were enrolled. Initially, participants were given hydrocortisone 50 mg every 6 h or placebo for 5 days with a reducing dose over the next 6 days. Fludrocortisone was not administered. Although the results are still to be published in full, the trial results have been presented at international meetings. We understand that a manuscript has been submitted for publication. From an abstract presentation, all-cause mortality was shown to be similar between the two arms regardless of ACTH responsiveness |48|: 33.5% and 31% in the hydrocortisone and placebo arms, respectively. Although the number of patients having reversal of shock was the same in both groups, the time to shock reversal was shorter in the hydrocortisone group but, interestingly, not significantly so in those who did not respond to ATCH. Rates of superinfection were significantly higher in those given corticosteroids, and the frequency of hospital-acquired new sepsis was also higher in those randomized to steroids. The study by Lipner-Friedman *et al.* is a recent publication of the retrospective CORTICUS data which looks specifically at plasma baseline cortisol and change in cortisol concentrations compared with outcome. Survival data on the use of hydrocortisone therapy are specifically excluded from this report. Non-survivors had higher baseline cortisol (29.5 ± 33.5 vs. $24.3 \pm 16.5 \mu g/dl$, $P = 0.03$) and also a smaller change in cortisol ($P = 0.006$).

INTERPRETATION. Corticosteroids do not affect mortality in sepsis, and indeed may lead to increased rates of new infection and sepsis. There has been increasing interest in the use of etomidate for tracheal intubation prior to mechanical ventilation and its possible effect on baseline cortisol and ACTH responsiveness. It transpires that many of the patients in the initial Annane *et al.* paper |16| had received etomidate. Interestingly, in the highlighted paper, etomidate was found to influence ACTH test results and was associated with a worse outcome.

Comment

This new evidence suggests that steroids do not have a role in the treatment of septic shock. There is growing criticism of the previous trials of corticosteroids in sepsis. For instance, it has become apparent that many of the enrolled patients had been given etomidate (a drug well known to suppress cortisol production for a long time after a single administration). It has also long been known that patients with sepsis who have higher baseline plasma cortisol concentrations have a worse mortality. Many of the meta-analyses that have been published in support of the use of corticosteroids have omitted certain papers in which the outcome was not favourable |49|.

Drotrecogin alfa (activated) for adults with severe sepsis and a low risk of death

Abraham E, Laterre P-F, Garg R, et al. for the Administration of Drotrecogin Alfa (Activated) in Early Stage Severe Sepsis (ADDRESS) Study Group. N Engl J Med 2005; **353**: 1332–41

BACKGROUND. The Surviving Sepsis campaign recommends the consideration of rhAPC in patients with a high risk of death based on the results of the PROWESS study |50|. This trial was stopped early after interim analysis demonstrated a significant survival benefit. A total of 1690 patients were treated. Treatment with activated protein C (APC) was associated with a reduction in relative risk of death of 19.4% (95% CI 6.6–30.5%). The observed mortality difference between treatment and placebo groups seemed to be limited to the patient population with the higher risk of mortality, as assessed by a baseline APACHE II score of greater than 24 |50|. The relative benefit to the sickest patients was even more pronounced when examining long-term survival. But in those patients with the lowest APACHE II scores, the observed mortality was greater in those patients exposed to APC. The ADDRESS study set out to test whether rhAPC was not useful and indeed potentially harmful to patients with lesser degrees of severe sepsis. The trial was terminated after enrolling 2640 patients because of a low likelihood of meeting the prospectively defined objective of demonstrating a significant reduction in the 28-day mortality rate with the use of rhAPC. There were no statistically significant differences between the placebo group and the rhAPC group in 28 day mortality or in in-hospital mortality (Fig. 14.3). However, the rate of serious bleeding was greater in the rhAPC group than in the placebo group during both the infusion and the 28-day study period.

INTERPRETATION. This study confirms that there is no benefit and a significant increase in risk of bleeding associated with the administration of rhAPC to patients with severe sepsis and an APACHE II score of less than 25.

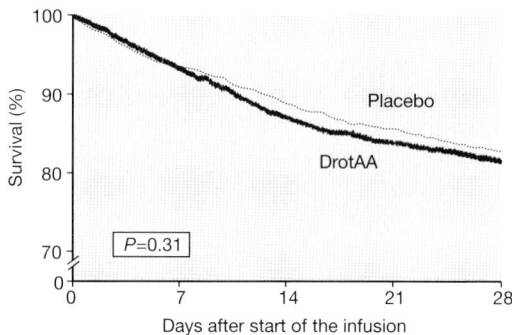

Fig. 14.3 Kaplan–Meier curves of survival of the 1316 patients with severe sepsis in the Drotrecogin Alfa (Activated) (DrotAA) group and 1297 patients in the placebo group (P = 0.31 by the log-rank test). Source: Abraham et al. (2005).

Comment

The rush to embrace rhAPC has been criticized in some quarters and this study emphasizes that its use should be undertaken only after due consideration of risks and benefits. A further study to examine the use of this agent is believed to be planned, which may provide more evidence to be considered.

Intensive insulin therapy in the medical ICU

Van den Berghe G, Wilmer A, Hermans G, *et al*. *N Engl J Med* 2006; **354**: 449–61

BACKGROUND. Intensive insulin therapy reduces morbidity and mortality in patients in surgical intensive care units (ICUs) |51|, but its role in patients in medical ICUs is unknown. This study randomized 1200 patients admitted to a medical intensive care unit to receive strict (4.4–6.1 mmol/l) or normal (insulin administered if glucose above 12 mmol/l) control of blood glucose. Whilst there was a significant decrease in new onset renal failure, time spent on mechanical ventilation, and decreased time to unit and hospital discharge, there was no significant decrease in mortality in the intention to treat analysis. *Post hoc* subgroup analysis of patients staying for 3 days or more did demonstrate a mortality benefit. A significant risk of hypoglycaemia occurred in the intensive group with an incidence of 18.7%.

INTERPRETATION. Whilst the group led by Van den Berghe previously demonstrated survival benefit with tight glucose control in a surgical ICU |51|, that single-centre trial was criticized as the patients were mainly cardiac surgery patients and had low APACHE II scores. As such, the applicability of the result to the majority of ICU patients is questionable. Furthermore, as the patients received such a large glucose load and correspondingly large amounts of insulin, the benefit seen in that study could have been due to either tight glycaemic control or to administration of insulin. In this study the protocol concentrates on tight glycaemic control without the glucose load and patients who are more likely to be comparable to the group of patients with severe sepsis. The overall intention to treat results showed no statistical difference ($P = 0.40$), but on retrospective subgroup analysis the group of patients staying in the ICU for 3 or more days did show a significant benefit from tight glycaemic control ($P = 0.02$) (Fig. 14.4). Of course, this implies, but is not stated in the paper, that those staying in the ICU for less than 3 days would have done significantly worse in the tight glycaemic control group.

Comment

This evidence casts some doubt on the recommendation that blood glucose should be maintained at less than 8.3 mmol/l, and further studies may be required. There appears to be differences depending on whether it is a surgical or medical admission and also on the length of ICU stay.

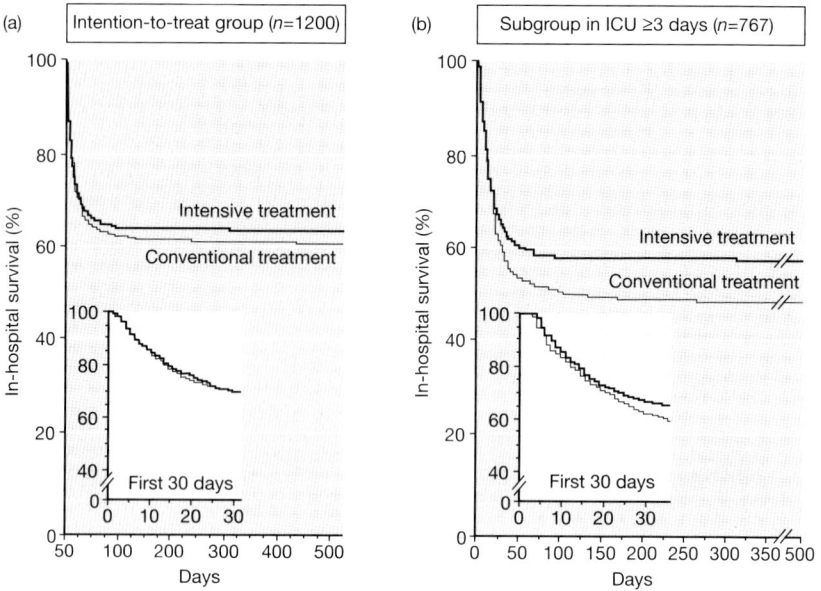

Fig. 14.4 Kaplan–Meier curves for in-hospital survival for the intent to treat group (a) ($P = 0.40$) and the subgroup staying in the ICU for 3 or more days (b) ($P = 0.02$). Source: Van den Berghe et al. (2006).

Conclusion

The Surviving Sepsis campaign is a noble cause; it is widely accepted that this spectrum of disease is both common and significant. Furthermore, the management of sepsis varies significantly and outcomes remain poor. The question as to whether a committee of 'experts' should generalize as to the management of individual patients is perhaps more contentious. Indeed, the role of certain sectors of the pharmaceutical industry in the formulation of these recommendations has been the subject of debate. If the recommendations provided were a distillation of good-quality clinical trials then this simply is good evidence-based medicine and all clinicians should be following the guidance anyway. However, as we have demonstrated, a significant proportion of the recommendations have little or no evidence base beyond 'expert opinion' – hardly the basis for a worldwide standard of care. Whilst the Surviving Sepsis campaign does encompass a wide variety of opinion, there are clearly some whose views are not included in the recommendations. One example would be to consider selective decontamination of the digestive tract (SDD). There are many who use this practice as a routine in their units believing that a strong evidence base exists to support it, and yet there is no mention of it anywhere in the Surviving Sepsis guidelines. Does this highlight a deficiency in the process or raise a question as to the effect of personal opinion on our ability to truly practise evidence-based medicine?

New evidence has come to light that leads us to rethink some of the Surviving Sepsis campaign's recommendations. It highlights the continuing search for the optimal management of sepsis that will enable us to improve the outcome of our patients. What is clear, however, is that merely labelling a patient as having sepsis or severe sepsis will result in an improvement in survival. It is this identification of such patients that is often difficult. Once the patient status has been established then timely and appropriate treatment can commence.

References

1. Harrison DA, Welch CA, Eddleston JM. The epidemiology of severe sepsis in England, Wales and Northern Ireland, 1996 to 2004: secondary analysis of a high quality clinical database, the ICNARC Case Mix Programme Database. *Crit Care* 2006; **10**: R42–52.

2. Angus D, Linde-Zwirble WT, Lidicker J, *et al.* Epidemiology of severe sepsis in the United States: analysis of incidence, outcome, and associated costs of care. *Crit Care Med* 2001; **29**: 1303–10.

3. Bone RC, Balk RA, Cerra FB, *et al.* Definitions for sepsis and organ failure and guidelines for the use of innovative therapies in sepsis. *Chest* 1992; **101**: 1644–55.

4. Heyland DK, Hopman W, Coo H, Tranmer J, McColl MA. Long-term health-related quality of life in survivors of sepsis. Short form 36: a valid and reliable measure of health-related quality of life. *Crit Care Med* 2000; **28**: 3599–605.

5. The Surviving sepsis campaign. Barcelona Declaration. Available at: http://www.survivingsepsis.com/hcp_barcelona.html.

6. Dellinger RP, Carlet JM, Masur HM, *et al.* Surviving Sepsis Campaign guidelines for the management of severe sepsis and septic shock. *Crit Care Med* 2004; **32**: 858–73.

7. Rivers E, Nguyen B, Havstad S, *et al.* Early goal-directed therapy in the treatment of severe sepsis and septic shock. *N Engl J Med* 2001; **345**: 1368–77.

8. Chawla LS, Zia H, Gutierrez G, Katz NM, Seneff MG, Shah M. Lack of equivalence between central and mixed venous oxygen saturation. *Chest* 2004; **126**: 1891–6.

9. Choi PTL, Yip G, Quinonez LG, Cook DJ. Crystalloids vs. colloids in fluid resuscitation: a systematic review. *Crit Care Med* 1999; **27**: 200–10.

10. Cook D, Guyatt G. Colloid use for fluid resuscitation: Evidence and spin. *Ann Intern Med* 2001; **135**: 205–8.

11. Schierhout G, Roberts I. Fluid resuscitation with colloid or crystalloid solutions in critically ill patients: a systematic review of randomized trials. *BMJ* 1998; **316**: 961–4.

12. Bellomo R, Chapman M, Finfer S, Hickling K, Myburgh J. Low-dose dopamine in patients with early renal dysfunction: a placebo-controlled randomised trial. Australian and New Zealand Intensive Care Society (ANZICS) Clinical Trials Group. *Lancet* 2000; **356**: 2139–43.

13. Kellum J, Decker J. Use of dopamine in acute renal failure: a meta-analysis. *Crit Care Med* 2001; **29**: 1526–53.

14. Gattinoni L, Brazzi L, Pelosi P, Latini R, Tognoni G, Pesenti A, Fumagalli R. A trial of goal-oriented hemodynamic therapy in critically ill patients. *N Engl J Med* 1995; **333**: 1025–32.

15. Hayes MA, Timmins AC, Yau EHS, Palazzo M, Hinds CJ, Watson D. Elevation of systemic oxygen delivery in the treatment of critically ill patients. *N Engl J Med* 1994; **330**: 1717–22.

16. Annane D, Sebille V, Charpentier C, *et al*. Effect of treatment with low doses of hydrocortisone and fludrocortisone on mortality in patients with septic shock. *JAMA* 2002; **288**: 862–71.

17. Bone RC, Fisher CJ, Clemmer TP. A controlled clinical trial of high-dose methylprednisolone in the treatment of severe sepsis and septic shock. *N Engl J Med* 1987; **317**: 653–8.

18. The Veterans Administration Systemic Sepsis Cooperative Study Group. Effect on high-dose glucocorticoid therapy on mortality in patients with clinical signs of sepsis. *N Engl J Med* 1987; **317**: 659–65.

19. Cronin L, Cook DJ, Carlet J, Heyland DK, King D, Lansang MA, Fisher CJ Jr. Corticosteroid treatment for sepsis: a critical appraisal and meta-analysis of the literature. *Crit Care Med* 1995; **23**: 1430–9.

20. Bernard GR, Vincent JL, Laterre PF, *et al*. Efficacy and safety of recombinant human activated protein C for severe sepsis. *N Engl J Med* 2001; **344**: 699–709.

21. Hébert PC, Wells G, Blajchman MA, *et al*. A multicenter, randomized, controlled clinical trial of transfusion in critical care. *N Engl J Med* 1999; **340**: 409–17.

22. Corwin HL, Gettinger A, Rodriguez RM, *et al*. Efficacy of recombinant human erythropoietin in the critically ill patient: a randomized double-blind, placebo-controlled trial. *Crit Care Med* 1999; **27**: 2346–50.

23. Corwin HL, Gettinger A, Pearl RG, *et al*. Efficacy of recombinant human erythropoietin in critically ill patients. *JAMA* 2002; **288**: 2827–35.

24. Warren BL, Eid A, Singer P, *et al*. High-dose antithrombin III in severe sepsis. A randomized controlled trial. *JAMA* 2001; **286**: 1869–78.

25. Amato MB, Barbas CS, Medeiros DM, *et al*. Effect of a protective-ventilation strategy on mortality in the acute respiratory distress syndrome. *N Engl J Med* 1998; **338**: 347–54.

26. Stewart TE, Meade MO, Cook DJ, *et al*. Evaluation of a ventilation strategy to prevent barotrauma in patients at high risk for acute respiratory distress syndrome. Pressure- and Volume-Limited Ventilation Strategy Group. *N Engl J Med* 1998; **338**: 355–61.

27. Brochard L, Roudat-Thoraval F, Roupie E, *et al*. Tidal volume reduction for prevention of ventilator-induced lung injury in acute respiratory distress syndrome. The Multicenter Trial Group on Tidal Volume reduction in ARDS. *Am J Respir Crit Care Med* 1998; **158**: 1831–8.

28. Brower RG, Shanholtz CB, Fessler HE, *et al*. Prospective, randomized, controlled clinical trial comparing traditional versus reduced tidal volume ventilation in acute respiratory distress syndrome patients. *Crit Care Med* 1999; **27**: 1492–8.

29. The Acute Respiratory Distress Syndrome Network. Ventilation with lower tidal volumes as compared with traditional tidal volumes for acute lung injury and the acute respiratory distress syndrome. *N Engl J Med* 2000; **342**: 1301–8.

30. Hickling KG, Walsh J, Henderson S, *et al.* Low mortality rate in adult respiratory distress syndrome using low-volume, pressure-limited ventilation with permissive hypercapnia: a prospective study. *Crit Care Med 1994*; **22**: 1568–78.

31. Bidani A, Tzouanakis AE, Cardenas VJ, *et al.* Permissive hypercapnia in acute respiratory failure. *JAMA* 1994; **272**: 957–62.

32. Drakulovic MB, Torres A, Bauer TT, Nicolas JM, Nogue S, Ferrer M. Supine body position as a risk factor for nosocomial pneumonia in ventilated patients: a randomized trial. *Lancet* 1999; **354**: 1851–8.

33. Esteban A, Alia I, Tobin MJ, *et al.* Effect of spontaneous breathing trial duration on outcome of attempts to discontinue mechanical ventilation. Spanish Lung Failure Collaborative Group. *Am J Respir Crit Care Med* 1999; **159**: 512–18.

34. Ely EW, Baker AM, Dunagan DP, *et al.* Effect on the duration of mechanical ventilation of identifying patients capable of breathing spontaneously. *N Engl J Med* 1996; **335**: 1864–9 .

35. Esteban A, Alia I, Gordo F, *et al.* Extubation outcome after spontaneous breathing trials with T-tube or pressure support ventilation. The Spanish Lung Failure Collaborative Group. *Am J Respir Crit Care Med* 1997; **156**: 459–65.

36. Brook AD, Ahrens TS, Schaiff R, *et al.* Effect of a nursing-implemented sedation protocol on the duration of mechanical ventilation. *Crit Care Med* 1999; **27**: 2609–15.

37. Kress JP, Pohlman AS, O'Connor MF, *et al.* Daily interruption of sedative infusions in critically ill patients undergoing mechanical ventilation. *N Engl J Med* 2000; **342**: 1471–7.

38. Mehta RL, McDonald B, Gabbai FB, *et al.* A randomized clinical trial of continuous vs. intermittent dialysis for acute renal failure. *Kidney Int* 2001; **60**: 1154–63.

39. Kellum J, Angus DC, Johnson JP, *et al.* Continuous versus intermittent renal replacement therapy: a meta-analysis. *Intensive Care Med* 2002; **28**: 29–37.

40. Cooper DJ, Walley KR, Wiggs BR, *et al.* Bicarbonate does not improve hemodynamics in critically ill patients who have lactic acidosis: a prospective, controlled clinical study. *Ann Intern Med* 1990; **112**: 492–8.

41. Mathieu D, Neviere R, Billard V, *et al.* Effects of bicarbonate therapy on hemodynamics and tissue oxygenation in patients with lactic acidosis: a prospective, controlled clinical study. *Crit Care Med* 1991; **19**: 1352–6.

42. Cade JF. High risk of the critically ill for venous thromboembolism. *Crit Care Med 1982*; **10**: 448–50.

43. Belch JJ, Lowe GD, Ward AG, *et al.* Prevention of deep vein thrombosis in medical patients by low-dose heparin. *Scot Med J* 1981; **26**: 115–7.

44. Samama MM, Cohen AT, Darmon JY, *et al.* A comparison of enoxaparin with placebo for the prevention of venous thromboembolism in acutely ill medical patients. Prophylaxis in Medical Patients with Enoxaparin Study Group. *N Engl J Med* 1999; **341**: 793–800.

45. Borrero E, Bank S, Margolis I, *et al.* Comparison of antacid and sucralfate in the prevention of gastrointestinal bleeding in patients who are critically ill. *Am J Med* 1985; **79**: 62–4.

46. Bresalier RS, Grendell JH, Cello JP, *et al.* Sucralfate versus titrated antacid for the prevention of acute stress-related gastrointestinal hemorrhage in critically ill patients. *Am J Med* 1987; **83**: 110–6.

47. Cook D, Guyatt G, Marshall J, *et al.* A comparison of sucralfate and ranitidine for the prevention of upper gastrointestinal bleeding in patients requiring mechanical ventilation. Canadian Critical Care Trials Group. *N Engl J Med* 1998; **338**: 791–7.

48. Sprung CL, Annane D, Briegel J, et al. Corticosteroid. Therapy of Septic Shock (CORTICUS) (Abstract). *Am J Resp Crit Care Med* 2007; **175**: A507 (abstract issue).

49. Bennett IL, Finland M, Hamburger M. The effectiveness of hydrocortisone in the management of severe infections. *JAMA* 1963; **183**: 462–5.

50. Bernard GR, Vincent JL, Laterre PF, *et al.* Efficacy and safety of recombinant human activated protein C for severe sepsis. *N Engl J Med* 2001; **344**: 699–709.

51. Van den Berghe G, Wouters P, Weekers F, *et al.* Intensive insulin therapy in critically ill patients. *N Engl J Med* 2001; **345**: 1359–67.

15

Glycaemic control in critical care

REBECCA CUSACK, BARBARA PHILIPS

Introduction

Hyperglycaemia is common in critically ill patients and is associated with a poor outcome from various medical and surgical conditions including acute myocardial infarction, stroke, exacerbations of chronic obstructive airways disease, cardiac surgery and critical illness [1–6]. Indeed, merely presenting in the accident and emergency department with an increased blood sugar may significantly increase the risk of in-hospital mortality [7]. In the critically ill patient it is described as an independent predictor of poor outcome. This raises the question: is hyperglycaemia a casual or causal factor?

The endocrine stress response of critical illness causes insulin resistance and hyperglycaemia. Gluconeogenesis is up-regulated secondary to increased circulating concentrations of glucagon, growth hormone, cortisol and cytokines. These hormonal changes promote lipolysis and proteolysis, increasing glycerol and amino acid availability for gluconeogenesis. Insulin resistance decreases the uptake of glucose into tissues dependent on the activity of glucose transporter 4 (GLUT 4), notably in adipose tissue and skeletal and heart muscle. The availability of glucose for insulin-independent tissues, such as brain, red blood cells and immune cells, is increased. This has previously been considered potentially beneficial, part of an adaptive response to critical illness, but the unregulated uptake of glucose via insulin-independent mechanisms in the presence of a superfluity of glucose may be the route of harm and glucose toxicity.

Until recently, blood glucose concentrations of 12 mmol/l were considered acceptable, but in 2001 the Leuven study [8] of surgical critically ill patients showed improved outcome for patients treated with intensive insulin therapy who achieved a blood glucose of between 4.4 and 6.1 mmol/l. There were marked decreases in morbidity and mortality. What could not be elucidated was whether the benefit was due to control of glucose or the anti-inflammatory, immune-modulatory effects of insulin. Intensive insulin regimens were subsequently implemented in many intensive care units but clinicians found tight glycaemic control surprisingly difficult to achieve. Importantly, a marked increase in the incidence of hypoglycaemia occurred. Aware of these issues, the Surviving Sepsis campaign |9| has recommended the control of blood glucose concentration to <8.0 mmol/l. This is not based on evidence but is a pragmatic solution which is untested. Other clinicians have questioned the cost benefits of developing and using such regimens, citing increased blood glucose testing and nursing time as potential problems. The following studies review the most recent evidence for and against tight glycaemic control and are selected in order to consider the following questions:

1   Is there evidence that glucose is toxic to cells and is this toxicity decreased by normoglycaemia?

2   Are the glucose-independent actions of insulin more important?

3   Are all critically ill patients the same? Are there identifiable groups of patients who would benefit or be harmed?

4   In implementation of tight glycaemic control, what is the risk of hypoglycaemia?

5   To what standard has the technology developed? Are our glucose monitoring systems adequate and how is treatment best titrated?

Intensive insulin therapy in the medical ICU

Van den Berghe G, Wilmer A, Hermans G, *et al*. *N Engl J Med* 2006; **354**: 449–61

BACKGROUND. In 2001, the Leuven surgical study looked at glycaemic control in critically ill patients on a surgical intensive care unit and showed an overall decrease in mortality from 8% to 4.6% with tight glycaemic control |8|. The decrease was impressive but the question remained: could this be extrapolated to all intensive care patients? In this study, the investigation was repeated in medical critically ill patients, who again were either treated conventionally or by a protocol aimed at achieving tight glycaemic control (blood glucose concentration 4.4–6.1 mmol/l).

INTERPRETATION. A total of 1200 patients were randomized, of whom 767 required >3 days' intensive care. Overall, there was no difference in outcome, with average blood glucose concentrations of approximately 8.6 mmol/l and 5.5 mmol/l in the control and treatment groups, respectively. In patients requiring >3 days' admission, mortality was significantly decreased (Fig. 15.1). However, in patients requiring <3 days there was a trend to increased mortality. In terms of morbidity, tight glycaemic control was associated with an overall reduction in newly acquired kidney injury, earlier weaning from the ventilator, earlier discharge from intensive care and earlier discharge from hospital (see Fig. 15.1).

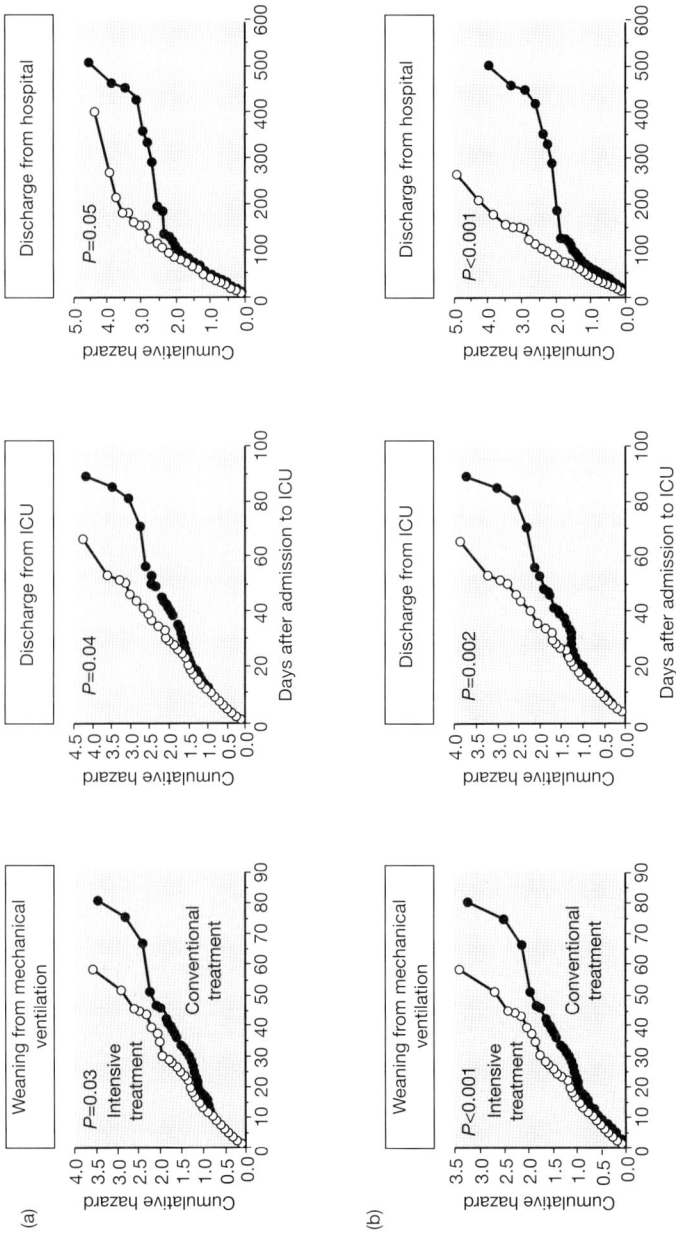

Fig. 15.1 The effect of tight glycaemic control on measures of morbidity in a medical intensive care unit. (a) All patients. (b) Subgroup of patients requiring 3 or more days in intensive care (n = 797). Time to weaning from mechanical ventilation, time to discharge from the intensive care unit (ICU), and time to discharge from the hospital are shown. P-values for the comparison between the two groups were calculated by proportional-hazards regression analysis with censoring for early deaths. Circles represent patients. Source: Van den Berghe et al. (2006).

Comment

This study provoked great debate. Protagonists of tight glycaemic control view the decrease in morbidity overall and in mortality of patients requiring >3 days' intensive care admission as evidence supporting the ongoing use of such protocols. Those less convinced of its merits highlight the lack of effect or even adverse mortality in patients requiring <3 days' stay as evidence against its use in all intensive care patients. The numbers of patients who died in this group were 56 in the tight glycaemic control group and 42 in the conventional group, the statistical significance depending on the test used. This as a crude mortality difference (chi-squared test) was significant at a *P*-value of 0.05; however, after being corrected for other risk factors for death (Acute Physiology and Chronic Health [APACHE] II score, liver necrosis and history of diabetes, renal impairment or cancer) the hazard ratio was 1.09 (CI 0.89–1.32, $P = 0.41$). Had the authors been trying to justify a positive result it is unlikely that a crude mortality would have been accepted as relevant. The corrected hazard ratio for mortality for patients requiring >3 days' admission was 0.84 (0.73–0.97, $P = 0.02$) favouring tight glycaemic control. The failure to show a positive result in all patients was disappointing but may be a reflection of the greater heterogeneity of medical critically ill patients. Other factors may have had a greater impact on outcome.

In common with the surgical Leuven study |8|, there was a marked decrease in morbidity. Notable effects included the significant decrease in newly acquired kidney injury and the decreased requirements for ventilation. Understanding the reasons for these changes may be a way of understanding the mechanisms of the effects.

Severity of insulin resistance in critically ill medical patients

Zauner A, Nimmerrichter P, Anderwald C, *et al*. *Metabolism* 2007; **56**: 1–5

BACKGROUND. The acute metabolic stress response to surgery and trauma is well described. Similar changes are presumed in critically ill medical patients but are less well investigated. This study measures insulin resistance and energy expenditure in 40 critically ill patients and 12 healthy volunteers. Insulin resistance was measured using isoglycaemic, hyperinsulinaemic clamps after an overnight fast, and energy expenditure by indirect calorimetry. Severity of illness was assessed by the APACHE III score.

INTERPRETATION. The critically ill medical patients were admitted with a wide variety of diagnoses. Age and body mass index (BMI) were similar in patients and control subjects. Patients had higher blood glucose concentrations before and during the tests than the volunteers but serum insulin concentrations achieved were similar. Hyperinsulinaemia caused a significant increase in the respiratory quotient and glucose oxidation rate, a decrease in the fat oxidation rate and no change to the resting energy expenditure. Insulin resistance was significantly greater in the critically ill patients than controls and was negatively correlated with APACHE III and BMI.

Comment

Insulin resistance may be an adaptive response to maintain glucose supplies to non-insulin-dependent and injured tissues or, alternatively, it may indicate that adaptive mechanisms are failing, i.e. the β-islet cells are unable to secrete sufficient insulin to maintain normoglycaemia within the inflammatory response. Either way the result is a surfeit of glucose. Insulin binds and acts through the insulin receptor and insulin-like growth factor-1 receptor via a series of post-receptor signals first, to trigger GLUT4 translocation to cell membranes and secondly, to mediate its nuclear and mitogenic effects |10|. Many of the post-receptor steps are affected by inflammatory mediators, which suppress the response to insulin and decrease cellular uptake of glucose in insulin-dependent tissues. Organs independent of the activity of insulin are therefore exposed to the excess glucose and uptake is unimpeded. Once within the cell glucose is immediately phosphorylated, creating a constant inward gradient that maintains the drive to take up glucose. In insulin-resistant tissues, this may be highly damaging. Intracellular glucose is proinflammatory, the amount that can complete glycolysis is limited by the inhibition of glyceraldehyde phosphate dehydrogenase (GAPDH) and increased glucose is diverted to the glucosamine pathway |11|. Intranuclear NF-κB is induced increasing the production of cytokines such as tumour necrosis factor-alpha (TNF- α), and interleukins 1β, 6 and 8 (IL-1β, IL-6 and IL-8). The effect of glucose on the production of reactive oxygen species (ROS) is complex. Increased pyruvate oxidation induced by maximal glycolysis increases the mitochondrial membrane potential, increasing mitochondrial ROS production and inhibiting GAPDH. However, whilst mitochondrial ROS production is increased, cytoplasmic ROS production may be enhanced or inhibited. Glucose plays a complex role in the oxidant signalling pathways affecting various systems and the cytoplasmic effect of hyperglycaemia will depend on the severity of the hyperglycaemia, the cell type, and the prevailing metabolic and inflammatory conditions |11|.

Survival benefits of intensive insulin therapy in critical illness

Impact of maintaining normoglycaemia versus glycaemia-independent actions of insulin

Ellger B, Debaveye Y, Vanhorebeek I. *Diabetes* 2006; **55**: 1096–105

BACKGROUND. The relative importance of tight glycaemic control and the glycaemic-independent actions of insulin in conferring any benefit to critically ill patients is uncertain. A rabbit model of acute stress was investigated. The animals were divided into four groups of glycaemic management, each with a varying glucose–insulin ratio: (1) normal insulin and normoglycaemia; (2) high

insulin and normoglycaemia; (3) normal insulin and hyperglycaemia; and (4) high insulin and hyperglycaemia. The impact of each regimen was studied on survival, myocardial contractility, endothelial function and liver, kidney and leucocyte function over a period of 7 days.

INTERPRETATION. Hyperglycaemia was associated with a lower survival than normoglycaemia, regardless of the dose of insulin administered (Fig. 15.2). Haemodynamics were broadly unaffected by the regimens, except for an increase in myocardial contractility with high insulin doses, but only if normoglycaemic. Liver and kidney function deteriorated in all groups as a result of the acute stress but recovered only in the normoglycaemic groups. The *ex vivo* test of endothelium-dependent relaxation of isolated aortic rings was impaired in all groups but relaxation to increasing acetylcholine concentrations was better in the normoglycaemic animals compared with those with hyperglycaemia. Insulin had no effect. Leucocyte function was impaired only in the hyperglycaemic, normal-insulin group.

Comment

Since the Leuven surgical study |8|, protagonists of tight glycaemic control have been divided into two groups: those who consider the benefit to be secondary to glucose control and those who favour the anti-inflammatory and immune modulatory effects of insulin. This intriguing animal study attempts to separate the glucose from the insulin effects. To prevent the endogenous stimulation of insulin, all animals were rendered insulin-deficient using alloxan and then managed within their allocated treatment group by infusion of glucose and insulin. Improvements were observed, whether insulin was implicated or not, only in the presence of normoglycaemia

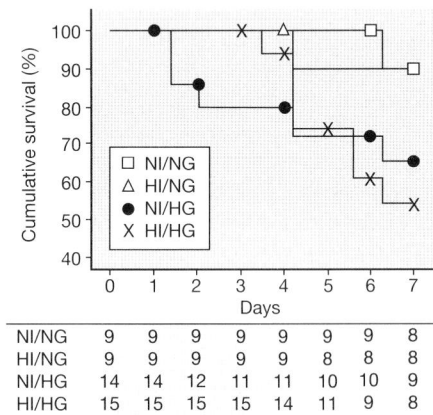

	0	1	2	3	4	5	6	7
NI/NG	9	9	9	9	9	9	9	8
HI/NG	9	9	9	9	9	8	8	8
NI/HG	14	14	12	11	11	10	10	9
HI/HG	15	15	15	15	14	11	9	8

Fig. 15.2 A comparison of glycaemic control and intensive insulin therapy showing the cumulative survival for animals managed by one of four regimens: NI, normoinsulinaemia; NG, normoglycaemia; HI, hyperinsulinaemia; HG, hyperglycaemia. Numbers of animals at risk are depicted below the graph. □, NI/NG; , △, HI/NG; •, NI/HG; ×, HI/HG; $n = 47$ total animals used. $P < 0.03$ for both normoglycaemic vs. both hyperglycaemic groups; no significant difference between NI/HG and HI/HG. Source: Ellger *et al.* (2006).

suggesting that glucose toxicity has greater impact than the protective actions of insulin. Kidney, liver, endothelial and innate immune dysfunction were all worsened by hyperglycaemia irrespective of the insulin administered.

The concept of acute glucose toxicity is one that is gaining support. Glucose is taken into non-insulin-dependent cells by facilitated glucose transporters, with the rate of uptake being dependent on the extracellular to intracellular glucose concentration gradient, the density of the transporters within the cell membrane and the kinetic properties of the individual transporters. The insulin-independent facilitated glucose transporters (GLUT 1, 2 and 3) are closely related proteins, which differ from each other in tissue distribution and affinity for glucose |12,13|. GLUT 1 is widely expressed. GLUT 2 is a low-affinity transporter found in kidney, small intestine, liver and lung and may be for glucose sensing rather than bulk glucose transport. GLUT 3 is a high-affinity glucose transporter found in neurones and the placenta. Normally, the expression of GLUT 1 and 3 are decreased as blood glucose concentrations increase but as insulin resistance develops and causes hyperglycaemia, acute stress mediators, including endothelin-1, pro-inflammatory cytokines, vascular endothelial growth factor and hypoxia, up-regulate GLUT 1 and GLUT 3 expression and glucose uptake is increased |10|.

Evaluation of short-term consequences of hypoglycemia in an intensive care unit

Vriesendorp TM, DeVries JH, van Santan S, *et al*. *Crit Care Med* 2006; **34**: 2714–18

BACKGROUND. The introduction of tight glycaemic control is thought to have increased the risk of hypoglycaemia in critically ill patients. Hypoglycaemia has been cited as one reason for not implementing tight glycaemic control on the premise of *first do no harm*. A retrospective cohort study of patients admitted to a single medical and surgical intensive care over 3 years investigated all the admissions for harm secondary to hypoglycaemia defined as a blood glucose concentration <2.5 mmol/l. Cases were identified from the database and matched with a control patient admitted to the unit concurrently. Outcome in terms of mortality and neurological deficit was investigated.

INTERPRETATION. Out of a total of 2272 patients who managed to achieve tight glycaemic control (4.5–8.0 mmol/l), 156 were found to have had 245 episodes of hypoglycaemia and 65 (41%) died, compared with 39 (27%) control subjects (hazard ratio for in-hospital death was 1.39 [95% CI 0.93–2.08]). Two cases of hypoglycaemic coma were reported in the discharge letters and one patient and one control had seizures within the study period.

Comment

The nested case–control design of this retrospective study is appropriate. The cases and control subjects were matched for age, sex, severity of illness and duration of intensive care admission before the episode of hypoglycaemia. Consequently, nine control subjects had to be excluded from the analyses because of a subsequent episode of hypoglycaemia, illustrating one of the difficulties with this sort of design. In addition, causality cannot be assessed, merely an association observed.

The study allows only limited interpretation of the results related to insulin use. Of the 156 patients with an episode of hypoglycaemia, 81% were treated with insulin but 19% were not. In the control group, 54% were treated with insulin. It is possible that insulin therapy increased the risk of hypoglycaemia, but this is not proven as its use was not protocol driven. We are, therefore, left uncertain about the clinical indications used. Nevertheless, the study was able to analyse a number of hypoglycaemic episodes and their consequences. The three patients who may have been harmed directly by hypoglycaemia were described in detail. The patient who developed seizures never received insulin, had repeated episodes of hypoglycaemia (lowest recorded 1.5 mmol/l) and eventually died. The other two patients did receive insulin and both had severe sepsis and repeated episodes of hypoglycaemia. In the Leuven medical study, 111 (18.7%) patients treated with insulin became hypoglycaemic (blood glucose <2.5 mmol/l) compared with 3.1% of patients receiving conventional therapy. Although no clinical events were directly associated with hypoglycaemia, it was later identified as an independent risk factor for death. There is an undoubted association between the use of insulin and an increased risk of hypoglycaemia. Hypoglycaemia may also be a marker of severity of illness and various predisposing factor have been identified, including the need for inotropic support, sepsis and a prior diagnosis of diabetes mellitus |14|.

Variability of blood glucose concentration and short-term mortality in critically ill patients

Egi M, Bellomo R, Stachowski E, *et al*. *Anesthesiology* 2006; **105**: 244–52

BACKGROUND. For patients with diabetes mellitus, increased blood glucose variability in addition to hyperglycaemia is predictive of complications |15|; this may also be true for acutely ill patients. This multicentre retrospective observational study looked at the variability in blood glucose during intensive care admission for all patients admitted to the units between January 2000 and October 2004. No specific glycaemic regimen was used; insulin was instigated at the discretion of the medical staff. The values used to measure variability included the standard deviation of blood glucose concentration (Glu_{SD}) and the coefficient of variability ($Glu_{CV} = Glu_{SD} \times 100$/mean blood glucose).

INTERPRETATION. A total of 7049 patients were studied, yielding a total of 168 837 blood glucose measurements. Overall mean glucose concentration was 8.4 mmol/l, Glu_{SD} 1.7 mmol/l and Glu_{Ave} 21%. In the comparison between survivors ($n = 6213$) and non-survivors ($n = 836$) both the Glu_{SD} and Glu_{CV} were significantly greater in the non-survivors (1.7 ± 1.3 vs. 2.3 ± 1.6 mmol/l and 20 ± 12 vs. 26 ± 13%, respectively). When the Glu_{SD} results were divided into four groups of increasing value, the difference between survivors and non-survivors was maintained (Fig. 15.3).

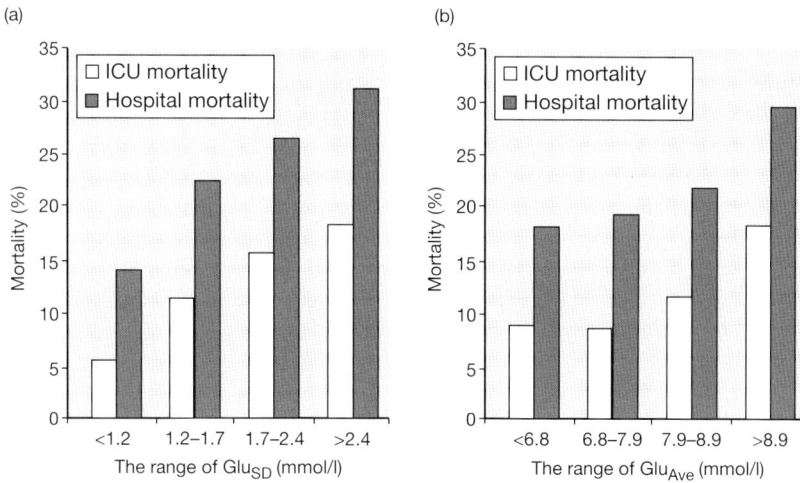

Fig. 15.3 (a and b) Relationship between blood glucose control and intensive care unit (ICU) and hospital mortality for 7049 patients divided into quartiles of either the standard deviation of glucose (Glu_{SD} = SD of blood glucose concentration) (a) or the mean blood glucose concentration (Glu_{Ave} = mean blood glucose concentration) (b). Source: Egi *et al.* (2006).

Comment

Although large numbers were investigated in this study, it is retrospective and caution should be exercised in its interpretation in case of unrecognized bias. Nevertheless, it raises the intriguing possibility that glucose variability is as important as hyperglycaemia in determining outcome. The standard deviation of blood glucose concentration and a calculated coefficient of variation were used as the measures of variation. These are appropriate measures but care is required in interpreting their meaning. The variation is measured around a set point: in this case it could be around high blood glucose concentrations, between high and low blood glucose concentrations, or indeed around low blood glucose concentrations. The authors found that blood glucose variability had greater predictive value for mortality than mean blood glucose. Although maximum blood glucose concentrations were given, minimum concentrations were not provided and, therefore, there is no indication of the incidence of hypoglycaemia. Glycaemic variability in diabetes mellitus may be an independent risk factor for diabetic complications |**15**|. Acute glucose variability is a strong predictor for free radical production when compared with postprandial area under the curve blood glucose concentrations, with a linear relationship between free radical production and the magnitude of glucose fluctuation |**16**|. It is hypothesized that this variability is important in the pathogenesis of microvascular complications. It is as yet unknown whether it is of any practical importance in critically ill non-diabetic patients.

Effect of glucose–insulin–potassium infusion on mortality in patients with acute ST-segment elevation myocardial infarction

The CREATE-ECLA Trial Group Investigators. *JAMA* 2005; **293**: 437–46

BACKGROUND. Glucose, potassium and insulin (GKI) regimens have been applied to the modulation of acute myocardial infarction since the 1960s under the premise that insulin suppresses the damaging proinflammatory response and high-dose glucose provides readily available energy for the struggling heart. This was a randomized controlled trial over 470 centres worldwide recruiting patients post ST-segment elevation myocardial infarction (STEMI). Patients received usual care alone (control) or usual care and a 24-h GKI regimen. The primary outcome was mortality from any cause at 30 days. Secondary outcome included composite measures of death or non-fatal cardiac arrest, death or cardiogenic shock, and death or reinfarction.

INTERPRETATION. In total, 20 201 patients were randomized to either GKI and usual care or usual care alone. At 30 days, there were no differences in any of the outcome measures between the groups. At 7 days, safety outcome was analysed and patients receiving the GKI regimen were more likely to develop hyperkalaemia (> 5.5 mmol/l), phlebitis and symptomatic hypoglycaemia. The mean admission blood glucose for all patients was 9.0 mmol/l. After randomization, the blood glucose in the GKI group increased to 10.4 mmol/l within 6 ho (8.2 mmol/l controls) and 8.6 mmol/l after 24 h (7.5 mmol/l controls). Increased mortality at 30 days was associated with higher baseline blood glucose concentrations.

Comment

This study concludes that it has reliably established that high-dose GKI infusion in patients with STEMI has no impact on mortality, cardiac arrest or cardiogenic shock. With such large numbers enrolled, the conclusion might appear sound. But before it is accepted without question it should be recognized that the blood glucose concentration in the study group was significantly higher than in the control group. The conclusion drawn can be relied upon only if it is accepted that the benefit expected would have been due to an insulin effect rather than the control of glucose.

In the DIGAMI-1 trial [17], GKI was shown to improve outcome from STEMI for patients with diabetes mellitus, but in this study good glycaemic control was an essential part of the regimen. The study group had significantly lower blood glucose than the control group. In DIGAMI-2 [18], designed to differentiate between glucose and insulin effect, there was no difference in blood glucose between groups and no benefit of GKI observed. These studies serve to illustrate further the conundrum of glucose control vs. insulin therapy. It could be concluded from this very large randomized trial that there is little evidence that high-dose insulin modulates the outcome from acute STEMI. But it remains to be seen if there is benefit from control of glucose and the avoidance of glucose toxicity.

Strict blood glucose control with insulin during intensive care after cardiac surgery: impact on 4-years survival, dependency on medical care, and quality of life

Ingels C, Debaveye Y, Milants I, et al. Eur Heart J 2006; **27**: 2716–24

BACKGROUND. In the Leuven surgical study |8| for patients randomized to tight glycaemic control, the in-hospital mortality was markedly decreased from 11% to 7%. The majority of these patients had undergone cardiac surgery. This study observes these cardiac surgery patients 4 years after the original investigation to examine whether the benefits in outcome are sustained. Long-term outcome was quantified as (1) 4-year survival; (2) incidence of hospital re-admission; (3) level of activity and medical care requirements; and (4) perceived health-related quality of life as assessed by the Nottingham Health Profile.

INTERPRETATION. Of the 1548 patients originally randomized, 970 cardiac patients were followed up at 4 years. More patients in the tight glycaemic control group required long-term care (12.8% vs. 5.9%). Overall mortality at 4 years was similar in each group but for patients requiring more than 3 days' intensive care, mortality in the tight glycaemic group was lower than in the control group (23.1% vs. 36.2%) (Fig. 15.4). Little difference was observed in terms of cardiac disability, pain, energy, sleep or physical mobility. Patients who had tight glycaemic control were more likely to score badly in terms of impact of health on family life, household activities and social life.

Comment

The mortality advantage of short-term glycaemic control appeared to be maintained over the 4 years. More of the patients in the tight glycaemic control group required transfer to another hospital, long-term facilities or rehabilitation, but the authors argue that these were the sicker individuals who would not have survived at all had they not received tight glycaemic control. At 4 years, these patients showed comparable medical dependency with the control group but were worse in terms of quality of social and family life scores. Medical dependency was measured by the incidence of re-admission to hospital and the Karnofsky score (range 0% [dead] to 100% [normal activity]; >60%: able to live independently). The most common causes of death within the 4-year follow-up were cardiovascular disease, malignancy and neurological complications.

The initial survival benefit was not related to cardiac complications but rather to a decrease in complications in other organs, notably decreased artificial ventilation requirements, and less renal impairment, transfusion requirement, liver impairment and critical illness polymyoneuropathy. The cardiac patients treated with tight glycaemic control also had decreased inflammation (based on C-reactive protein concentrations).

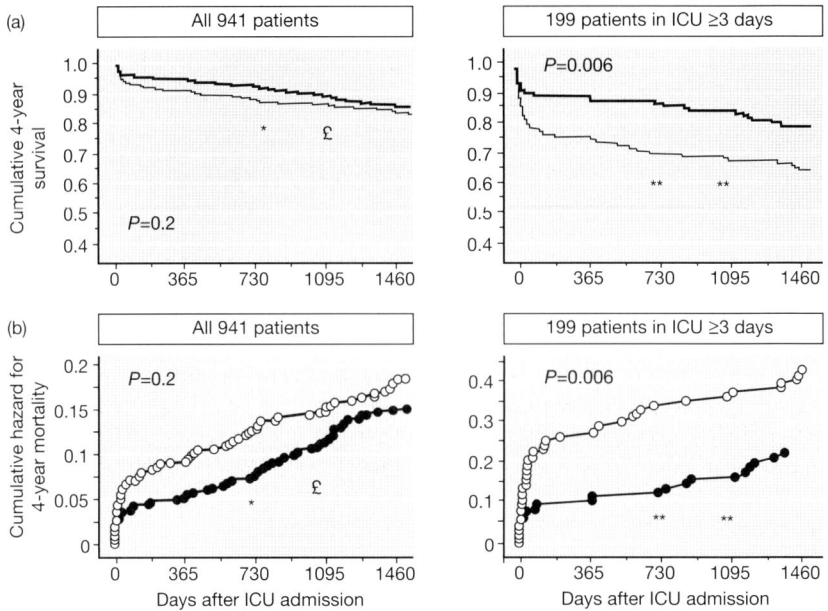

Fig. 15.4 Kaplan–Meier survival curves and cumulative hazard plots of the time course of mortality from inclusion in the study until 4 years later, of all 941 patients who had been admitted to ICU after cardiac surgery and of those 199 patients who required at least a third day of intensive care and of whom long-term follow-up data were available. Thick lines and filled circles represent patients in the intensive insulin group and thin lines and open circles the patients in the conventional insulin group. *P*-values were obtained by log-rank Mantel–Cox test. The symbols indicate levels of significance after 2 and 3 years, respectively. £*P* = 0.1; *P<0.05; **P<0.01. Source: Ingels *et al.* (2006).

This study does have its limitations. It was a pre-planned study based on the original Leuven surgical study |8| but was unblinded and, therefore, open to bias. It considered only cardiac surgery patients, and although these were the majority of the original study (970 patients out of a total of 1548 surgical ICU admissions), the results cannot be directly extrapolated to all surgical critically ill patients. The questionnaires used were incomplete; patients had to agree to answer the questions and some refused.

Nevertheless, this is one of very few studies looking at the long-term impact of intensive care management and it was able to show a lasting benefit of a very simple critical care intervention.

Association of hypoglycaemia, hyperglycaemia and glucose variability with morbidity and death in the paediatric intensive care unit

Wintergerst KA, Buckingham B, Gandrud L, *et al*. *Paediatrics* 2006; **118**: 173–9

BACKGROUND. Although most studies investigating hyperglycaemia and its implications have been based in adult critical care settings, a number have looked at infants and children. As with adults, hyperglycaemia is associated with a poor outcome in a number of paediatric critical care settings |19|. In this study, consideration was given to the variability in blood glucose measurements, including both hypoglycaemia and hyperglycaemia. It was a retrospective single-centre study reviewing electronic data from March 2003 to March 2004. During this period, there had been no formal blood glucose control protocols, the management of blood glucose being at the discretion of the clinician in charge.

INTERPRETATION. With the exclusion of children with known diabetes mellitus, a total of 1094 patients with 50 deaths were included in the analyses. Both hyperglycaemia and hypoglycaemia were common; 61% had blood glucose recorded > 8.3 mmol/l and 18.7% < 3.6 mmol/l. A glucose variability index was calculated from the difference in sequential glucose measurements and the time between measurements. Patients with the greatest variability in blood glucose concentrations had the highest length of intensive care stay and the highest mortality. In addition, patients with the highest blood glucose concentrations were most likely also to have the lowest blood glucose concentrations and the highest mortality.

Comment

The relationship between hyperglycaemia and poor outcome in the adult intensive care population has been recognized for some time but only recently appreciated in the paediatric patient |19|. In 947 non-diabetic paediatric intensive care patients, hyperglycaemia was found to be common and the risk of death increased as blood glucose concentration increased. In this study, the authors were interested in the blood glucose concentration variability in addition to hyperglycaemia. It was a retrospective study, with the attendant risks of concealed bias and difficulty in attributing causality to findings. However, it included over 1000 admissions to the paediatric intensive care unit from various medical and surgical specialties. In common with the previous study, a relationship was observed between hyperglycaemia and poor outcome, but even more striking was the relationship between glucose variability and mortality. In the previously discussed study by Egi and colleagues, glucose variability was measured using the standard deviation of the mean. In this study, variability over time was taken into account and the authors were able to illustrate an association with hypoglycaemia and poor outcome, suggesting that the greatest effect of variability was over a wide range of glucose concentrations. Glucose variability also had the strongest association with length of stay on the intensive care unit. Unfortunately, as this is a retrospective study, it is impossible to determine whether the variability is a cause or consequence of the severity of illness.

A number of questions arise from these findings. Which is more likely to cause metabolic chaos, sustained hyperglycaemia or sudden changes in blood glucose? Evidence from patients with diabetes mellitus might suggest the latter |15,16|. Is exogenous administration of glucose harmful, especially the administration of strong glucose solutions? It is often unclear from these studies how hypoglycaemia was managed. Hypoglycaemia is a medical emergency but perhaps the administration of high concentrations of exogenous glucose is harmful. These questions warrant investigation.

Intensive insulin therapy in mixed medical/surgical intensive care units. Benefit versus harm

Van den Berghe G, Wilmer A, Milants I, et al. Diabetes 2006; 55: 3151–9

BACKGROUND. The original Leuven surgical study |8| showed an impressive decrease in mortality for patients managed with tight glycaemic control. But in the medical study (van den Berghe et al., 2006), this advantage was not observed for all patients, although a significant decrease in mortality was seen for the patients requiring > 3 days' intensive care. Concerns have since risen regarding the safety of tight glycaemic control, particularly if applied to a mixed medical and surgical intensive care population. This study looks at the pooled data from the two original studies with the aim of assessing the impact of tight glycaemic control on various subgroups of patients differentiated by their underlying medical condition.

INTERPRETATION. The amalgamation of the two studies generated 2478 patients. Morbidity and mortality were significantly decreased by tight glycaemic control. For patients requiring <3 days' admission to intensive care, there was no difference between the groups in terms of morbidity or mortality. The only subgroup that did not benefit from tight glycaemic control in terms of mortality were patients with a prior history of diabetes mellitus; no difference between treatments was then observed. Intensive insulin therapy did markedly increase the risk of hypoglycaemia and it was associated with an increased mortality. This was greatest in patients with spontaneous hypoglycaemia.

Comment

The advantage of this methodology is that a large population can be assessed ($n = 2748$). Of course, this was not an intention of the original study designs and, although the protocols for each study were similar, they were separated in time and experience. The results should, therefore, be interpreted with caution. One of the aims of the exercise was to clarify the impact of short-term tight glycaemic control which had caused a non-significant increase in mortality in medical patients requiring <3 days' intensive care. On pooling the data, the difference in in-hospital mortality for short-stay patients disappeared, although this is hardly surprising given that the differences involved were small. One argument against short-term tight glycaemic control is that much of the overall advantage observed (decreased ventilator requirements, decreased acute kidney injury, decreased polymyoneuropathy) is of complications that require time to develop: the benefit of tight glycaemic control may only be seen in long-stay patients.

The pooled data allowed closer inspection of the hypoglycaemia data. In the surgical study, 39 patients became hypoglycaemic in the treatment group compared with six control subjects. In the medical study, 111 treatment patients and 19 control subjects became hypoglycaemic. This represents 11.3% of the pooled intervention group developing severe hypoglycaemia (defined as blood glucose concentrations <2.2 mmol/l). No data are available for the number of patients developing less severe hypoglycaemia (2.2–4.0 mmol/l). Hypoglycaemia was more common in patients receiving most nutrition, although an explanation for this is not offered: it may be related to problems managing the insulin regimen. Hypoglycaemia in both control and treatment groups was associated with increased mortality. Hypoglycaemia was observed in 11 patients not receiving insulin and mortality was significantly higher for these patients. Three survivors with hypoglycaemia showed long-term neurological deficits, but these patients had known underlying neurological problems and there was no evidence that the outcome was directly related to hypoglycaemia.

Multicentric, randomized, controlled trial to evaluate blood glucose control by the model predictive control algorithm versus routine glucose management protocols in intensive care unit patients

Plank J, Blaha J, Cordingley J, *et al. Diabetes Care* 2006; **29**: 271–6

BACKGROUND. One of the major concerns with implementing protocols aimed at the management of hyperglycaemia in non-diabetic critically ill patients is the avoidance of hypoglycaemia. Questions arise regarding the frequency and reliability of glucose testing required for safe use and the manipulation of insulin infusions. In this study, an algorithm aimed at predicting blood glucose concentrations rather than responding to measurements is investigated. Cardiac surgery patients were investigated across three units, aiming to achieve a constant blood glucose concentration of 4.4–6.1 mmol/l, using a fully automated model. Arterial blood was analysed every hour for blood glucose to describe the glucose profile.

INTERPRETATION. Sixty patients were randomized either to receive the study protocol or conventional control of blood glucose, all aiming to achieve a blood glucose of 4.4–6.1 mmol/l. Patients in the control group were maintained in the target range for only 19% of the time, compared with 52% for patients receiving the study protocol. No hypoglycaemic episodes were documented for either group, indicating a tendency to under treat hyperglycaemia. The average blood glucose concentrations achieved were 6.5 (5.7–8.0) mmol/l for the study group and 7.2 (5.4–13.0) mmol/l for conventional controls.

Comment

The clinical reality of tight glycaemic control is that it is very difficult to do well. The pooled data from the study by van den Berghe and colleagues (2006) clearly illustrate this. Despite study conditions and highly motivated staff, the rate of severe hypoglycaemia in the tight glycaemic control group was high (11.3%), and only 69.3% of patients were managed at the targeted blood glucose concentration of <6.1 mmol/l (compared with 6.3% in the control group). Of the remaining treatment group patients, 27.7% achieved blood glucose concentrations of 6.1–8.3 mmol/l and 3.0% remained >8.3 mmol/l. In this study, only 52% were maintained in the target range, although this compared with 19% of the controls. Hypoglycaemia was defined as <3.0 mmol/l and no episodes were observed in the treatment group. The protocol, however, did demand hourly blood glucose analysis, and it is possible that many regimens would be improved by increasing the frequency of analysis. Unfortunately, this is unlikely to be practical in terms of nursing time and, therefore, unlikely to be achieved in day-to-day practice. The idea of predicting insulin requirements rather than reacting to blood glucose concentrations is attractive. The system used required input to an algorithm of glucose concentration, carbohydrate intake and insulin dosage. The aim was to predict insulin requirements so that hyperglycaemia was corrected gradually, hypoglycaemia was avoided or treated rapidly, or normoglycaemia was maintained. How easy such a system would be to use in critically ill patients with sepsis remains to be seen. However, the patients in this study were all cardiac intensive care patients and, thus, a relatively homogeneous group |20|.

Conclusion

Both the Leuven surgical |8| and medical studies showed that morbidity and mortality benefit from tight glycaemic control for patients requiring prolonged intensive care admission. However, both protocols involved the administration of intensive insulin regimens, and it remains unclear whether the benefits were due to control of glucose or to the immune modulating effects of insulin.

The concept of glucose as a direct toxin to cells is gaining merit. Cell membranes are impermeable to glucose. Uptake of glucose into cells occurs via either secondary active transport (sodium glucose-linked transporters) or facilitated transport (glucose uptake transporters GLUT 1, 2, 3 and 4). The distribution of transporters varies between tissues depending on requirements. Once within the cell, glucose is either utilized for energy via glycolysis, limited only by the production of mitochondrial ROS, or used in cell signalling pathways. Many of these latter pathways are proinflammatory and may be damaging if sustained.

Insulin resistance in critical illness is both peripheral (adipose cells, skeletal and heart muscle) and hepatic |10,21|. Excess exogenous insulin can overcome peripheral insulin resistance by increasing translocation of GLUT 4 to the cell membrane and the expression of hexokinase II. But it has less impact on hepatic insulin resistance, with little change observed in the expression of either glucokinase or phosphoenolpyruvate carboxykinase. The evidence for a significant benefit from insulin therapy independent of its actions on glucose is poor; intensive insulin regimens only appear to confer benefit if glucose concentrations are also controlled |22,23|.

Evidence for glucose toxicity also comes from an interesting study of snap frozen liver and muscle biopsies taken from patients dying in the Leuven surgical study |22|. Liver but not muscle mitochondrial morphology and function was significantly impaired in samples from patients with hyperglycaemia. It was attributed to unopposed uptake of glucose into liver cells through GLUT 2 transporters, compared with the restricted glucose uptake through GLUT 4 in insulin-dependent muscle cells. Tight glycaemic control decreases the requirement for ventilatory and renal support and the risk of critical illness polymyoneuropathy. All these systems are dependent on insulin-independent glucose uptake and, thus, may be directly vulnerable to glucose toxicity.

Morbidity associated with hyperglycaemia may also be secondary to infection |3,24,25|. Hyperglycaemia is known to impair several immune pathways |26|, and it is possible that some complications observed are secondary to sepsis rather than glucose toxicity *per se.*

Overall, evidence supports the implementation of tight glycaemic control. It is simple and cost-effective |27| but unfortunately it is not easy to achieve without the risk of significant hypoglycaemia . The compromise suggested in the Surviving Sepsis campaign |9| may help prevent hypoglycaemia but may also prevent full benefit being realized. Blood glucose concentrations have a circadian rhythm |28| and critical illness causes marked blood glucose variability. Good regimens for tight glycaemic control are urgently required, which need technology that allows accurate and frequent point of care testing. Individual algorithms also need to be developed, which are predictive rather than reactive to blood glucose changes |20,29|.

References

1. Capes SE, Hunt D, Malmberg K, Pathak P, Gerstein HC. Stress hyperglycemia and prognosis of stroke in nondiabetic and diabetic patients: a systematic overview. *Stroke* 2001; **32**: 2426–32.

2. Capes SE, Hunt D, Malmberg K, Gerstein HC. Stress hyperglycaemia and increased risk of death after myocardial infarction in patients with and without diabetes: a systematic overview. *Lancet* 2000; **355**: 773–8.

3. Baker EH, Janaway CH, Philips BJ, Brennan AL, Baines DL, Wood DM, Jones PW. Hyperglycaemia is associated with poor outcomes in patients admitted to hospital with acute exacerbations of chronic obstructive pulmonary disease. *Thorax* 2006; **61**: 284–9.

4. Doenst T, Wijeysundera D, Karkouti K, Zechner C, Maganti M, Rao V, Borger MA. Hyperglycemia during cardiopulmonary bypass is an independent risk factor for mortality in patients undergoing cardiac surgery. *J Thorac Cardiovasc Surg* 2005; **130**: 1144.

5. Whitcomb BW, Pradhan EK, Pittas AG, Roghmann MC, Perencevich EN. Impact of admission hyperglycemia on hospital mortality in various intensive care unit populations. *Crit Care Med* 2005; **33**: 2772–7.

6. Freire AX, Bridges L, Umpierrez GE, Kuhl D, Kitabchi AE. Admission hyperglycemia and other risk factors as predictors of hospital mortality in a medical ICU population. *Chest* 2005; **128**: 3109–16.

7. Umpierrez GE, Isaacs SD, Bazargan N, You X, Thaler LM, Kitabchi AE. Hyperglycemia: an independent marker of in-hospital mortality in patients with undiagnosed diabetes. *J Clin Endocrinol Metab* 2002; **87**: 978–82.

8. van den Berghe G, Wouters P, Weekers F, Verwaest C, Bruyninckx F, Schetz M, *et al.* Intensive insulin therapy in the surgical intensive care unit. *N Engl J Med* 2001; **345**: 1359–67.

9. Dellinger RP, Carlet JM, Masur H, Gerlach H, Calandra T, Cohen J, *et al.* Surviving Sepsis Campaign guidelines for management of severe sepsis and septic shock. *Crit Care Med* 2004; **32**: 858–73.

10. Langouche L, Vanhorebeek I, Van den Berghe G. Therapy insight: the effect of tight glycemic control in acute illness. *Nat Clin Pract Endocrinol Metab* 2007; **3**: 270–8.

11. Leverve X. Hyperglycemia and oxidative stress: complex relationships with attractive prospects. *Intensive Care Med* 2003; **29**: 511–14.

12. Brown GK. Glucose transporters: structure, function and consequences of deficiency. *J Inherit Metab Dis* 2000; **23**: 237–46.

13. Joost HG, Thorens B. The extended GLUT-family of sugar/polyol transport facilitators: nomenclature, sequence characteristics, and potential function of its novel members (review). *Mol Membr Biol* 2001; **18**: 247–56.

14. Vriesendorp TM, van Santen S, DeVries JH, de Jonge E, Rosendaal FR, Schultz MJ, *et al.* Predisposing factors for hypoglycemia in the intensive care unit. *Crit Care Med* 2006; **34**: 96–101.

15. Brownlee M, Hirsch IB. Glycemic variability: a hemoglobin A1c-independent risk factor for diabetic complications. *JAMA* 2006; **295**: 1707–8.

16. Heine RJ, Balkau B, Ceriello A, Del Prato S, Horton ES, Taskinen MR. What does postprandial hyperglycaemia mean? *Diabet Med* 2004; **21**: 208–13.

17. Malmberg K, Norhammar A, Wedel H, Ryden L. Glycometabolic state at admission: important risk marker of mortality in conventionally treated patients with diabetes mellitus and acute myocardial infarction: long-term results from the Diabetes and

Insulin-Glucose Infusion in Acute Myocardial Infarction (DIGAMI) study. *Circulation* 1999; **99**: 2626–32.

18. Malmberg K, Ryden L, Wedel H, Birkeland K, Bootsma A, Dickstein K, Efendic S, Fisher M, Hamsten A, Herlitz J, Hildebrandt P, Macleod K, Laakso M, Torp-Pedersen C, Waldenström A. Intense metabolic control by means of insulin in patients with diabetes mellitus and acute myocardial infarction (DIGAMI 2): effects on mortality and morbidity. *Eur Heart J* 2005; **26**: 650–61.

19. Faustino EV, Apkon M. Persistent hyperglycemia in critically ill children. *J Pediatr* 2005; **146**: 30–4.

20. Meijering S, Corstjens AM, Tulleken JE, Meertens JH, Zijlstra JG, Ligtenberg JJ. Towards a feasible algorithm for tight glycaemic control in critically ill patients: a systematic review of the literature. *Crit Care* 2006; **10**: R19.

21. Andreelli F, Jacquier D, Troy S. Molecular aspects of insulin therapy in critically ill patients. *Curr Opin Clin Nutr Metab Care* 2006; **9**: 124–30.

22. Vanhorebeek I, De Vos R, Mesotten D, Wouters PJ, De Wolf-Peeters C, van den Berghe G. Protection of hepatocyte mitochondrial ultrastructure and function by strict blood glucose control with insulin in critically ill patients. *Lancet* 2005; **365**: 53–9.

23. van den Berghe G, Wouters PJ, Bouillon R, Weekers F, Verwaest C, Schetz M, Vlaseelaers D, Ferdinande P, Lauwers P. Outcome benefit of intensive insulin therapy in the critically ill: insulin dose versus glycemic control. *Crit Care Med* 2003; **31**: 359–66.

24. Vriesendorp TM, Morelis QJ, Devries JH, Legemate DA, Hoekstra JB. Early post-operative glucose levels are an independent risk factor for infection after peripheral vascular surgery. A retrospective study. *Eur J Vasc Endovasc Surg* 2004; **28**: 520–5.

25. Philips BJ, Redman J, Brennan A, Wood D, Holliman R, Baines D, *et al.* Glucose in bronchial aspirates increases the risk of respiratory MRSA in intubated patients. *Thorax* 2005; **60**: 761–4.

26. Turina M, Fry DE, Polk HC Jr. Acute hyperglycemia and the innate immune system: clinical, cellular, and molecular aspects. *Crit Care Med* 2005; **33**: 1624–33.

27. Krinsley JS, Jones RL. Cost analysis of intensive glycemic control in critically ill adult patients. *Chest* 2006; **129**: 644–50.

28. Egi M, Bellomo R, Stachowski E, French CJ, Hart G, Stow P. Circadian rhythm of blood glucose values in critically ill patients. *Crit Care Med* 2007; **35**: 416–21.

29. Pittas AG, Siegel RD, Lau J. Insulin therapy and in-hospital mortality in critically ill patients: systematic review and meta-analysis of randomized controlled trials. *J Parenter Enteral Nutr* 2006; **30**: 164–72.

16

Hypothermia after cardiac arrest

JERRY NOLAN

Introduction

After cardiac arrest, successfully restoring spontaneous circulation is only the first stage towards the ultimate goal of producing a neurologically intact survivor. Unless the cardiac arrest has been brief, most survivors will be comatose initially and require admission to an intensive care unit (ICU). The cerebral ischaemia and hypoxia that occurs during cardiac arrest and cardiopulmonary resuscitation (CPR) is compounded by reperfusion injury that occurs when spontaneous circulation is restored. These insults provoke a cascade of chemical reactions that will cause transient or permanent neurological injury. Many of these mechanisms are also responsible for the systemic inflammatory response and associated multiple organ dysfunction, known as the post-cardiac arrest syndrome, which develops in many of these patients |1|.

About one-third of the comatose and mechanically ventilated patients admitted to ICU after cardiac arrest will survive to hospital discharge |2|. Among deaths in ICU after out-of-hospital cardiac arrest, two-thirds are due to neurological injury |3|. Most of those dying in ICU after in-hospital cardiac arrest die from multiple organ failure, but a quarter of deaths are attributed primarily to a neurological cause |3|.

Mild hypothermia is neuroprotective both before and after brain ischaemia through several mechanisms, including reduced production of excitotoxins and free radicals; suppression of apoptosis; and other anti-inflammatory actions |4,5|. Two randomized clinical trials showed improved outcome in adults who remained comatose after initial resuscitation from out-of-hospital ventricular fibrillation (VF) cardiac arrest and who were cooled within minutes to hours after return of spontaneous circulation (ROSC) |6,7|. Patients in these studies were cooled to 33°C |6| or to the range of 32–34°C |7| for 12–24 h.

External or internal techniques can be used to initiate and maintain cooling |6–13|. An infusion of 30 ml/kg of 4°C saline decreases core temperature by approximately 1.5°C |10,11,13|. Intravascular cooling enables more precise control of core temperature than external methods |12,14|, but there is no evidence to show that the cooling method influences survival. Multiple studies in animals indicate the importance of initiating cooling as soon as possible and for an adequate duration (e.g. 12–24 h) |15,16|. After out-of-hospital cardiac arrest it seems rational to initiate cooling on scene (Kim *et al.*, 2007) |7|.

Complications of mild therapeutic hypothermia include increased infection, cardiovascular instability, coagulopathy, hyperglycaemia, shivering and electrolyte abnormalities such as hypophosphataemia and hypomagnesaemia |17,18|. Shivering is treated by increasing sedation and the use of intermittent or continuous neuromuscular blockade. Seizures or myoclonus are common in survivors of cardiac arrest, and continuous neuromuscular blockade could mask seizure activity.

Following an advisory statement by the International Liaison Committee on Resuscitation (ILCOR) |19|, implementation of mild hypothermia after cardiac arrest has been slow (Laver *et al.*; Merchant *et al.*), but it is the author's impression that this has increased significantly over the last 2 years. The optimum target temperature, rate of cooling, duration of hypothermia and rate of rewarming have yet to be determined; further research is essential.

This review will focus on clinical studies of hypothermia after cardiac arrest published in 2006 and 2007. The studies are grouped into practical application, implementation and outcome.

Practical application of hypothermia

Efficacy and safety of endovascular cooling after cardiac arrest: cohort study and Bayesian approach

Holzer M, Mullner M, Sterz F, *et al. Stroke* 2006; **37**: 1792–7

BACKGROUND. The two initial randomized controlled trials of therapeutic hypothermia were restricted to comatose survivors of out-of-hospital VF cardiac arrest |6,7|. There are relatively few data to support the use of hypothermia after cardiac arrest from other rhythms and after in-hospital cardiac arrest; despite this, many clinicians are using hypothermia in these groups of patients. The two initial prospective trials used external methods to cool. Endovascular cooling is used by some ICUs but there are few safety data on this technique. In this retrospective cohort study the authors have investigated the use of hypothermia outside the confines of these prospective trials. They have studied the safety and efficacy of endovascular cooling in survivors of witnessed cardiac arrest from any rhythm, in or out of hospital.

INTERPRETATION. The authors evaluated 1038 consecutive comatose patients who were admitted to an emergency department of a tertiary hospital between 1991 and 2004. Ninety-seven of these patients were treated with endovascular cooling (Icy and Coolgard 3000, Alsius Corporation, Irvine, CA, USA) and the remaining 941 (the controls) were treated with standard post-resuscitation therapy. Forty-one of the cooled patients were given additional cold fluid during induction of hypothermia. In the cooled group, temperature was monitored continuously from a probe incorporated into a urinary catheter; the target temperature was 33°C, which was maintained for 24h; and patients were rewarmed slowly at 0.5°C per hour. Thirty days after cardiac arrest, 51 (53%) of the cooled group had a good outcome (cerebral performance category [CPC] 1 or 2) compared with 320 (34%) of the control group (odds ratio 2.15, 95% CI 1.38–3.35; $P = 0.0003$). After adjusting for baseline differences using a multivariate model, the odds ratio increased to 2.56 (95% CI 1.57–4.17; $P<0.001$). A safety analysis of endovascular cooling was undertaken using a frequency matching technique: the matching criteria were out-of-hospital VF cardiac arrest lasting more than 1 min. On this basis, bradycardia was more common in the cooled group (15% vs. 3%; $P = 0.025$) but there were no other statistical differences in adverse events. Pneumonia occurred more frequently in the cooled group (27% vs. 19%) but this was not statistically significant ($P = 0.23$).

Comment

This study provides some useful safety data on the use of endovascular cooling and reinforces the findings of other investigators who have shown that this technique enables precise temperature control. Although these data are encouraging, the study has several weaknesses which we must consider when assessing the strength of the conclusions. Patients were not randomized to the treatment group, which makes selection bias a strong possibility. Indeed, there are clear baseline differences between the two groups and although the authors have used two statistical techniques (multivariable and Bayesian analysis) to adjust for this, it is highly likely that undetected confounders continue to influence the results. It is very likely that patients deemed likely to have a poor outcome were less likely to be selected for cooling.

There were relatively few cooled patients, which limits the ability to detect uncommon but clinically significant side-effects. In 14 of the 97 cooled patients, cooling was stopped early (at a median of 11.7h after start of cooling). In two of these patients, cooling was stopped because of bleeding from the catheter site; one of these patients had received thrombolytic drugs and the other had undergone angioplasty. Reperfusion therapy, either percutaneous coronary intervention (PCI) or thrombolysis, is frequently indicated in the post-resuscitation phase. After both of these interventions bleeding will be impaired: blood loss from the insertion of a large-bore (9 F) cooling catheter is predictable.

The authors have not compared endovascular cooling with external cooling methods; this will be disappointing for many clinicians, who want to know which cooling strategy to use. Clinicians also want to know if they should cool comatose survivors of in-hospital cardiac arrest and non-VF cardiac arrest. In-hospital cardiac arrest patients were included in this study, but they accounted for only 8% of the cooled group. Only 28 (29%) of the cooled patients had been resuscitated from non-VF cardiac arrest. Thus, although the authors comment that their results are more generalizable than those of the initial prospective studies |**6,7**|, there are too few patients outside of the out-of-hospital VF cardiac group to enable reliable conclusions to be made.

Therapeutic hypothermia after cardiac arrest: unintentional overcooling is common using ice packs and conventional cooling blankets

Merchant RM, Abella BS, Peberdy MA, *et al*. *Crit Care Med* 2006; **34**: S490–S494

BACKGROUND. The frequency of complications caused by induced hypothermia will increase if the temperature is reduced to less than the lower limit of the target range (normally 32°C). In comparison with endovascular cooling, external cooling is considered generally to be more difficult to titrate, making it more difficult to keep the temperature in the target range |20|. The authors of this study have used a retrospective chart review in three hospitals (two in the USA and one in the UK) to measure the prevalence of overcooling and temperature variability in 32 post-cardiac arrest patients who were surface cooled.

INTERPRETATION. All 32 patients were treated primarily with surface cooling using a mattress/blanket or ice bags, although some were also cooled with boluses of intravenous fluid at 4°C. The target temperature was 33°C and temperature was recorded with either a bladder or tympanic thermometer. Fourteen of the 32 patients were cooled after in-hospital cardiac arrest and the remainder after out-of-hospital cardiac arrest. Significant problems with overcooling (lasting for more than 1 h) were identified: two-thirds of the patients reached temperatures of <32°C, and a quarter of them reached temperatures of <3°C. Temperatures of <30°C were reached by 4 (13%) of the 32 patients. Rebound hyperthermia (temperature of >38°C at 12–18 h after the end of active rewarming) developed in 7 (22%) of 32 patients.

Comment

Temperature control is difficult during surface cooling. There is inevitably a lag in the equilibration between peripheral and core body temperature. This lag has to be anticipated by nurses and doctors treating the patient, otherwise the core temperature will swing widely above and below the target temperature. Some automatic surface cooling systems that monitor core temperature continuously have in-built algorithms that are designed to anticipate the lag between peripheral and core temperature but these are imperfect. In any case, factors such as the patient's weight, the underlying inflammatory response, and variable venous and arterial vasodilatation will influence the lag time. Overcooling will increase the risk of complications, such as arrhythmias, bleeding and infection. Any rebound hyperthermia occurring during rewarming is potentially even more harmful: the risk of a poor neurological outcome increases for each degree of body temperature >37°C |21|. Many of these patients will have a profound systemic inflammatory response and will develop significant pyrexia unless active cooling is continued. In practice, this means closely controlled rewarming at about 0.25°C/h. If active cooling systems (internal or external) have been used to maintain hypothermia, it is rational to leave them in place for 48–72 h and attempt to maintain a temperature of 36.5–37°C.

Although precise temperature control is considered important, we await firm evidence that outcome is improved by this strategy. In this study by Merchant and colleagues, of those with overcooling to less than 32°C, 6 of 20 (30%) survived to hospital discharge; of those without overcooling, 7 of 12 (58%) survived to hospital discharge (not statistically significant). Even if these differences had been statistically significant, it would be impossible to eliminate other confounders that could account for them. For example, a patient with a poor cardiac output and poor peripheral perfusion is more likely to have a greater lag in equilibration between core and peripheral temperatures and is, therefore, more likely to be overcooled. The most important take-home message from this study is that we need more research to establish the best cooling methods.

Pilot randomized clinical trial of prehospital induction of mild hypothermia in out-of-hospital cardiac arrest patients with a rapid infusion of 4°C normal saline

Kim F, Olsufka M, Longstreth WT Jr, et al. Circulation 2007; **115**: 3064–70

BACKGROUND. Two small pilot in-hospital studies have demonstrated that the intravenous infusion of 30 ml/kg of 4°C fluid will decrease core temperature by 1.7°C without causing pulmonary oedema or electrolyte abnormalities |10,22|. One study of 13 post-cardiac arrest patients has demonstrated a similar temperature decrease with cold intravenous fluid given in the pre-hospital phase |11|. Animals studies indicate that post-resuscitation hypothermia is more effective the earlier it is started |23|. In comatose survivors of out-of-hospital cardiac arrest it would seem sensible to start the infusion of cold intravenous fluid before arriving at hospital. The aims of this study by Kim and co-workers from Seattle were to assess the feasibility, safety and effectiveness of pre-hospital cooling with rapid infusion of up to 2l of 4°C normal saline. Patients initially resuscitated from out-of-hospital cardiac arrest were randomized to receive standard care or intravenous cooling. The effect on oesophageal temperature was determined before hospital arrival. All cardiac arrest rhythms were included in the study but those patients with cardiac arrest caused by trauma were excluded. On arrival at hospital, patients were treated according to physicians' preferences – this meant that cooling was continued in some cases but not in others.

INTERPRETATION. A total of 125 patients were included in the study; 51 (41%) of these had been resuscitated from VF cardiac arrest. Of the 63 patients randomized to cooling, 49 (78%) received an infusion of 500 to 2000 ml of cold saline before hospital admission; of these, 12 patients received the full 2l. In those randomized to cooling, the mean oesophageal temperature at hospital arrival was 34.7°C, which was 1.1°C lower than the temperature at randomization. The mean oesophageal temperature at hospital arrival in the standard care group was 35.7°C, which was 0.2°C higher than the temperature at randomization. Field cooling did not prolong the pre-hospital time and there were no complications associated with the infusion of cold fluid. The heart rate and systolic blood pressure on hospital admission were higher in the cooled group. The initial arterial blood gas analysis showed a significantly lower pH in the cooled group (7.14 vs. 7.23 [$P = 0.031$]). There was a trend towards improved survival to discharge in the patients randomized to field cooling when the initial rhythm was VF (19/29 [66%] vs. 10/22 [45%]); however, for non-VF rhythms the trend favoured the non-cooled group (survival to hospital discharge 2/34 [6%] vs. 8/40 [20%]). Of the 97 patients who were admitted to hospital, 60 were treated with hypothermia using surface cooling.

Comment

This study has been undertaken by a highly regarded and experienced group of resuscitation researchers. They have shown that pre-hospital cooling with 4°C intravenous fluid is feasible and not associated with adverse effects on blood pressure, heart rate or pulmonary oedema. A greater decrease in temperature is seen with higher volumes of fluid, but on the basis of this study and others |10,11,22|, infusion of 2l of 4°C fluid will decrease core temperature by 1.7–2.0°C. Interestingly, the authors did not reference the only other study of pre-hospital cooling with intravenous fluid in post-cardiac arrest patients |11|. The reduced pH in the cooled group almost certainly reflects the excess chloride associated with the infusion of normal saline, although the authors do not report the chloride values. Other investigators have used Ringer's lactate and did not report a problem with acidaemia |10,11|. The significance of the acidaemia caused by normal saline is unknown but use of Ringer's lactate should eliminate the problem.

A limitation of this trial is that only a few of the patients in the cooled group received all the 2l of fluid; however, this reflects the reality of clinical practice – there simply would not be time to infuse this volume into all patients. A study designed primarily to assess the impact of cold fluid on outcome should include use of an equal volume of non-cooled fluid in the control arm (as the authors point out); this would then enable us to determine whether any differences were caused by the temperature and not simply the effect of infusing volume. These investigators are about to start a large prospective randomized trial assessing long-term survival after pre-hospital induction of hypothermia with cold intravenous fluid (ClinicalTrials.gov identifier NCT00391469). Meanwhile, the use of cold intravenous fluid is a simple and effective way to initiate cooling. Directors of emergency medical services (EMS) systems should consider ways that they can carry cold intravenous fluid for patients resuscitated from cardiac arrest.

Cold infusions alone are effective for induction of therapeutic hypothermia but do not keep patients cool after cardiac arrest

Kliegel A, Janata A, Wandaller C, et al. Resuscitation 2007; **73**: 46–53

BACKGROUND. Infusions of cold fluid are effective for inducing hypothermia (Kim et al., 2007) |10,11,13| but are not generally used for maintenance of hypothermia. This was a prospective, observational cases series of 20 patients admitted to an emergency department after cardiac arrest of presumed cardiac aetiology. Patients were sedated with midazolam and fentanyl, and rocuronium was given by continuous infusion to prevent shivering. Cooling was induced with 30 ml/kg 4°C crystalloid (normal saline or lactated Ringer's solution, depending on serum electrolytes) given over 30 min. If the target temperature of 32–34°C was not achieved, additional cold fluid boluses of 10 ml/kg were given up to 6-hourly. Other cooling techniques were used if, despite the cold fluid, the temperature increased above 34°C.

INTERPRETATION. Two-thirds (13 of 20) of the patients reached the target temperature within the required 60 min in a mean time of 30 (± 16) min. The other seven patients required additional endovascular cooling after 60 min to enable the target temperature to be achieved. Of the 13 patients who reached target temperature with cold fluid alone, nine (about two-thirds) could not be maintained in the target range with cold fluid alone – they required additional endovascular cooling to maintain hypothermia. No patient developed pulmonary oedema.

Comment

Although the target temperature could be reached with cold fluid alone in two-thirds of the patients, the majority rewarmed within hours and required additional endovascular cooling. This study demonstrates that additional cooling techniques are required to reliably maintain hypothermia. In practice, cold intravenous fluid should be used to induce hypothermia but an alternative technique, either internal or external, should be used to maintain hypothermia.

The authors suggest that continuous muscle relaxation is necessary to prevent shivering that could then cause rewarming. This is not a universal view among those with expertise in cooling after cardiac arrest. Continuous infusions of muscle relaxants could mask convulsions that would require urgent treatment to avoid brain injury. Shivering can usually be controlled with adequate sedation and bolus doses of muscle relaxants – infusions of muscle relaxants are required rarely.

Feasibility and efficacy of a new non-invasive surface cooling device in post-resuscitation intensive care medicine

Haugk M, Sterz F, Brassberger M, *et al. Resuscitation* 2007; **75**: 76–81.

BACKGROUND. There are several different external cooling systems available for inducing and maintaining hypothermia after cardiac arrest. In this study, Haugk and colleagues have investigated the efficacy of the Arctic Sun System (Medivance Incorporated, Louisville, CO, USA). This comprises a thermoregulatory control unit that circulates water through four or five self-adhesive hydrogel pads. The pads are applied to the patient's skin over the back, abdomen and thighs, and incorporate insulated channels for the water to circulate through. Temperature-controlled water flows through the pads under negative pressure at a rate of 2–3 l/min per set of pads. A convenience sample of 27 patients was included in this study. All the patients had been resuscitated after witnessed out-of-hospital cardiac arrest and were admitted to an emergency department in Vienna, Austria.

INTERPRETATION. Time from admission to target temperature (33°C bladder temperature) was just over 4 h. The median cooling rate was 1.2°C/h, although individual cooling rates ranged from 0.4°C/h to 5.3°C/h. This wide range probably reflects the range in patient weight (45–136 kg). Temperature was maintained for 24 h between 32 and 34 °C in all the patients and controlled rewarming at 0.4°C/h was achieved successfully. There were no skin problems associated with prolonged application of the pads.

Comment

Although other investigators have reported on the use of the Arctic Sun system for inducing hypothermia, this is the first report of its use in post-resuscitation cooling. In this relatively small study, the Arctic Sun system appeared to function acceptably. The heat transfer pads are relatively bulky, but in the authors' opinion, this did not create any major problems. A randomized trial comparing cooling with the Arctic Sun system to conventional surface cooling in post-resuscitation patients is currently recruiting patients (ClinicalTrials.gov identifier NCT00282373) and may provide more useful data. The critical question is whether temperature control with an external system compared with an internal system results in a significant difference in any important outcome (i.e. survival, neurological recovery, adverse effects). A study of endovascular cooling compared with 'conventional' external cooling after out-of-hospital cardiac in Paris is currently recruiting patients (ClinicalTrials.gov NCT00392693). In the UK, the disposable costs for the Arctic Sun and for the Alsius endovascular cooling system are very similar (approximately £500 per patient). It is not clear whether this reflects research and development and production costs, or simply a price selected on what the market will pay. However, as usage increases, these costs should decrease significantly. Until more data are available, the clinician will have to weigh up the convenience of endovascular cooling with the non-invasiveness of surface cooling.

Implementation

From evidence to clinical practice: effective implementation of therapeutic hypothermia to improve patient outcome after cardiac arrest

Oddo M, Schaller MD, Feihl F, Ribordy V, *et al. Crit Care Med* 2006; **34**: 1865–73

BACKGROUND. Following the publication of evidence-based guidelines, implementation into clinical practice requires overcoming a variety of barriers, which slows the process significantly |24|. Oddo and associates from Lausanne, Switzerland, report on the implementation of therapeutic hypothermia in the ICU of a university hospital. This retrospective study included comatose patients resuscitated from out-of-hospital cardiac arrest of any rhythm. The authors analysed 55 consecutive patients (2002 to 2004) treated with external cooling (ice bags and cold circulating water blanket) to a target temperature of 33°C and maintained for 24 h; they were compared with a historical control group of 54 consecutive patients (1999 to 2002) treated conventionally. The primary endpoint was good outcome (cerebral performance category [CPC] 1 or 2 – defined in Table 16.1) at hospital discharge.

INTERPRETATION. In the patients treated with hypothermia, the median time to achieve the target temperature was 5 h after admission to the emergency department. In the patients resuscitated from VF cardiac arrest, a good outcome was achieved in 24 of 43 (55.8%) patients in the hypothermic group vs. 11 of 43 (25.6%) patients in the control group ($P = 0.004$). The outcome following non-VF cardiac arrest was very poor: 2/12 had a good outcome in the hypothermia group vs. 0/11 in the control group. The authors used multivariable binary logistic regression in an attempt to eliminate confounders and determine the true influence of hypothermia on outcome. Following this analysis, only

Table 16.1 The Glasgow–Pittsburgh Cerebral Performance Category (CPC) definitions

CPC 1	Conscious. Alert; able to work and lead a normal life
CPC 2	Moderate cerebral disability. Conscious; sufficient cerebral function for part-time work in sheltered environment or independent activities of daily life
CPC 3	Severe cerebral disability. Conscious; dependent on others for daily support because of impaired brain function
CPC 4	Coma, vegetative state
CPC 5	Death

Source: adapted from Ref. 30.

two independent predictors were retained as statistically significant for determining a good outcome: a treatment group odds ratio (OR) 5.56, 95% CI 2.0–16.7 in favour of hypothermia; and the time from collapse to ROSC. Infections and arrhythmias were equally common in both groups: infection: 34.5% in hypothermia group vs. 42.6% in the control group; and arrhythmia: 36.4% in hypothermia group vs. 42.6% in the control group.

Comment

This study shows that therapeutic hypothermia can be successfully implemented outside the confines of a strictly regulated prospective controlled trial. However, the use of a historical control group severely limits the conclusions that can be drawn from the outcome data. Although the authors have used multivariate analysis in an attempt to eliminate confounders, there will almost certainly be differences in the way these two groups were treated that have not been accounted for. The authors dismiss a Hawthorne effect associated with the introduction of hypothermia, but it is entirely possible that a highly 'visible' treatment, such as hypothermia, increases the intensity and quality of the rest of the patient's ICU treatment and could account for an improvement in outcome. The authors inserted pulmonary artery catheters (PACs) in all the cooled patients to enable 'continuous reliable monitoring of central temperature'. It is no longer conventional practice to insert PACs and this is a rather invasive way of monitoring temperature. The use of PACs introduced an unnecessary extra cost to the hypothermia group. The authors also report an increase in length of stay in the hypothermia group (median 4.5 days vs. 2 days, $P = 0.013$). It is not clear whether this reflects the use of therapeutic hypothermia or other changes in practice that have occurred since the control was treated.

Therapeutic hypothermia utilization among physicians after resuscitation from cardiac arrest

Merchant RM, Soar J, Skrifvars MB, et al. Crit Care Med 2006; **34**: 1935–40

BACKGROUND. In 2003, a survey among US physicians on the use of therapeutic hypothermia after cardiac arrest indicated that most (87%) had not used it; the commonest reason cited was insufficient data |25|. The authors of this original survey were joined by other investigators and together they devised a web-based survey that was distributed to physicians in several countries. The authors were seeking to evaluate the current use of therapeutic hypothermia, the reasons for non-implementation, and the cooling techniques used. Using e-mail, members of the Society for Academic Emergency Medicine, the American Thoracic Society and the American Heart Association were contacted, along with a group of critical care physicians in the UK and Finland.

INTERPRETATION. Of the 13 272 surveys distributed to physicians, 2248 (17%) were completed; 91% of these respondents practised in the USA. Of all the replies, 74% of US respondents and 64% of non-US respondents had never used therapeutic hypothermia.

The most commonly cited reasons for not using hypothermia were: not enough data; not part of Advanced Cardiac Life Support (ACLS) guidelines; and too technically difficult to use. Most respondents using hypothermia primarily cooled patients after VF (82%) for both in-hospital and out-of-hospital cardiac arrests. Most respondents used surface cooling via a mattress/blanket (82%) or ice packs (58%). Endovascular cooling was used by 15% of the 440 US-based physicians responding to this question and by 27% of 66 non-US respondents.

Comment

Although this study provides an interesting snapshot of therapeutic hypothermia practice, its reliability is limited severely by the response rate of just 17%. Respondents are far more likely to be hypothermia enthusiasts, which implies that this survey almost certainly overestimates the uptake of therapeutic hypothermia, particularly in the USA. The US physicians were contacted using the databases of large medical societies, whereas those in the UK and Finland represented pre-selected groups of physicians – the latter were far more likely to be interested in therapeutic hypothermia. Having indicated the potential biases in this study, it is interesting to note that two other surveys, one from the UK (Laver *et al.*, 2006, discussed below) and one from Germany |26| both demonstrate that about 25% of ICUs have implemented therapeutic hypothermia.

The lack of detailed practical guidance on the use of hypothermia, along with lack of data indicating which of the many available cooling techniques is best, probably accounts for much of the hesitancy in implementing this therapy.

Therapeutic hypothermia after cardiac arrest. A survey of practice in intensive care units in the United Kingdom

Laver SR, Padkin A, Atalla A, *et al. Anaesthesia* 2006; **61**: 873–7

BACKGROUND. There have been several surveys on the implementation of therapeutic hypothermia to treat post-cardiac arrest patients (Merchant et al., 2006) |25,26|; all of these have suffered from poor response rates. Laver and co-investigators have surveyed the uptake of therapeutic hypothermia among UK ICUs. In an attempt to maximize the response rate, the survey was undertaken by telephone. All 256 UK ICUs listed in the Critical Care Services Manual 2004 were contacted and the consultant on call for the day was asked to take part in the survey. The standardized questions focused on whether hypothermia was used and, if so, how often; the reasons for non-implementation; and the methods used to induce and maintain hypothermia.

INTERPRETATION. Six of the units were deemed ineligible because they took only elective patients. The response rate was 98.4% and 67 (28.4%) of the 246 ICUs reported that they had cooled patients after cardiac arrest, although the majority of these had treated fewer than 10 patients. The reasons for non-implementation are listed in Table 16.2. Of the ICUs that had implemented hypothermia, over half would consider cooling patients who had been resuscitated from non-VF cardiac arrest and about two-

Table 16.2 Reasons given for not using therapeutic hypothermia for unconscious patients following cardiac arrest. Some ICUs provided more than one reason

Reason	Number of responses (%*)
Logistics/resource issues	45 (26)
No local consensus/not enough evidence	40 (23)
Unaware of the evidence	24 (14)
Discussed but not yet implemented	17 (10)
Other	29 (16)
No reason given	51 (29)

*Percentage of the 176 ICUs with no current intention of implementing therapeutic hypothermia.
Source: Laver et al. (2007).

thirds would consider cooling patients after in-hospital cardiac arrest, as well as those resuscitated from out-of-hospital cardiac arrest.

Comment

By using a telephone survey the response rate is much higher and the results should be more reliable. The limitations of this technique are that the person responding may not be completely familiar with the normal practice of the ICU and, unless the interviewer is careful to standardize the questions, they could unconsciously or consciously influence the responses. This survey showed that endovascular cooling was used rarely: this might be a reflection of lack of funding. 'Resources issues' was the commonest reason cited for lack of implementation in general. This survey was completed in June 2005 but was not published until late in 2006. Such publication delay is inevitable but, to some extent, the information is out of date as soon as it is published. It is this author's impression, however, that the use of therapeutic hypothermia in UK ICUs is now much more common – a repeat of this survey would usefully confirm or refute this.

As one of the authors on this paper, I acknowledge that there is a potential conflict of interest with my comments.

Outcome

Clinical application of mild therapeutic hypothermia after cardiac arrest

Arrich J. Crit Care Med 2007; **35**: 1041–7

BACKGROUND. Although prospective controlled trials are the gold standard for assessing the impact of a new therapy, in the context of resuscitation they are often difficult to achieve, not least because, in the absence of interest from pharmaceutical companies, it can be difficult to secure adequate funding. Resuscitation registries – large databases containing anonymized data – may enable useful information to be gleaned about a variety of resuscitation interventions. The European Resuscitation Council Hypothermia After Cardiac Arrest Registry (ERC HACA-R) was established to monitor developments after publication of the ILCOR recommendation on hypothermia after cardiac arrest |19|. The ERC HACA-R was opened to licensed medical practitioners in Europe and data entry was web-based. The registry was intended for all patients who presented after cardiac arrest with ROSC, whether or not they received hypothermia. Participating sites had control and responsibility for the quality of their data within the registry. Arrich and the ERC HACA-R Study Group report on the first 650 patients entered into this registry. Their primary objectives were to assess adherence to the ILCOR recommendations on therapeutic hypothermia and to determine adverse events, survival rate and neurological outcome associated with this therapy.

INTERPRETATION. Between May 2003 and June 2005, data on 650 patients from 19 sites were entered into the registry. Of these, 462 (79%) received therapeutic hypothermia: 347 (59%) were cooled with an endovascular device; and 114 (19%) were cooled with other methods such as ice packs, cooling blankets and cold fluids. The median cooling rate was 1.1 °C/h; 15 (3%) of the cooled patients had an episode of bleeding and 28 (6%) had at least one reported arrhythmia within 7 days after cooling. There were no reported deaths caused by cooling. Over 80% of the patients had been resuscitated from out-of-hospital cardiac arrest and approximately two-thirds had an initial rhythm of VF or pulseless ventricular tachycardia (VT). Unfavourable outcome (defined by a cerebral performance category score of > 2 – see Table 16.1) was more common in the normothermic group (68%) compared with the hypothermic group (55%). Among those with an initial rhythm of pulseless electrical activity (PEA) or asystole, 19% survived to discharge in the normothermic group compared with 35% in the hypothermia group (P = 0.23); however, 81% from each group had an unfavourable outcome.

Comment

This study reports the greatest number of post-cardiac arrest patients treated with hypothermia to date. It includes by far the greatest number of endovascularly cooled patients. Although the data provide an interesting insight into the application of hypothermia in post-cardiac arrest patients, there are significant limitations to the conclusions that can be drawn. The registry was funded by the Alsius Corporation (Irvine, CA, USA), manufacturer of the Coolgard 3000 system, and this is reflected in the large proportion of patients that had been cooled endovascularly. The high proportion of patients that had been cooled using any method also reflects the interests of the participating sites. Thus, the cooled and non-cooled patients are far from being matched groups, which makes outcome comparisons between groups highly unreliable. What can be learnt from this study is that the incidence of adverse events associated with therapeutic hypothermia in general, and endovascular cooling in particular, is relatively low. We still lack data to show any survival benefit for hypothermia after cardiac arrest from non-VF rhythms – although this study appears to be encouraging in this respect, the unmatched groups make any conclusion unreliable.

Implementation of a standardized treatment protocol for post resuscitation care after out-of-hospital cardiac arrest

Sunde K, Pytte M, Jacobsen D, *et al*. *Resuscitation* 2007; **73**: 29–39

BACKGROUND. Therapeutic hypothermia is just one component of a bundle of care that should be used to treat the post-cardiac arrest syndrome |1|. Other important therapies include early coronary reperfusion (percutaneous intervention or thrombolysis) |27,28|, controlled ventilation to achieve normal arterial blood oxygen and carbon dioxide tensions, cardiovascular support with vasoactive drugs and, if necessary, an intra-aortic balloon pump, and intensive control of blood glucose. Sunde and colleagues from Oslo, Norway have reported the outcome of post-cardiac arrest patients treated with a standardized resuscitation protocol and compared them with a historical group control.

INTERPRETATION. All patients with out-of-hospital cardiac arrest of cardiac aetiology admitted to the authors' ICU from September 2003 to May 2005 were studied prospectively and compared with a control group of patients that had been admitted from February 1996 to February 1998. In the control period 15/58 (26%) survived to hospital discharge with a favourable neurological outcome compared with 34/61 (56%) in the intervention period (OR 3.61, 95% CI 1.66–7.84; $P = 0.001$). There were dramatic differences in the treatment given to patients in the intervention and control periods (Table 16.3). None of the patients in the control period were treated with therapeutic hypothermia compared with 40 of the 52 (77%) comatose patients in the intervention period. Of the cooled patients, 29 (73%) were treated with endovascular cooling (Alsius Corporation, Irvine, CA, USA). They also used the Arctic Sun surface cooling system if the endovascular device was unavailable.

Table 16.3 In-hospital treatment in the control (1996–8) and intervention (2003–5) periods, presented as absolute numbers (%) or mean ± SD (fluid balance)

	Control period ($n = 58$)	Intervention period ($n = 61$)	P-value
Reperfusion therapy	2 (3)	30 (49)	<0.001
Therapeutic hypothermia	0	40 (66)	<0.001
Inotropic drugs	29 (50)	43 (80)	0.022
Intra-aortic balloon pump	0	8 (15)	0.006
Glyceryl trinitrate	31 (53)	0	<0.001
Fluid balance day 1 (ml)	2300 ± 1211	3455 ± 1594	<0.001
Insulin	4 (7)	27 (44)	<0.001

Source: Sunde *et al.* (2007).

Comment

Although this is a comparatively small study and uses a historical control group, it provides us with very important messages. The differences between the intervention and control periods in the treatment given and the outcomes achieved are dramatic. The authors seem to have a relatively high proportion of post-VF cardiac arrest patients in both of their groups; 90% of the patients in the intervention group had an initial rhythm of VF and this might partly account for their very impressive survival figures in comparison with many other studies. The authors highlight six factors that probably contribute to these improved outcomes: new treatment strategies, such as hypothermia and early reperfusion therapy, could generate a Hawthorne effect with a general improvement in quality of care for these patients.

Early reperfusion with percutaneous coronary intervention is an important contributor to improved outcome |27,28|, and this demands availability of interventional cardiologists at all times; many healthcare systems, particularly in the UK, will not achieve this. Based on the evidence in this review, therapeutic hypothermia is an important component of post-resuscitation care.

A standardized treatment protocol or 'bundle of care' has been deemed important for other critically ill patients |29|, and is no less important for treating the post-cardiac arrest syndrome. Maintenance of an adequate blood pressure is important if cerebral perfusion is to be optimized. These patients may develop significant vasodilatation caused by the release of various cytokines that contribute to the post-cardiac arrest syndrome |1|. Maintenance of a mean arterial pressure of 65–70 mm Hg may require an infusion of noradrenaline.

An improvement in the quality of pre-hospital CPR could account for some of the improvement in outcome in the intervention period. Strengthening of all links in the chain of survival is fundamental to improving outcome after cardiac arrest.

Attention to the quality of care in the post-resuscitation phase should improve outcome for these patients. In the future, information provided by analysing the Intensive Care National Audit and Research Centre Case Mix Programme in the UK should enable this hypothesis to be tested.

Conclusion

After the first prospective controlled trials of 12–24 hours of therapeutic hypothermia for comatose survivors of VF cardiac arrest |6,7|, there have been no further randomized trials comparing this intervention with 'standard care'. Despite the existing evidence and inclusion in guidelines, the uptake of mild hypothermia by ICUs around the world is variable (Merchant *et al.*, 2006; Laver *et al.*, 2006). Some clinicians remain sceptical about the evidence: they indicate that there are just two relatively small, unblinded, controlled trials – one of which used pseudo-randomization to allocate treatments |7|, and the other enrolled just 8% of all the patients assessed for eligibility |6|. There is little doubt that, rightly or wrongly, the enthusiasts for post-cardiac arrest therapeutic hypothermia are implementing this therapy largely on the basis of evidence from animal data and two small trials. Furthermore, many are extrapolating outside of the inclusion criteria used in the original trials (i.e. they are including cardiac arrests with non-VF initial rhythms and in-hospital cardiac arrests). Unfortunately, intensive care clinicians and emergency physicians rarely have high-level data on which to base their practice – they often use therapies with relatively little evidence base. Our cardiology colleagues are more fortunate – their interventions are invariably based on evidence generated from trials involving thousands of patients. There are plans for a large multicentre European trial that will compare cooling started in the pre-hospital phase with that delayed until hospital admission (F Sterz, personal communication). A second phase of the trial may even compare different target temperatures, including a group with strict normothermia. The latter will address a question raised by some experts: the control group in the original HACA (hypothermia after cardiac arrest) trial were actually hyperthermic |6| – would the difference in outcome have occurred if the control group had been maintained at strict normothermia?

Does the evidence published in 2006 and 2007 assist the clinician in deciding whether or not to implement therapeutic hypothermia after cardiac arrest? The implementation studies indicate that a significant minority are already using this therapy (Merchant *et al.*, 2006; Laver *et al.*, 2006). None of the studies highlighted in this review reports a significant increase in complications associated with hypothermia and this may give some reassurance to clinicians. However, there is a strong possibility of selection bias in any studies that lack randomization. Whether we are using therapeutic hypothermia or not, it is vitally important that we continue to collect data on all post-cardiac arrest patients. In the absence of large randomized, controlled trials, high-quality registries may provide the information we need. If we can correct for case mix, it may be possible to show whether interventions such as therapeutic hypothermia are improving outcome. In the UK, ICNARC has recently amended its Case Mix Programme to include more information on post-cardiac arrest patients (e.g. the initial arrest rhythm is now documented) – this may enable better comparison of outcomes between ICUs.

The implementation of a standardized treatment protocol for post-resuscitation care, as described by Sunde *et al.* (2007), is arguably the most important study in this review of 2006 and 2007. The level of evidence it provides is relatively low, but the message is very strong – implementation of this bundle of care is associated with a significantly better outcome. It is difficult to pick out the relative contributions of each component: until we have this information we should probably apply all of these post-resuscitation therapies, and continue to monitor outcomes.

References

1. Adrie C, Adib-Conquy M, Laurent I, *et al.* Successful cardiopulmonary resuscitation after cardiac arrest as a "sepsis-like" syndrome. *Circulation* 2002; **106**: 562–8.

2. Nolan JP, Laver SR, Welch CA, Harrison DA, Gupta V, Rowan K. Outcome following admission to UK intensive care units after cardiac arrest: a secondary analysis of the ICNARC Case Mix Programme Database. *Anaesthesia* 2007; **62**: 1207–16.

3. Laver S, Farrow C, Turner D, Nolan J. Mode of death after admission to an intensive care unit following cardiac arrest. *Intensive Care Med* 2004; **30**: 2126–8.

4. Liu L, Yenari MA. Therapeutic hypothermia: neuroprotective mechanisms. *Front Biosci* 2007; **12**: 816–25.

5. Gunn AJ, Thoresen M. Hypothermic neuroprotection. *NeuroRx* 2006; **3**: 154–69.

6. Hypothermia After Cardiac Arrest Study Group. Mild therapeutic hypothermia to improve the neurologic outcome after cardiac arrest. *N Engl J Med* 2002; **346**: 549–56.

7. Bernard SA, Gray TW, Buist MD, *et al.* Treatment of comatose survivors of out-of-hospital cardiac arrest with induced hypothermia. *N Engl J Med* 2002; **346**: 557–63.

8. Hachimi-Idrissi S, Corne L, Ebinger G, Michotte Y, Huyghens L. Mild hypothermia induced by a helmet device: a clinical feasibility study. *Resuscitation* 2001; **51**: 275–81.

9. Busch M, Soreide E, Lossius HM, Lexow K, Dickstein K. Rapid implementation of therapeutic hypothermia in comatose out-of-hospital cardiac arrest survivors. *Acta Anaesthesiol Scand* 2006; **50**: 1277–83.

10. Bernard S, Buist M, Monteiro O, Smith K. Induced hypothermia using large volume, ice-cold intravenous fluid in comatose survivors of out-of-hospital cardiac arrest: a preliminary report. *Resuscitation* 2003; **56**: 9–13.

11. Virkkunen I, Yli-Hankala A, Silfvast T. Induction of therapeutic hypothermia after cardiac arrest in prehospital patients using ice-cold Ringer's solution: a pilot study. *Resuscitation* 2004; **62**: 299–302.

12. Al-Senani FM, Graffagnino C, Grotta JC, *et al.* A prospective, multicenter pilot study to evaluate the feasibility and safety of using the CoolGard System and Icy catheter following cardiac arrest. *Resuscitation* 2004; **62**: 143–50.

13. Kliegel A, Losert H, Sterz F, *et al.* Cold simple intravenous infusions preceding special endovascular cooling for faster induction of mild hypothermia after cardiac arrest – a feasibility study. *Resuscitation* 2005; **64**: 347–51.

14. Diringer MN, Reaven NL, Funk SE, Uman GC. Elevated body temperature independently contributes to increased length of stay in neurologic intensive care unit patients. *Crit Care Med* 2004; **32**: 1489–95.

15. Agnew DM, Koehler RC, Guerguerian AM, *et al.* Hypothermia for 24 hours after asphyxic cardiac arrest in piglets provides striatal neuroprotection that is sustained 10 days after rewarming. *Pediatr Res* 2003; **54**: 253–62.

16. Sterz F, Safar P, Tisherman S, Radovsky A, Kuboyama K, Oku K. Mild hypothermic cardiopulmonary resuscitation improves outcome after prolonged cardiac arrest in dogs. *Crit Care Med* 1991; **19**: 379–89.

17. Polderman KH, Peerdeman SM, Girbes AR. Hypophosphatemia and hypomagnesemia induced by cooling in patients with severe head injury. *J Neurosurg* 2001; **94**: 697–705.

18. Polderman KH. Application of therapeutic hypothermia in the intensive care unit. Opportunities and pitfalls of a promising treatment modality – Part 2: Practical aspects and side-effects. *Intensive Care Med* 2004; **30**: 757–69.

19. Nolan JP, Morley PT, Vanden Hoek TL, Hickey RW. Therapeutic hypothermia after cardiac arrest. An advisory statement by the Advancement Life support Task Force of the International Liaison committee on Resuscitation. *Resuscitation* 2003; **57**: 231–5.

20. Keller E, Imhof HG, Gasser S, Terzic A, Yonekawa Y. Endovascular cooling with heat exchange catheters: a new method to induce and maintain hypothermia. *Intensive Care Med* 2003; **29**: 939–43.

21. Zeiner A, Holzer M, Sterz F, *et al.* Hyperthermia after cardiac arrest is associated with an unfavorable neurologic outcome. *Arch Intern Med* 2001; **161**: 2007–12.

22. Kim F, Olsufka M, Carlbom D, *et al.* Pilot study of rapid infusion of 2 L of 4 degrees C normal saline for induction of mild hypothermia in hospitalized, comatose survivors of out-of-hospital cardiac arrest. *Circulation* 2005; **112**: 715–19.

23. Kuboyama K, Safar P, Radovsky A, Tisherman SA, Stezoski SW, Alexander H. Delay in cooling negates the beneficial effect of mild resuscitative cerebral hypothermia after cardiac arrest in dogs: a prospective, randomized study. *Crit Care Med* 1993; **21**: 1348–58.

24. Bosse G, Breuer JP, Spies C. The resistance to changing guidelines – what are the challenges and how to meet them. *Best Pract Res Clin Anaesthesiol* 2006; **20**: 379–95.

25. Abella BS, Rhee JW, Huang KN, Vanden Hoek TL, Becker LB. Induced hypothermia is underused after resuscitation from cardiac arrest: a current practice survey. *Resuscitation* 2005; **64**: 181–6.

26. Wolfrum S, Radke PW, Pischon T, Willich SN, Schunkert H, Kurowski V. Mild therapeutic hypothermia after cardiac arrest – a nationwide survey on the implementation of the ILCOR guidelines in German intensive care units. *Resuscitation* 2007; **72**: 207–13.

27. Hovdenes J, Laake JH, Aaberge L, Haugaa H, Bugge JF. Therapeutic hypothermia after out-of-hospital cardiac arrest: experiences with patients treated with percutaneous coronary intervention and cardiogenic shock. *Acta Anaesthesiol Scand* 2007; **51**: 137–42.

28. Garot P, Lefevre T, Eltchaninoff H, *et al.* Six-month outcome of emergency percutaneous coronary intervention in resuscitated patients after cardiac arrest complicating ST-elevation myocardial infarction. *Circulation* 2007; **115**: 1354–62.

29. Dellinger RP, Carlet JM, Masur H, *et al.* Surviving Sepsis Campaign guidelines for management of severe sepsis and septic shock. *Crit Care Med* 2004; **32**: 858–73.

30. Cummins RO, Chamberlain DA, Abramson NS, *et al.* Recommended guidelines for uniform reporting of data from out-of-hospital cardiac arrest: the Utstein style. A statement for health professionals from a task force of the American Heart Association, the European Resuscitation Council, the Heart and Stroke Foundation of Canada, and the Australian Resuscitation Council. *Circulation* 1991; **84**: 960–75.

Declaration of interest

Jerry Nolan is an editor for the journal *Resuscitation*. Some of the studies reviewed in this chapter were published in the journal.

Acronyms/abbreviations

ACC	American College of Cardiology	COURAGE	Clinical Outcomes Utilization Revascularization and Aggressive Drug Evaluation
ACLS	Advanced Cardiac Life Support		
AEC	airway exchange catheter		
AED	automated external defibrillator	CPAP	continuous positive airway pressure
AHA	American Heart Association	CPB	cardiopulmonary bypass
AIMS	anaesthetic information management system	CPOE	computerized physician order entry
ALI	acute lung injury	CPR	cardiopulmonary resuscitation
ALS	advanced life support	CRBI	catheter-related bloodstream infection
APC	anaesthetic preconditioning		
ARDS	acute respiratory distress syndrome	CVD	cardiovascular disease
		DVT	deep venous thrombosis
ASA	American Society of Anesthesiologists	ECG	electrocardiogram
		EEG	electroencephalogram
ATP	adenosine triphosphate	EIT	electric impedance tomography
BIPAP	biphasic positive airway pressure		
		EMS	emergency medical service
BIS	bispectral index		
BMI	body mass index	EWS	early warning score
BNP	brain natriuretic peptide	FDA	Food and Drugs Administration
CABG	coronary artery bypass graft		
		FFP	fresh-frozen plasma
CARP	Coronary Artery Revascularization Prophylaxis	FRC	functional residual capacity
		Hb	haemoglobin
		HDL	high-density lipoprotein
CCS	Canadian Cardiovascular Society	HPV	hypoxic pulmonary vasoconstriction
		HRS	hepatorenal syndrome
CI	confidence interval	ICU	intensive care unit
CJD	Creutzfeldt–Jakob disease	IDS	intubation difficulty score

IHD	ischaemic heart disease	PCA	patient-controlled analgesia
i.m.	intramuscular		
IPPV	intermittent positive-pressure ventilation	PCI	percutaneous coronary intervention
ITV	impedance threshold valve	PEEP	positive end-expiratory pressure
LCI	lung clearance index	PONV	postoperative nausea and vomiting
LDB	load-distributing band		
LDL	low-density lipoprotein	QI	quality improvement
LMA	laryngeal mask airway	QSAR	quantitative structure-activity relationship
LOS	length of stay		
MACE	major adverse cardiac event	RCRI	revised cardiac risk index
		RCT	randomized controlled trial
MDN	mean dilution number		
MH	malignant hypothermia	ROC	receiver operator characteristic
MHRA	Medicines and Healthcare products Regulatory Agency	ROSC	return of spontaneous circulation
MI	myocardial infarction	RR	relative risk
MIGET	multiple inert gas elimination technique	SIRS	systemic inflammatory response syndrome
MIH	mild induced hypothermia	SMI	silent myocardial ischaemia
MPI	myocardial performance index	SP	substance P
		TIVA	total intravenous anaesthesia
NIPPV	non-invasive positive-pressure ventilation	TNF	tumour necrosis factor
NNT	number needed to treat	TRICC	Transfusion Requirements in Critical Care
OPCAB	off-pump coronary artery bypass		
OR	odds ratio	TRP	transient receptor potential
OSA	obstructive sleep apnoea		
OSAI	outpatient surgery admission index	UFH	unfractionated heparin
		VAP	ventilator associated pneumonia
PACU	post-anesthesia care unit		
PAD	public access defibrillation	WMD	weighted mean difference

Index of papers reviewed

Abella BS, Edelson DP, Kim S, *et al*. CPR quality improvement during in-hospital cardiac arrest using a real-time audiovisual feedback system. *Resuscitation* 2007; 73: 54–61. **230**

Abraham E, Laterre P-F, Garg R, *et al.* **for the Administration of Drotrecogin Alfa (Activated) in Early Stage Severe Sepsis (ADDRESS) Study Group.** Drotrecogin alfa (activated) for adults with severe sepsis and a low risk of death. *N Engl J Med* 2005; 353: 1332–41. **350**

Anderson NK, Jones AD, Martin EE, *et al*. Anaesthetic care of the trauma patient: development of a web-based resource. *AANA J* 2007; 75: 49–56. **262**

Arrich J. Clinical application of mild therapeutic hypothermia after cardiac arrest. *Crit Care Med* 2007; 35: 1041–7. **388**

Axelsson C, Nestin J, Svensson L, *et al*. Clinical consequences of the introduction of mechanical chest compression in the EMS system for treatment of out-of-hospital cardiac arrest – a pilot study. *Resuscitation* 2006; 71: 47–55. **234**

Beckers SK, Skorning MH, Fries M, *et al*. CPREzy™ improves performance of external chest compressions in simulated cardiac arrest. *Resuscitation* 2007; 72: 100–7. **229**

Berkenstadt H, Yusim Y, Katznelson R, *et al*. A novel point-of-care information system reduces anaesthesiologists' errors while managing case scenarios. *Eur J Anaesthesiology* 2006; 23: 239–50. **282**

Biro P, Baatig U, Henderson J, *et al*. First clinical experience of tracheal intubation with the SensaScope®, a novel steerable semirigid video stylet. *Br J Anaesth* 2006; 97: 255–61. **295**

Bitterman N. Technologies and solutions for data display in the operating room. *J Clin Monitoring Comput* 2006; 20: 165–73. **253**

de Boer HD, van Egmond J, van de Pol F, *et al*. Time course of action of sugammadex (Org 25969) on rocuronium-induced block in the rhesus monkey, using a simple model of equilibrium of complex formation. *Br J Anaesth* 2006; 97: 681–6. **174**

Boyle J. Wireless technologies and patient safety in hospitals. *Telemedicine and e-Health* 2006; 12: 373–82. **249**

Bradley P. A history of simulation in medical education and possible future directions. *Med Ed* 2006; 40: 254–62. **270**

Brown JR, Birkmeyer NJO, O'Connor GT. Meta-analysis comparing the effectiveness and adverse outcomes of antifibrinolytic agents in cardiac surgery. *Circulation* 2007; 115: 2801–13. **33**

Byford AJ, Anderson A, Jones PS, *et al*. The hypnotic, electroencephalographic, and antinociceptive properties of nonpeptide ORL1 receptor agonists after intravenous injection in rodents. *Anesth Analg* 2007; 104: 174–9. **195**

General index

A

A118G polymorphism, effect on morphine efficacy 190–1
abdominal hysterectomy, use of local anaesthetic 119
ACADEMIA study 228
ACGME (Accreditation Council for Graduate Medical Education) duty hour standards 332, 333
acute coronary syndromes
　anti-platelet drug therapy 9–11
　GKi regimens, use after STEMI 366–7
　intensive medical therapy 6–9
acute lung injury (ALI)
　lung-protective ventilation 53, 66
　in oesophagectomy 54
　ventilatory strategy 15
acute respiratory distress syndrome (ARDS)
　ventilation guidelines in severe sepsis 341–3
　ventilatory strategy 15
ADDRESS (Administration of Drotrecogin Alfa (Activated) in Early Stage Severe Sepsis) 350–1
adenoidectomy, ambulatory 122–3, 124
adrenaline, use with vasopressin in cardiac arrest 312
adverse effects
　of anti-fibrinolytic drugs 31, 34, 35
　of nitrous oxide 109
　of sugammadex 167–8, 170, 172–4, 182
　of vasopressin 314–15
　see also medical errors
Airtraq 291–3
airway exchange catheter (AEC) 17–18
airway management training, use of simulators 208
AirWay Scope 293–4
albumin levels, as predictor of postoperative pulmonary complications 12
allodynia, role of HCN channels 147–8
alpha-2-adrenoceptor agonists, cardioprotection 89–90
alveolar coagulation, effect of ventilatory strategy 56–7

alveolar overventilation 53
ambulatory anaesthesia 101–2, 124
　anti-emetic prophylaxis 120–2
　intraoperative awareness 110–11
　knee arthroscopy, spinal anaesthesia 114–16
　nitrous oxide 109–10
　outpatient surgery admission index (OSAI) 107–8
　paediatric tonsillectomy and adenoidectomy 122–3
　patients with obstructive sleep apnoea 102–7
　postoperative pain management
　　perineural infusion 116–17
　　PROSPECT initiative 117–20
American Heart Association (AHA)
　ACC/AHA guidelines
　　cardiac risk assessment 71–2
　　perioperative cardiac evaluation 18–19
　Guidelines for Cardiopulmonary Resuscitation 310
American Society of Anaesthesiologists (ASA), OSA guidelines 102–7
aminocaproic acid 30, 31
　adverse effects 34, 35
　comparison with other anti-fibrinolytic agents 33–4
anaemia, preoperative, relationship to postoperative outcomes 42–5
anaesthetic agents, cardioprotection 79–82
anaesthetic information management systems (AIMSs) 259–61
anaesthetic pharmacology 131–4
anaesthetic postconditioning 6
anaesthetic preconditioning 4–5
anaesthetic state 131
analgesia 132
　administration techniques 155
　　depots of buprenorphine prodrugs 156–7
　　fentanyl, iontophoretic transdermal system 160–2
　　morphine, single-dose epidural formulation 157–9
　patient-controlled 116–17, 160–2

CLINICAL PUBLISHING

The Year in
Anaesthesia and Critical Care

VOLUME 1

ISBN: 978-1-904392-66-8

KEEPING UP TO DATE IN ONE VOLUME